Dr. Nurse

Dr. Nurse

Science, Politics, and
the Transformation of American Nursing

DOMINIQUE A. TOBBELL

The University of Chicago Press
Chicago and London

The University of Chicago Press, Chicago 60637
The University of Chicago Press, Ltd., London
© 2022 by The University of Chicago
Published 2022
Printed in the United States of America

31 30 29 28 27 26 25 24 23 22   1 2 3 4 5

ISBN-13: 978-0-226-82288-4 (cloth)
ISBN-13: 978-0-226-82290-7 (paper)
ISBN-13: 978-0-226-82289-1 (e-book)
DOI: https://doi.org/10.7208/chicago/9780226822891.001.0001

Library of Congress Cataloging-in-Publication Data

Names: Tobbell, Dominique A., 1978– author.
Title: Dr. nurse : science, politics, and the transformation of American nursing /
    Dominique A. Tobbell.
Other titles: Science, politics, and the transformation of American nursing
Description: Chicago : The University of Chicago Press, 2022. |
    Includes bibliographical references and index.
Identifiers: LCCN 2022015129 | ISBN 9780226822884 (cloth) | ISBN 9780226822907
    (paperback) | ISBN 9780226822891 (ebook)
Subjects: LCSH: Nursing—United States—History—20th century. | Nursing—
    Study and teaching (Graduate)—United States—History. | Nursing—Study and
    teaching—United States—History. | Nurses—Education—United States—
    History—20th century.
Classification: LCC RT4 .T63 2022 | DDC 610.73071/173—dc23/eng/20220509
LC record available at https://lccn.loc.gov/2022015129

♾ This paper meets the requirements of ANSI/NISO z39.48-1992 (Permanence of Paper).

To Beth Klakoski

Contents

Introduction

The U.S.'s more than three million nurses represent the largest segment of the U.S. health care workforce. They are referred to as the backbone of the American health care system, spending significantly more time interacting with patients than any other member of the health care team.[1] They provide care in a variety of health care settings including hospitals, community health clinics, long-term care facilities, and in individual homes. As the World Health Organization notes, "Nurses and midwives are often the first and only point of care in their communities."[2] The nursing model of care, which centers on the nurse-patient relationship and on improving health among individuals and communities, is underpinned by a distinctive body of knowledge. For the past sixty years and more, nurses have conducted research, contributing to that body of knowledge that has shaped health care practice, informed health policy, and improved health outcomes.

Yet, in the early twenty-first century, many people, including those who work in health care, are still surprised to hear that nurses do research, and that this research is underpinned by a distinct body of knowledge—nursing science.[3] Furthermore, relative to other types of health science research, nursing research is poorly funded.[4] And nurse scientists—nurses who have also earned a PhD (either in nursing or one of the biomedical, behavioral, or social sciences)—often reflect on the importance of identifying themselves as scientists rather than as nurses, in order to be taken seriously as researchers and avoid conflict with their physician research collaborators.[5] In other words, despite more than half a century of experience as researchers, nurses' status as scientists is still contested. *Dr. Nurse* describes and analyzes what I am calling the "academic project"—the efforts of American nurses to establish nursing as an academic discipline and nurses as valued researchers in the decades after World War II—and considers why, in the early twenty-first century, that academic project remains incomplete.

This history provides a valuable perspective on major changes that have taken place in American health care in the second half of the twentieth century. From the 1950s through the 1980s, these academic nurses engaged in an epistemological project to construct a science of nursing—distinct from that of the related biomedical or behavioral sciences—that would provide the basis of nursing practice. They did so not only to develop science-based nursing practice amid the broadscale changes in patient care initiated by the introduction of new medical innovations, but also to secure their roles within the postwar research university. In doing so, academic nurses transformed nursing practice into a valuable site of knowledge production and demonstrated the ways in which the application of this knowledge was integral to improving patient outcomes and health care delivery. Indeed, as nurses conducted research to reduce hospital-based infections and adverse drug interactions, and to improve end-of-life care, pain management, and the management of chronic illness and disability, their research was shaped by an emergent quality assessment movement within health care and the burgeoning patient movement, both of which sought to transform the ways in which biomedical research was conducted and health care delivered.

To be sure, as historian Susan Reverby has described, academic nurses held and mobilized differing meanings of science during the first half of the twentieth century, and this continued to be the case in the decades after World War II.[6] The multiple and changing meanings that academic nurses held of nursing science were both political and epistemological. On the one hand, academic nurses understood the development of nursing science as a political process to justify nursing's positioning within universities and academic health centers. On the other hand, they conceptualized nursing science as a process of knowledge development and application to practice. As I attend to the shifting definitions and meanings of nursing science that my historical actors mobilized, however, I rely on a definition of nursing science that reflects the overall process of research, knowledge production, and application of knowledge into practice and policy.

Nursing's academic project also took shape as academic health centers (AHCs) emerged as a defining feature of postwar biomedicine. AHCs are institutional umbrellas that combine a university's health science schools, biomedical research institutes, and affiliated teaching hospitals and clinics. In the postwar decades, as concerns mounted about rising health care costs, shortages of health care professionals, and regional inequities in health care access, policymakers looked to academic health institutions to solve the fundamental disparities between health care needs and health care services created by the country's market-oriented health care system. In response, public and private universities throughout the U.S. reorganized their health science schools into centrally administered AHCs in an effort to efficiently and cost-effectively integrate health care education, delivery, and research. Through the federally funded Area Health Education Centers on their campuses, AHCs attempted to coordinate the supply and distribution of health care professionals within a region. With each health science school theoretically granted equal administrative status, AHCs were designed to dismantle the disciplinary silos that had previously characterized the health sciences, where the educational needs of nursing and public health were routinely subordinated to those of medicine. AHCs were therefore intended to promote interdisciplinarity in research and education, and a team approach to clinical practice—by integrating nursing, medical, dental, pharmacy, public health, and allied health care. By the late 1970s, AHCs had emerged as a dominant institution in American health care.[7]

Nursing, Hospitals, and Patient Care after World War II

By the 1940s, hospitals were the site and symbol of specialized, high-technology medicine.[8] A series of wartime innovations had affirmed the importance of the laboratory-based biomedical sciences to the practice of medicine. Included among these innovations were the production of penicillin, the development of better blood replacement techniques, and improvements in resuscitation therapy that helped prevent and treat shock. These and other innovations helped change the demand for and nature of hospital care in the postwar decade. The introduction of antibiotics, for example, transformed previously life-threatening infectious diseases into short-term illnesses, and enabled many infectious diseases to be treated in outpatient settings. As a result, demand for hospital care of infectious diseases declined.[9] In contrast, the availability of antibiotics, blood plasma, and shock-prevention techniques increased opportunities and demand for complex surgeries, and "enabled lives to be saved that would previously have been lost."[10] And as chronic diseases like cancer and cardiovascular disease replaced infectious diseases as the leading cause of morbidity and mortality in the U.S., demand for their diagnosis and treatment also increased.[11]

The central role of the hospital in the provision of health care—and the increased need for hospital services—was also facilitated by the federal government. In 1946, President Harry Truman signed into law the Hospital Survey and Reconstruction Act (commonly called Hill-Burton by the bill's sponsors). The Hill-Burton Act provided federal grants and federal tax incentives to states and local communities to develop and expand hospitals and other health facilities. Between 1946 and 1960, the total number of hospitals in the country increased by 962.[12]

The employment-based system of health insurance expanded after the war, which also contributed to increased demand for hospital services as access to a growing range of procedures and services was made affordable to those with insurance coverage.[13] Although, as the historian Rosemary Stevens explains, "insurance targeted the most expensive services, not the most common."[14] This meant that while hospitalized services and procedures provided by specialist physicians were reimbursed, primary care and other out-of-hospital services typically were not.[15] Access to health insurance—either employer-financed or privately purchased—was heavily circumscribed by race. The insurance industry had a long history of discriminatory practices, either denying coverage or raising premiums to Black Americans.[16] In addition, widespread racial discrimination in employment and occupational segregation pushed Black Americans and other people of color into job categories that rarely provided health insurance benefits, reinforcing the profound racial disparities in health care access already experienced by Black Americans and other people of color.[17] But for the majority of Americans, access to health insurance—and thus coverage of hospital care—grew significantly in the postwar decades. For example, by 1945, only about a quarter of Americans had health insurance.[18] Fifteen years later, however, by 1960, 72 percent of the population carried some form of health insurance.[19] The increased availability of health insurance together with the expansion of hospitals under Hill-Burton, significantly increased demand for hospital services after World War II. Between 1946 and 1952, hospital admissions increased by 25 percent.[20]

As the demand for hospital services increased, so, too, did demand for hospital nurses. Throughout the 1930s, the majority of hospital nursing labor was provided by student nurses. In the 1940s, graduate nurses had replaced students as the main hospital nursing workforce. By the late 1940s, approximately 53 percent of white nurses were employees of hospitals, while the remainder worked either in private duty nursing or public health nursing.[21] For Black nurses, the employment situation was very different. As the historian Darlene Clark Hine has documented, the segregated system of health care and widespread racial discrimination meant that very few Black nurses worked in hospitals at this time and were instead concentrated in private duty or public health nursing.[22] Hospital nurses, though, faced low wages, long workdays, and a lack of economic security. Perhaps not surprisingly, hospital administrators "struggled to find and keep the necessary nurses to staff their hospitals."[23] A series of studies conducted in the late 1940s and early 1950s documented the crisis in hospital nursing and predicted that between 50,000 and 75,000 new graduate nurses were needed each year.[24] But rather than tackle discriminatory hiring practices, salaries, or working conditions— issues that might have improved job satisfaction among, and thus expand retention of, nurses—nurse leaders, hospital administrators, and other health care leaders focused only on how to produce more nurses.[25] These efforts centered on expanding and reforming nursing education.

Nursing's Academic Project

Through the mid-twentieth century, the majority of American nurses were trained in hospital training schools (or diploma programs) in which nurse training and practice was predicated on the medical model and which emphasized regimented, procedure-based training.[26] However, the increasing complexity of patient care in the decades after World War II made clear the limits of that educational model. Major surgical innovations introduced in the 1950s, which included open-heart, vascular, and large-scale abdominal surgeries, exposed patients to new types of postsurgical complications such as shock and respiratory failure. The arrival of new medical technologies like kidney dialysis and electronic fetal monitors, and the availability of increasingly powerful pharmaceuticals with oftentimes equally powerful side effects, also contributed to the increasing complexity of patient care. In this context, nurses realized they often lacked the knowledge, education, and authority to respond safely and effectively to patients' needs.[27] In response, nurse leaders sought to transform nursing education so as to better prepare professional nurses for the ever more complicated nature of treatment. They also called on nurses to engage in sustained and systematic research in order to generate the knowledge needed to improve nursing practice.

To this end, in the decades after World War II, nurse scholars and educators were engaged in an effort to establish nursing as an academic discipline by raising the educational level of nurses, creating and demarcating the boundaries of a distinct science of nursing, and establishing nursing PhD programs to prepare new generations of nurse scientists able to conduct the clinical research necessary to improve patient care. For these nurse scholars and educators, establishing nursing as an academic discipline was essential if nurses were to better care for the changing health and illness needs of the population.

This academic project took place in the context of the changing political economy of American universities. As the federal government became the primary patron of basic research after the war, universities increasingly prioritized research—and the acquisition of federal research funding—over teaching and service.[28] At the same time, the federal government and its policymakers ensured that graduate education (particularly at the doctoral level) became an integral component of the research enterprise.[29] Nursing's academic project also occurred at the same time that many American academic health institutions were being conceptualized or reconfigured as AHCs. Nursing faculty thus sought to adapt to the postwar research economy by shifting their focus to securing external funding, engaging in research, establishing themselves as the producers and disseminators of expert knowledge, and securing the academic status of their discipline—nursing science—within the postwar research university and academic health center. In this context, nursing science served not only as a way for academic nurses to transform nursing practice and health policy, but also as a means by which they could secure nursing's legitimacy and status within universities and AHCs.

Nursing's academic project entailed several components. Beginning in the 1950s, nurse educators introduced new models of undergraduate nursing education, located on university and colleges campuses, that replaced the regimented, procedure-based training of hospital-based diploma programs. These new baccalaureate programs were premised on liberal education and integrated the physical, biological, and social sciences. By emphasizing the nursing model of care—and rejecting the medical model of nursing practice—these new baccalaureate programs prepared professional nurses for their work as independent and expert practitioners. Innovations in graduate nursing education also took place during these decades.[30] By the 1960s, increasingly complex, specialized patient care had created new roles for nurses who had undergone advanced clinical training, at the master's degree level, in various nursing specialties, such as psychiatric nursing, pediatric nursing, and geriatric nursing. The nurse practitioner movement of the 1960s and 1970s also expanded the demand for clinical master's programs.[31]

Each of these innovations was predicated on the belief that nursing was grounded in a body of knowledge that was specific to nursing. Rather than relying on the knowledge claims and theories of the biomedical or behavioral sciences, a key aspect of nursing's academic project was for nurse researchers and theorists to build a science of nursing. This entailed debates over the degree to which this new science would draw upon the theoretical precepts of the existing sciences and the degree to which it would be founded upon the development of new theories that were unique to nursing. As they did so, academic nurses engaged in critical boundary and legitimation work: the process of selecting the requisite credentials of researchers, the types of research questions to be asked, and the methods and theoretical perspectives to be used for the purpose of drawing epistemic boundaries between nursing science and the existing biomedical and behavioral sciences.[32]

The effort by academic nurses to create a science of nursing occurred in parallel with the effort by academic physicians to establish a science of clinical medicine grounded in the new discipline of clinical epidemiology. This new clinical science centered on producing scientific evidence of therapeutic interventions—of what worked and what didn't work—and using that evidence (rather than subjective clinical judgment) to direct clinical decision-making.[33] It also took place amid an emergent—and related—quality assessment movement in health care, which aimed to systematically measure the outcome of patient care so as to determine which clinical interventions worked and which didn't, and to hold physicians accountable for those outcomes.[34] The goal of the quality assessment movement was to restructure the "health care delivery system characterized by idiosyncratic and often ill-informed judgments" into one premised on "evidence-based medical practice, regular assessment of the quality of care, and accountability."[35]

The efforts of academic nurses to develop a science that would underpin and inform nursing practice must be understood in this broader context. While academic physicians focused on constructing an empirical and statistically derived clinical science, academic nurses worked instead to construct a science of nursing that was not only empirical but also theoretical. Academic nurses did so in part because, as sociologist Andrew Abbott has observed, the development of an abstract system of knowledge demarcates the "borders of professional jurisdiction with utmost clarity," making "obvious what is and what is not part of the professionally claimed universe of tasks."[36] According to Abbott, the degree of abstraction shapes the strength of a profession's jurisdictional claims. For this generation of academic nurses, theory offered the highest level of abstraction and thus, they believed, was the best path forward to demarcating the boundaries of nursing science and securing nursing's academic legitimacy.[37]

By the end of the 1970s, nurse researchers and nurse theorists had determined the boundaries and empirical focus of nursing science: the interaction between people, their environment, and their health, and the influence of nursing interventions on enabling and supporting people as agents in the pursuit of their health goals. By emphasizing a health perspective rather than a disease perspective, by considering the patient holistically, and by prioritizing the agency of the patient in shaping their health, nursing and its science sought to stand apart from the reductionist model of medicine that emphasized disease, diagnosis, and cure. This was particularly important at a time when the women's health movement and a growing patient-consumer move-ment were criticizing the medical profession and the system of health care it lionized, for being reductionist, dehumanizing, and paternalistic.[38]

The work of academic nurses to develop a science of nursing also took shape in the midst of a burgeoning feminist critique of science.[39] This cri-tique, as Evelyn Fox Keller summarized in 1987, "argued that modern science evolved under the influence of a consciously chosen conjunction of scientific norms and masculine ideas," which led to "a sexual division of emotional and intellectual labor that effectively excludes most women from scientific profes-sions and simultaneously excludes all those values that have been tradition-ally regarded as 'feminine' from the practice of science." Feminist critics thus called "into question the grounds on which some values have been judged 'scientific' and others 'unscientific,'" and revaluated the "criteria for 'good' science."[40] In turn, some feminist scholars called for a complete revisioning of science and the enactment of feminist science grounded in women's suppos-edly distinctive ways of knowing. These included the feminine characteristics of caring, holism, and maternal thinking, which had "purportedly been ex-cluded from the practices of dominant forms of science."[41]

Yet, the overwhelming majority of nurse scientists did not see their epis-temological project as part of the feminist critique of science. They were not challenging or even questioning the assumptions or practices of science. They were also not interested in doing science that challenged or undermined race-based oppressions. This is an important aspect of more recent feminist science studies scholarship, with implications for understanding the ways in which nursing has been integral to the racism embedded within the health care system and the biomedical and nursing knowledge that underpins it.[42] Instead, nurse scientists were arguing for equality in access to doing science-as-it-was-currently-done, so-called normal science. This is not surprising, given the extensive scholarship on feminist science studies that documents this as a common strategy of women scientists throughout the twentieth cen-tury.[43] But unlike the many women scientists who, in the decades after World War II, sought access to already-established scientific disciplines, nurses were working to build an entirely new scientific discipline. That they saw the cre-ation of an abstract knowledge system underpinned by nursing *theory* as key to gaining entry to so-called normal science is just part of the story. The other important piece of this history is that in the process of seeking access to nor-mal science, this early generation of nurse scientists claimed nursing's histori-cally gendered labor as a site of knowledge production—labor that has all too often been regarded as inconsequential by feminist science studies scholars. Indeed, despite the extensive scholarship on gender and science in general, and feminist science in particular, nurses remain, as Julie Fairman and Patricia D'Antonio first noted back in 1999, "merely a footnote to this vibrant discussion."[44]

Even as feminist science studies scholars asserted that part of the feminist project in science was to value reproductive and caring labor and the experiential knowledge attached to and generated by it, they dismissed nursing as an appropriate site of analysis, seeing it as merely subordinate to medicine.[45] However, as the following chapters make clear, nursing *is* a critical site of gender and feminist analysis. Although the overwhelming majority of nurse scientists did not lay claim to possessing distinctive *feminist* ways of knowing, they nevertheless constructed a system of abstract knowledge (the epitome of normal science) that emphasized *nursing's* distinctive perspective, rooted as it was in holism, caring, and an emphasis on environment—all qualities that some feminists have argued *are* distinctively feminist ways of knowing.[46] While this early generation of nurse scientists struggled to establish their scientific legitimacy, they nevertheless established nursing practice as an important site of knowledge production and sought to demonstrate the ways in which application of this knowledge was integral to improving patient outcomes and health care delivery.

Another core component of nursing's academic project was the establishment of PhD programs in nursing. While many nurses had earned doctorates in schools or departments of education and, increasingly from the early 1960s, in the basic or behavioral sciences, the development of the *nursing* research doctorate—the PhD—for the first time prepared nurses within nursing schools to *do* nursing science, that is, to conduct research aimed at producing new nursing knowledge that would, ultimately, advance nursing practice. By contributing to the production of new nursing knowledge, nurse scientists would not only help advance patient care, they would also secure membership in the "community of scholars."[47] In this way, nursing faculty would no longer be just teachers but would become full-fledged members of academe and as such should be accorded equal intellectual and institutional status with their university peers. This was especially important in the political economy of the postwar American university in which research—and the acquisition of federal research funding—was prioritized over teaching and service.[48]

While nurse educators, researchers, and theorists argued that the nursing PhD was essential to nursing's academic project, nurse educators and health planners also argued that the nursing PhD was critical to building the nursing workforce. Indeed, the emergence of nursing's academic project coincided with growing state, regional, and national concerns among health care leaders and policymakers about impending shortages of health care workers, including nurses. Beginning in the early 1960s, health policymakers joined nursing educators in calling for the increased production of doctorally prepared nurses. By producing more nurses with PhDs, schools of nursing could improve the quality of and expand the scale of master's, baccalaureate, and associate degree–level education. Nurse educators thus framed their arguments for the nursing PhD not only in terms of a new type of disciplinary knowledge but also in the context of urgent nursing workforce concerns.

But even as some nursing leaders promoted nursing's academic project, others argued that it weakened nursing education by divorcing it from the realities and needs of nursing practice. Furthermore, others within nursing argued that academic nursing's "emphasis on 'credentialism'" was undermining the nursing workforce by denigrating nurses who had been trained in hospital-based diploma programs and creating obstacles to educational and social mobility for the scores of nurses (including the majority of nurses of color) educated in diploma and associate degree programs.[49] In this way, the ideas of a handful of academic nurses located at elite institutions nevertheless impacted the majority of nurses who were not part of an academic setting. The so-called debates over entry into practice reflected in the efforts of academic nurses, the American Nurses Association (ANA), and several state nursing associations to establish the bachelor of science in nursing (BSN) as the basis for licensure during these decades, was one such way. After all, the efforts to raise the entry-level credentials into professional nursing were a direct result of nursing's academic project and were a matter of great concern for diploma and associate degree graduates (and the hospital training schools and community colleges that trained them). As a result, diploma and associate degree graduates were under constant pressure during the late 1960s and 1970s to upgrade their educational credentials in order to keep their jobs or move up the career ladder.

Nurses of color faced significant barriers to educational mobility. Throughout these decades, nursing education in the South remained segregated, and in the North it was heavily circumscribed by racial discrimination. Even after passage of the Civil Rights Act in 1964 formally ended segregation and made discrimination by race in employment and education illegal, ongoing systemic racism meant that Black, Indigenous, and other people of color continued to face exclusion from access to higher education in nursing.[50] The debates over nursing's academic project took place amid broader shifts in higher education, particularly the increasing commitment of education policymakers to significantly expand access to and diversify institutions of higher education.[51]

During these formative years of nursing's academic project, access to the status of professional nurse was thus heavily circumscribed by race and gender. Only those able to advance through the educational hierarchy to attain the formal educational credentials of first a BSN, then a master of science in nursing (MSN), and eventually a doctorate were invited to contribute to the science of nursing. This meant that those with access to nursing's epistemological project were primarily white and female. Nursing's epistemological project, and the broader academic project of which it was a part, was thus a racialized and gendered project, the roots of which dated back to the introduction of trained nursing in the late nineteenth century.[52] These legacies continue into the present, as people of color are still significantly underrepresented within academic nursing. Such racial inequities significantly undermine nursing's ability to address ongoing racial health disparities and structural racism in health care.[53]

Another consequence of nursing's academic project was an essential severing of the relationship between nursing education and nursing's practice base. In hospital diploma programs, education and practice occurred in the same space and were overseen by the hospital's nursing service. In baccalaureate programs, by contrast, education took place on university or college campuses and was directed by nursing faculty, while nursing practice took place in the university's teaching hospitals, overseen by the hospital's nursing service. Nursing faculty rarely held clinical appointments in the teaching hospital's nursing service. Indeed, for some nurse educators, a strict separation between education and practice was seen as essential to establishing nursing as an academic discipline. The education-service gap (as it came to be called), however, had profound implications for nursing's academic project: the nursing content of baccalaureate and graduate curricula was often divorced from the realities and needs of clinical practice; nurses in practice complained that nurse scientists were not asking research questions relevant to practice and nurse theorists were failing to develop and test their theories in practice settings. By the 1960s, the unification of nursing education and service was seen as critical to nursing's academic project. To this end, a small but growing group of nurse educators began calling for the establishment of academic leadership in nursing. Predicated on the medical model of professional education, nursing faculty would participate in the tripartite academic mission of research, education, *and* practice, and nursing schools would have responsibility for and authority over the quality of nursing education, care, and research that took place in teaching hospitals and clinics. Academic leadership in nursing would, they argued, lead to improvements in nursing education, ensure the clinical relevance of nursing research and theory development, and secure nursing's equal status among the other health professions within academic health centers.

Dr. Nurse describes the impetus for and implementation of nursing's academic project, revealing the knowledge claims, strategies, and politics involved in the work of academic nurses as they negotiated their roles and nursing's place within universities and academic health centers, and situating them alongside nursing's workforce needs and persistent debates about what level of education is needed to be a professional nurse. In doing so, it places nursing's academic project in the context of the changing political economy of American universities; the civil rights and women's movements; and the public's growing dissatisfaction with an increasingly expensive, reductionist, and paternalistic health care system. How nurses constructed their discipline determined which types of knowledge and knowledge workers would be valued, and managed the educational pathways into professional nursing matters in the present, as nurses and other health care professionals are called to reckon with the racism embedded within the health care system, and address the racial inequities that have resulted.[54]

Academization of the Practice Professions

Nursing was not the only practice profession engaged in an effort to establish its academic standing and undergo a process of academization. As historian Jonathan Harwood explains, academization describes "the shift of educational institutions toward a stronger 'science orientation' "[55] and "the process whereby knowledge which is intended to be useful gradually loses close ties to practice while becoming more tightly integrated with one or other body of scientific knowledge."[56] During these same decades, engineering, computing, clinical psychology, and pharmacy were embroiled in similar scientific and political debates as they undertook their own academic projects. For example, as historians of engineering have documented, the American engineering profession had been engaged in a process of academization since the 1920s, which intensified in the postwar years as engineering science became the dominant emphasis in postwar engineering education.[57] As Nathan Ensmenger describes, the emergence of computer science as an academic discipline in the period between 1955 and 1975 required the first generation of computer scientists "to clearly define the body of theory that was at the center of their discipline." This entailed a significant degree of boundary work with the academic disciplines upon which computer science drew for its people and its content. It also led to significant tensions with practitioners—those working as computer programmers—particularly regarding the balance of theory and practice in computer science education.[58]

In the health sciences, the fields of clinical psychology and pharmacy were also engaged in a process of academization after World War II. As historians of psychology have documented, clinical psychologists initially developed the "scientist-practitioner" training model, which was widely adopted by university psychology departments in the 1950s and 1960s. In this model, clinical psychologists were educated in PhD programs where they received training in clinical practice as well as research design, methodology, and analysis. Despite the early success of the "scientist-practitioner" training model, by the mid-1960s, some leaders within clinical psychology had become critical of the model. As increasing numbers of clinical psychologists entered private practice, the rationale for the integrated "scientist-practitioner" model was declining. In its place, clinical psychologists began calling for the establishment of a separate doctoral program that emphasized advanced clinical training. The subsequent debates over the appropriate training model for clinical psychologists led to the development of the professional doctorate, the PsyD. By the mid-1970s, the PsyD had emerged as a legitimate graduate program for training practitioners of clinical psychology.[59]

Pharmacists, like nurses, were engaged in a decades-long debate over educational reform and the academic requirements for entry into professional practice. As historians of pharmacy have shown, during the postwar decades, pharmacy educators led an educational reform movement intended to shore up the academic underpinnings of their profession and raise the professional status of the pharmacist within the health care system. But throughout the 1950s and 1960s, practicing pharmacists charged educators with overemphasizing the scientific basis of industrial techniques and not adequately preparing students for careers in actual pharmacy practice.[60] By the 1960s, as physicians struggled to make sense of the ever-growing array of new drugs on the market, pharmacists took on new clinical roles. In hospitals, they established themselves as drug information experts and played an increasingly critical role within the health care team, while community pharmacists began providing drug information and counseling to patients.[61] In this context, the movement for academic reform—in this instance, the push to expand clinical education and establish the PharmD as the entry-level degree for the profession—gained greater traction. Nevertheless, it took until 1992 for pharmacists to finally resolve the entry into practice debate, implementing plans to eliminate the baccalaureate degree in pharmacy and establish the entry-level PharmD as the minimum entry-level degree program for pharmacy.[62]

As nursing embarked on its academic project, it drew upon the experiences of these other practice disciplines, particularly engineering and clinical psychology. During the 1960s and 1970s, nurse leaders focused on securing their academic legitimacy through the establishment of PhD programs. But beginning in the late 1970s, a handful of nurse educators began experimenting with a professional doctorate, one comparable to the professional doctorates in medicine, dentistry, and—increasingly—pharmacy. By the early 2000s, nursing leaders argued that nursing's professional doctorate, the doctor of nursing practice (DNP), should replace clinical master's degrees and designate entry into *advanced* nursing practice. This distinguished nursing from medicine, dentistry, and pharmacy, whose professional doctorates designated preparation for entry-level generalist professional practice. Ultimately, then, nursing followed its own path to academization. By placing nursing's academic project in this broader context of the academization of the practice disciplines after World War II, *Dr. Nurse* identifies the common strategies used by the practice professions to demarcate the boundaries of their disciplines and to justify the establishment of doctoral programs in their fields. It also reveals the different strategies used by nursing—and the particular set of challenges nurses faced—in drawing its boundaries and establishing itself as an academic discipline in the second half of the twentieth century. In doing so, it sheds light on the limits, consequences, and future of nursing's academic project.

Knowledge, Politics, and Policy in American Health Care

Histories of American nursing education have focused, primarily, on the period between the late nineteenth and mid-twentieth centuries.[63] This scholarship has shown that throughout the history of trained nursing, professional politics have indelibly shaped nursing's relationship with science.[64] Historians of nursing and health care have also demonstrated the intellectual and political work nurses have done to transform patient care and the American health care system during the mid- and late twentieth century.[65] Much of this work has centered on the emergence of advance practice nursing in the second half of the twentieth century.[66] *Dr. Nurse* builds on this critical scholarship.

This book is grounded in three central arguments. First, nursing's academic project has existed in tension with nursing's workforce needs and, as such, is situated within the politics of state health policymaking. On the one hand, the need for more nurses was used effectively by nurse educators to argue for support for doctoral education in nursing in order to prepare enough nurse faculty to teach expanded numbers of students. On the other hand, the effort to raise the educational level of nurses and limit educational pathways into nursing (by attempting, first, to eliminate the diploma training schools and then later, to question the need for associate degree programs) has been opposed by those who see these multiple pathways as critical to ensuring both upward mobility for diverse populations within nursing and for increasing workforce numbers. As nurse leaders sought to balance nursing's academic imperatives against workforce needs, it placed nursing's academic project and the politics of nursing education more broadly, within the context of state health policymaking.

Despite massive infusions of federal funding into health science research and health care in the postwar decades, by the 1960s the U.S. had no mechanism for matching biomedical research and workforce production with the country's health care needs. In the absence of a comprehensive national health policy, state-supported academic health centers became sites in which federal and state health policies intersected and were implemented in local settings. Since the 1950s, state governments have relied on schools of medicine, nursing, dentistry, public health, pharmacy, and veterinary medicine to respond to the health care needs of state residents. In exchange for state funding, academic institutions have been required to produce enough of the "right type" of health care professionals willing to work in the state. As state-supported schools of nursing sought to reform nursing education, state legislators called on them to produce more nurses able to meet the states' growing health care needs. As a result, state-supported schools throughout the country were sites in which federal, state, institutional, and interprofessional politics intersected in the making of the American nursing workforce and the creation of state health policies.

Second, nursing's academic project has been shaped by the gendered politics of academia and the gendered interprofessional politics of health care. Nursing's academic project was premised on rejecting the medical model in favor of a nursing model that integrated the biomedical, behavioral, and social sciences and prioritized a holistic, patient-centered approach to practice. As part of this, academic nurses, through the development and application of nursing science, sought to position nurses as agents of change needed to reform the reductionist and paternalistic health care system, even as nurses of color and feminist nurses questioned their willingness to engage in substantive reform. Furthermore, by the 1960s, many of nursing's academic leaders realized what had been lost by a wholesale rejection of the medical model. In particular, by opposing the medical model of professional education, which charged medical faculty with responsibility for education, research, and practice, academic nursing lost its connection (both structurally and, many argued, intellectually) to nursing's practice base. At the same time, the absence of nursing faculty from teaching hospitals meant they had little contact with physicians, which disadvantaged them as they sought to claim their rightful place as equals within the interprofessional health care team. As academic nurses worked to rebuild the connection between education and practice and establish academic nursing as parallel and complementary to academic medicine, they confronted resistance from physicians and hospital administrators all too comfortable with the gendered and hierarchical status quo within academic health centers.

Finally, the history of nursing's academic project is valuable for understanding current health policy and the politics of health professions education, particularly as it relates to tackling ongoing nursing shortages.[67] Indeed, the tension between the need to raise the educational level of nurses even as the U.S. faces a nursing shortage persists today. In 2010, the Institute of Medicine (IOM) report, *The Future of Nursing: Leading Change, Advancing Health*, called for the proportion of nurses with baccalaureate degrees to increase from 50 percent to 80 percent and for the number of nurses with doctoral degrees to double by 2020.[68] The associate degree, however, remains a critical entry point into nursing, particularly for people from rural and underserved areas. By favoring the baccalaureate as the entry point to nursing, nursing leaders and health planners risk undermining a vital pathway into nursing, particularly for underrepresented populations, which could, in turn, undermine efforts to stem the nursing shortage and increase diversity in the nursing workforce.

The history of nursing's academic project also provides important insights into contemporary efforts to promote health professions education that is interdisciplinary, interprofessional, and patient centered. For example, in 2003, the IOM's *Health Professions Education* called for "a major overhaul" of clinical education. In particular, the IOM urged that all health professionals be "educated to deliver patient-centered care as members of an interdisciplinary team, emphasizing evidence-based practice, quality improvement approaches, and informatics."[69] This report provided the context in which nurse leaders, at the turn of the twenty-first century, advocated a new vision for the education of advanced practice nurses: the establishment of practice-focused doctoral programs—the doctor of nursing practice (DNP)—to "prepare graduates for the highest level of nursing practice."[70] After some initial and at times heated debate, nursing leaders now regard the DNP as the entry into advanced nursing practice. This very recent history of the DNP—and the longer history of nursing's academic project in which it is situated—offers important lessons and context for the ongoing debates about the need for, and value added of, practice-based doctorates in other health-related professions, including audiology, physical therapy, and occupational therapy.[71]

Dr. Nurse draws together and analyzes archival sources from university-based nursing schools, regional nursing organizations, nurse leaders, state governments, and the published nursing literature, as well as oral histories with nurse educators and nurse researchers who were involved in nursing's academic project. In particular, this book is based on research in the archives of several American nursing schools that attempted to establish, and in some cases succeeded in establishing, nursing PhD programs during the 1960s and 1970s, and oral history interviews with nursing faculty at some of those schools. The nursing schools at Case Western Reserve University, University of Illinois Chicago, and Wayne State University were among the first cohort (after Teachers College, Columbia University and New York University established their doctoral programs in the 1920s and 1930s) to establish nursing PhD programs in the United States during the 1960s and 1970s, while the nursing schools at the University of California, Los Angeles (UCLA), the University of Florida, the University of Minnesota, and the University of Pennsylvania all struggled to establish nursing PhD programs during these decades. Collectively, these schools provide a diverse perspective on the contested institutional politics of nursing's academic project.

In addition to being regionally diverse, these schools also reflect the distinct experiences and challenges encountered by nursing schools that had long been part of state-funded institutions, which in the postwar decades sought to transform their health professional schools into AHCs (e.g., the University of Minnesota), as well as newer nursing schools that were from the start integrated within newly established AHCs (e.g., the University of Florida and UCLA). Although the experiences of private nursing schools are considered (particularly Case Western Reserve University and the University of Pennsylvania), the focus in *Dr. Nurse* is on the experiences of state-funded nursing schools. Since World War II, state governments have expected state-funded academic health institutions to produce sufficient numbers of health care professionals able to meet the health care needs of the state's residents. Even when private academic health institutions have received state support, neither their constitutions nor their priorities have been shaped by the land-grant mission of state institutions. As such, state-funded nursing schools (in contrast to private schools) have had to balance the expectation of legislators against the disciplinary and professional interests of its faculty. To this end, the archival materials from state-funded nursing schools are considered alongside material from state government archives and state legislative records. Finally, this book is also based on an analysis of the personal papers and published work of nurse researchers, nurse educators, and nurse leaders from the 1950s through the 1980s, to identify the major intellectual, social, and political themes, issues, and debates among—and sources of conflicts confronted by—American nurses as they worked to establish nursing as an academic discipline during these decades.

The chapters in *Dr. Nurse* are organized both chronologically and thematically. Chapter 1 describes the impetus for nursing's academic project and the tensions it created—between bedside nurses and academic nurses, hospital-trained and university-educated nurses, and university-educated nurses and physicians. The chapter focuses on the educational reforms implemented during the 1950s and 1960s, situating those reforms in the context of state health policymaking. Using the nursing schools at UCLA and the University of Minnesota as case studies, this chapter highlights the intersections of professional, institutional, and state politics embedded within nursing's academic project.

But nursing's academic project was about more than just politics. As chapter 2 details, the first generation of academic nurses were also engaged in an epistemological project. This chapter focuses on the efforts of nurse theorists and researchers from the 1950s through the 1970s to demarcate the boundaries of nursing science and claim nursing's empirical domain as person, health, environment. Nursing's epistemological project took shape in the midst of the feminist movement. Yet, nurse scientists did not see their project as part of the feminist critique of science. Rather, they were arguing for equality in access to doing science-as-it-was-currently-done. In other words, they wanted to do "masculine" science. Nevertheless, their efforts were not taken seriously by the broader culture of science and medicine. While there is gender at work here, it was also about the ways in which nurse scientists were choosing to do science. The research that nurse scientists conducted from the 1960s through the early 1980s primarily involved small-scale observational studies and utilized qualitative research methods. But this was at a time when the broader culture of biomedicine regarded large-scale, randomized, controlled trials and clinical epidemiological studies as the gold standard of biomedical research. That nurses were not using the research methods that were most highly valorized in the biomedical culture thus impacted the effectiveness of their efforts.

Chapter 3 situates nursing's academic project within the context of the changing political economy of American universities which, by the 1960s, prioritized research—and the acquisition of federal research funding—over teaching and service. In response, nursing leaders sought to secure the legitimacy of nursing as a research discipline and establish PhD programs so as to capitalize on new federal funding opportunities and secure the academic status of nursing schools.

The next two chapters use the history of academic nursing as a lens through which to understand the impact of AHCs on health professions education and health care delivery. Chapter 4 does so by showing the ways in which the federal/state layer cake of health and higher educational policies shaped nursing education and research in the 1960s and 1970s. In particular, as academic nurses sought to raise the educational preparation of nurses to the baccalaureate and graduate level, the graduates of diploma and associate degree programs were under pressure to upgrade their educational credentials. These nurses, however, frequently confronted significant financial, institutional, and social barriers to achieving so-called educational mobility. During the 1970s, graduates of diploma and associate degree (AD) programs, along with representatives from state nursing organizations, pressured state legislators to push state-funded nursing schools to establish programs that would facilitate nurses' movement from the lower levels of the educational hierarchy through the higher levels. They did so as policymakers at both the federal and state level instituted policies aimed at expanding access to higher education, particularly for women and minorities.

Chapter 5 examines the efforts of academic nurses to secure leadership roles in the delivery and governance of health care within AHCs. In particular, it details the history of the academic nursing practice movement, which sought to bring academic nursing closer to the structural model of academic medicine and establish integrated models of nursing education, research, and practice. This chapter reveals the limits of this approach. Most significantly, academic nurses, unlike their colleagues in medicine, could not be reimbursed for nursing care services. The model also led to the development of a two-tier system within nursing schools in which the faculty who engaged in academic practice were often ineligible for tenure, while the research and nonclinical teaching faculty were eligible for tenure. The model also proved limited in facilitating interprofessional collaboration—an often-articulated but rarely enacted goal of AHCs—because professional nursing education continued to take place at the undergraduate level while physician education took place at the graduate level. The limited success of academic nursing practice in the 1970s and early 1980s, ultimately undermined nursing's academic project and contributed to calls among a growing number of nursing leaders in the 1990s and early 2000s to establish the doctor of nursing practice. The conclusion ties together the major themes of the book, and considers why, in the early twenty-first century, nursing's academic project remains incomplete. It also examines the implications of this history not only for understanding the broadscale changes that took place in American health care in the late twentieth century but also for interrogating ongoing issues in health care.

By centering on the knowledge claims, strategies, and politics involved in the work of academic nurses as they negotiated their roles and nursing's place within AHCs, and situating them alongside nursing's workforce needs, *Dr. Nurse* provides insights on the history of AHCs and the new ecosystem of knowledge production and application they were part of. In particular, *Dr. Nurse* reveals the ways in which state-supported AHCs have, throughout their short history, existed in tension with the states that fund them, the state and federal health policies that direct them, and the health science professions that constitute their core.

The Need for Educational Reform

The 1950s and 1960s were decades of change for the American health care system and the nursing profession. The postwar decades witnessed the introduction of new diagnostic and therapeutic technologies, the expansion of private health insurance and public health care provision, and the massive growth of both the biomedical research enterprise and the infrastructure for and provision of health care delivery. Throughout these decades, physicians and health policymakers emphasized the primacy of acute, high-tech, interventionist curative medicine centered in hospitals and specialty clinics. But as chronic diseases replaced acute diseases as the major causes of mortality and morbidity, the limits of high-tech medicine and the need for and growing importance of preventive, palliative, or long-term care became increasingly apparent.

During the 1950s and 1960s, nursing, too, was primarily hospital-based. Indeed, through the mid-twentieth century, the majority of American nurses were trained in hospital training schools (also called diploma programs) in which nurse training and practice was, as historian Julie Fairman describes, "rule based, activity oriented, and relied heavily on the repetition of procedures rather than scientific or social theory-based decision-making."[1] Throughout the United States during the 1950s and 1960s, however, a new generation of nurse educators sought to create greater professional autonomy for the nurse by introducing new models of education that emphasized science-based learning and clinical thinking over technical expertise and functional practice. The functional method had been introduced in the 1930s and relied on nurses having knowledge of procedures (technical competence), without having "an intellectual understanding of the knowledge needed for larger patient-focused principles or goals."[2] As these reformers worked to develop nursing's own scientific base, they recognized that a growing proportion of nursing care was taking place outside of the hospital. To better prepare nurses for the provision of increasingly complex patient care both inside and outside the hospital, nurse educators introduced a new nursing model of care. This nursing model was premised on understanding the biopsychosocial dimensions of health so as to improve the health and well-being of individuals and communities. As part of this, the nursing model centered on the nurse-patient relationship and sought to empower patients as agents of change in their own health care. These educational reformers also sought to create new clinical roles for the nurse, based on advanced graduate education. As these educational reforms were gradually implemented throughout the country, the primary site of nursing education shifted from hospital-based diploma schools to colleges and universities.[3]

The introduction of education reform at nursing schools did not pass uncontested. Indeed, within a few years of being implemented, curriculum reforms introduced at university-based nursing schools were causing problems for faculty, students, and administrators alike. Nurse educators confronted resistance from an older generation of nurses who feared becoming "second-class citizens" in increasingly academic nursing schools, and from academic health institutions all too comfortable with the gendered hierarchy on which the traditional model of nursing education was predicated. Nor was the introduction of reform a uniform process. Rather, the character and politics of education reform at any one institution depended on the personalities involved and the local culture and politics of the specific institution. Using the University of California, Los Angeles (UCLA) and the University of Minnesota as case studies, this chapter describes the generational conflicts this new cadre of nurse educators confronted *within* schools of nursing, and the institutional politics it struggled with as it sought to secure greater institutional status for the schools among the universities' other health science units.[4]

This chapter also situates the politics of nursing education reform within the broader context of state health policymaking and the politics of state-supported academic health institutions in the United States in the decades after World War II. Even as the federal government invested heavily in health sciences research and health care, it did not introduce any policies or practices to ensure that biomedical research and health workforce production was meeting the country's health care needs. In the absence of a comprehensive national health policy in the U.S., state-supported academic health institutions, like those at UCLA and the University of Minnesota, became sites in which federal and state health policies intersected and were implemented in local settings. As these nursing schools sought to reform nursing education, state legislators called on them to produce greater numbers of professional nurses able to meet the states' growing health care needs. As a result, these nursing schools, along with other state-supported schools throughout the country, were sites in which federal, state, institutional, and interprofessional politics intersected in the making of the American nursing workforce and the creation of state health policies.

The Need for Better Educated Nurses

In the late 1940s, almost all nurses were educated in 1,100 hospital-based schools of nursing.[5] These hospital training schools (also called diploma programs) were three years long and typically included six months of "classroom work in the physical, biological, medical, and social sciences, and in nursing and allied arts."[6] The focus of the diploma programs, however, was procedure-oriented clinical training that emphasized learning by repetition. Students spent from thirty to forty-eight hours a week on hospital service, practicing techniques and procedures repeatedly so that they became rote, and learning "standard methods of doing the [clinical] work: ward management, medical diagnosis and treatment, and sanitation."[7] Graduates of hospital training schools earned a diploma and were entitled to sit for the state licensing exam, which would certify them as a registered nurse.

But while students gained technical competence—the skills to apply specific procedures to generalized situations—in hospital training programs, they were not being educated to understand, think through, and respond to the specific clinical needs of individual patients. In the 1930s, a handful of nursing faculty, including Virginia Henderson at Teachers College, Columbia University (and later at Yale University), began to challenge this traditional model of nursing education.[8] These challenges intensified—and the cohort of educational reformers grew—after World War II.

The postwar push for educational reform was in part the result of postwar changes in patient care. In particular, the increasing complexity of patient care in the postwar hospital made clear the limits of the diploma program model of nursing education. As noted earlier, the introduction of antibiotics contributed to the decline in infectious diseases, with chronic diseases like cancer and cardiovascular disease replacing them as the leading cause of morbidity and mortality in the U.S. The introduction of open-heart surgery and other complex surgical procedures in the 1950s exposed patients to new types of post-surgical complications (such as shock, respiratory failure, wound infections, and wound drainage problems). And the availability of increasingly potent pharmaceuticals, and—by the 1960s—the arrival of new medical technologies such as kidney dialysis and electronic fetal monitors, contributed to the increasing complexity of patient care. As a result, by the 1950s and 1960s, as historians Julie Fairman and Joan Lynaugh describe, "the patient care situation in the hospital . . . was very dynamic. On any single unit patient conditions varied widely and changed rapidly. Often, inexperienced nurses faced new emergency situations with little assistance or appropriate knowledge." All too often, nurses responsible for critically ill and dying patients found themselves without the availability, knowledge, or authority to provide appropriate care.[9]

But it wasn't just that nurses felt unprepared "to make rapid, complex clinical decisions," they also did not "quite understand how their patients made decisions or behaved in particular ways."[10] Nurses struggled, in particular, to understand the behaviors, attitudes, and decisions of patients whose religious, ethnic, racial, or national backgrounds were different from their own. In the 1940s and 1950s, as it was for the entire twentieth century, nurses were overwhelmingly female, white, and middle class, and white nurses struggled, in particular, to understand their patients of color. And yet, as the sociologist Frances Cooke Macgregor wrote in 1960, it was imperative that nurses understood the ways in which "diversities in ethnic and regional background, religion, class membership, and psychological makeup . . . play an important role in patients' reactions to illness and hospitalization, and in their attitudes and responses toward management, treatment, and rehabilitation . . . [and] in the quality of interaction between the nurse and the patient."[11]

Diploma programs, like the hospitals in which they were located, were predicated on the medical model in which disease is defined in biological terms (without consideration of psychological, social, or cultural factors) and clinical assessment and decision-making are based on the diagnosis and treatment of definable syndromes or cluster of symptoms. The medical model is itself predicated upon knowledge generated in the laboratory sciences including anatomy, physiology, biochemistry, pharmacology, and—from the 1950s—molecular biology. In this model, the development of new biomedical knowledge through well-controlled experimental studies in the laboratory contributes understanding of the cause, prevention, diagnosis, and treatment of disease.[12] The medical model conveys, as historians Patricia D'Antonio and Julie Fairman explain, "the primary organizing principles of systems that make access to patients and resource utilization decisions dependent on discrete disease diagnoses and treatments."[13]

Despite the dominance of the medical model, by the 1940s, some medical and nursing leaders were seeking to move both medicine and nursing beyond "merely . . . treating disease entities," and to treat "patients as 'total persons.'"[14] They did so as they came increasingly to recognize "that many of the causal factors of illness, recovery and relapse are social, psychological, and cultural, as well as physiological" and that the social and behavioral sciences could make important contributions to patient care.[15]

In the 1940s and 1950s, a handful of medical schools sought to broaden the scope of medical education to encompass the behavioral and social sciences, as well as institute comprehensive care programs that allowed students "to study a patient in relation to his family, occupation, and environment."[16] At the University of Minnesota, for example, the medical school instituted a Comprehensive Clinic program in 1960 in which every new clinic patient was assigned a medical student who became "the patient's doctor . . . taking the patient around to the various specialties as need be, and summarizing the whole thing."[17] The medical student then followed the patient throughout the patient's entire clinic experience. The medical school terminated the program in 1967, "not because it wasn't successful," (it was) as the program's director, Richard Magraw recalled, but because "it was swimming against the current" of subspecialization in medicine. Faculty in the "various specialties," Magraw continued, "wanted more time [with students and in the medical curriculum] and thought this [the Comprehensive Care Clinic] was sort of a waste of student time."[18] The fate of the Comprehensive Care Clinic at the University of Minnesota was not unique; comprehensive care programs at medical schools throughout the country encountered similar resistance. Instead, the imperatives of tertiary and highly specialized care came to dominate both medical education and medical practice. And the biomedical sciences, in turn, dominated the medical curriculum, with few schools in the postwar decades offering "formal courses built exclusively on a social science foundation."[19]

Yet, while medical educators all but dismissed the value of the social and behavioral sciences for medical education, nurse educators embraced it. They did so not only because they realized that "total patient care cannot be achieved unless those in charge are scientifically trained and knowledgeable in the science of human behavior," but also because they recognized that "the average physician is still not being provided with the necessary knowledge of the psychological, cultural, and social components of health and illness."[20] By integrating the social and behavioral sciences into nursing education and practice then, nurses could claim distinctive knowledge, skills, and expertise, rooted in an understanding of patient behavior and attitudes, which they—and not physicians—would contribute to the improvement of patient care.[21]

Nursing Education after World War II

Substantial changes took place in American nursing education after World War II. These changes were led in part by sociologist Esther Lucille Brown

and nurse educators Hildegard Peplau and Virginia Henderson, who offered compelling critiques of nursing education based on new, theoretically
grounded definitions of nursing practice. In 1948, on behalf of the National
Nursing Council and with funding from the Russell Sage Foundation, Brown
published *Nursing for the Future*, a thorough survey of the qualitative and
quantitative status of nursing practice and education. Brown's report called
for all forms of professional nursing education to be placed within institutions of higher education, and for university-based nursing schools to be autonomous and granted the same status as the university's other professional
schools. Brown argued that only institutions of higher education could provide students with both the liberal arts education and technical training required for the adequate education of professional nurses. In particular, the
liberal arts would provide students with "a foundation that permits continuing growth of many kinds," including "insights into one's own motivation, the
behavior of others, and cultural patterns that condition human behavior;"
historical and anthropological perspectives "of contemporary social institutions and their functions;" and effective communication, data collection, and
analytical skills.[22] A second study published that same year by economist Eli
Ginzberg also called for the relocation of nursing schools from hospitals to
universities and colleges.[23]

Henderson's and Peplau's critiques of nursing education were influenced
by the Brown report but were also based on their experiences with diploma
and baccalaureate degree programs, and their disillusionment with the traditional model of nursing practice. For Henderson, "the regimentalized patient care" that nurses traditionally performed "and the concept of nursing as
merely ancillary to medicine" were outdated concepts that should be replaced.
Nursing, redefined, would primarily complement "the patient by supplying
what he needs in knowledge, will, or strength to perform his daily activities
and also to carry out the treatment prescribed for him by the physician."[24] In
this way, nursing would finally become "patient-centered," whereby the patient
and particularly his or her needs—not the medical diagnosis nor physician-
delegated tasks—are the "central" concern of nursing, and the patient "understand[s], accept[s], and participate[s]" in their health care.[25] In order to
practice such patient-centered nursing, the nurse would need to know and
understand the patient, "to 'get inside his skin.'" She would do so by listen-
ing to the patient and the patient's family and friends, and by being aware
of her own relationship with the patient and ensuring it is "a construc-
tive, or therapeutic one," which in turn would depend on the nurse's "self-
understanding."[26] Nursing education, Henderson contended, should therefore be reformulated to prepare nurses for their new role as an "expert and

an independent practitioner." Such education "must be organized around the nurse's major function rather than that of the physician" in order to prepare the nurse to identify, understand, and respond to the particular needs of each individual patient. It was time, Henderson argued, to replace the regimented, procedure-based, hands-on training of the diploma model with "a liberalizing education, a grounding in the physical, biological, and social sciences, and the ability to use analytic processes."[27]

Peplau, who like Henderson held a theoretically grounded and patient-centered view of nursing practice, advocated the implementation of advanced graduate nursing education to prepare nurses for expertise in specialist clinical areas such as psychiatric nursing. Beginning in the mid-1950s, Peplau advocated that psychiatric nurses should have expertise as psychotherapists.[28] This psychiatric nursing expertise was to be grounded in psychoanalytic and psychotherapeutic theory and interpersonal relations theory, and based on a psychodynamic model of nursing. By developing "specific interpersonal techniques useful in intervening in specific pathological behavior of patients," taught at the master's level, the psychiatric nurse would establish a therapeutic relationship with patients.[29] As historian Kylie Smith argues, Peplau's model challenged the paternalism of existing models of nursing care, "which saw the nurses' role as to do for the patient what they were unable to do for themselves," and instead required the nurse to "facilitate the patient's own experience."[30] While the psychiatric nurse engaged in specialized clinical practice, Peplau maintained, the technical work of nursing should fall to the general duty nurse.

For Brown, Henderson, and Peplau alike, then, the behavioral and social sciences would be integral to the new, collegiate-based model of nursing education. The social and behavioral sciences would help the nurse focus on the "total patient," increase understanding of the patient, and improve nurse-patient communication. Sociology, social psychology, and cultural anthropology—those sciences "that have in common the study of why people behave as they do" and which share the "view that all aspects of human behavior are interrelated and interdependent" were thought to be most important to nursing.[31] As Brown saw it, anthropology, sociology, and social psychology, in particular, offered potential solutions to nursing's "struggl[e] with the problem of patients as people."[32] Brown referred, in particular, to questions that had long "plagued all nursing services," such as "why some patients are unconsciously overlooked and neglected" and why "patients often labeled 'uncooperative' or 'demanding'" are subsequently "viewed as unworthy of little more than technical care."[33]

The social and behavioral sciences were seen as especially important for helping nurses better understand and care for patients from different racial, ethnic, or religious backgrounds than themselves. Nurses needed "knowledge of sociopsychological and cultural factors and the attitudes and behaviors fostered by them" so as to prevent communication barriers and "fear of differences, social distance, prejudice, hostility, stereotyping," and other such negative reactions that would interfere with patient care.[34] These social sciences would also, Brown hoped, help nurses to identify and understand the impact of a nurse's relationship with other members of the hospital staff, "the social system of the ward, the hierarchically structured nursing service, and even the hospital as a whole" on "the quality of nurse-patient relationships" and, ultimately, patient care.[35]

Beginning in the 1950s, then, nurse educators introduced new models of undergraduate nursing education, located on university and colleges campuses, that replaced the regimented, procedure-based training of hospital-based diploma programs. Although the first baccalaureate nursing program was introduced in 1909 and many university-based nursing schools offered baccalaureate programs in nursing, these early programs typically prepared RNs (those trained in diploma programs) for careers in advanced practice, nursing administration, or nursing education. In a few programs, students would earn a baccalaureate degree after completing two years of liberal arts study alongside three years of hospital-based training. Beginning in the 1950s, nurse educators reformulated baccalaureate programs as entry-level general nursing programs.

These new BSN programs were premised on liberal education and integrated the biomedical, behavioral, and social sciences, emphasizing nursing theory and patient-centered practice.[36] In some cases, nursing schools hired social scientists to teach these new courses (discussed in more detail in chapter 3). For example, Virginia Dunbar, dean at New York University School of Nursing, hired the anthropologist Frances Cooke Macgregor. At the University of Florida College of Nursing, Dean Dorothy Smith hired both a psychologist and an anthropologist to serve on the faculty. At the University of Washington, Dean Mary Tschudin hired sociologists and psychologists to the faculty, and at the University of California, San Francisco (UCSF), Dean Helen Nahm hired sociologists to the faculty, including Anselm Strauss. It was in this context that several nurses began to develop nursing-specific theories that defined nursing's expert and independent role and could be used to structure the undergraduate curriculum reforms (see chapter 2). By emphasizing the nursing model of care—and rejecting the medical model of nursing practice—these new BSN programs prepared professional nurses for their work as independent and expert practitioners.

The nursing model of care is reflected in the innovative approach taken by Smith at the University of Florida to transform nursing education and practice. As part of a broader set of institutional and educational reforms (discussed in chapter 5), Smith introduced the nursing history—a patient data form. The nursing history was a "tool" that "provide[d] a first step in arriving at a more scientific and less intuitive methodology for nursing practice."[37] It enabled nurses to collect information from patients in an organized, systematic way in order to identify the patient's strengths and nursing care needs and formulate a nursing care plan.[38] As former faculty member Betty Hilliard reflected, the nursing history was "a parallel history of the medical one, but it wasn't disease oriented, it was patient-oriented."[39]

The nursing history was Smith's effort to identify and operationalize nurses' "*clinical thinking*" (emphasis in original).[40] For Smith, clinical thinking was the process by which a clinician makes a diagnostic or prognostic prediction after taking the patient's history, completing an examination of the patient, making "inferences based on a rapid and mostly pre-conscious cross checking against each of the knowledge models," and determining the "preferred method of treatment" based on these inferences.[41] Smith used Virginia Henderson's definition of nursing to delineate the unique functions and clinical nursing problems encountered by professional nurses, and thus to identify the types of data the nurse would need to collect from a patient in order to make a nursing diagnosis and develop a nursing care plan.[42] Henderson defined nursing's unique role as assisting "the individual, sick or well, in the performance of those activities contributing to health or recovery (or to a peaceful death) that he would perform unaided if he had the necessary strength, will or knowledge. And to do so in such a way as to help him gain independence as rapidly as possible."[43] To this end, the nursing history guided nurses to document the patient's understanding of their illness and the events leading up to it; the patient's expectations regarding their illness, treatment, and recovery; and what the patient considered important, particularly regarding what would help the patient "feel secure, comfortable, protected, safe, [and] cared for." The nursing history would also guide the nurse in the "process of clinical thinking based on obtained data" (which included the patient's vital statistics and social history) "and appropriate parameters of knowledge."[44] The nurse would then use the data in the nursing history to formulate a nursing care plan.

For Smith, the nursing history was to be instrumental in the clinical education of nursing students. After all, it helped identify the "specific parameters of knowledge needed by the baccalaureate nurse" and the "sciences basic to nursing practice." In addition, it also made clear that "repetition in the clinical program should be in the use of the knowledge—not in the knowledge itself." For example, she argued, the nursing students "must practice over and over again the skills of assessing patients' nursing needs with different people with different conditions in different settings and from different socio-economic backgrounds."[45] In addition, the students "must practice the writing of nursing orders and the implementing of these orders. They must do these over and over again until the method becomes familiar to them."[46] To this end, nursing students would complete nursing histories on each patient they saw, turning them into the faculty who would then evaluate them.[47] In turn, the nursing history helped clarify the clinical function of the academic nursing faculty. Indeed, to help students develop clinical thinking skills, Smith argued, the faculty must themselves "be expert" in those skills—"of assessment, goal setting, methodology to reach the goals, evaluatory [sic] procedures and in a knowledge basis for all these skills," as well as in the "application of knowledge to the solving of clinical nursing problems."[48]

As Fairman has argued, the nursing history "made visible the work of nurses and helped other professions understand that nurses had something important to say and could contribute to patient care decisions."[49] In this way, Smith intended the nursing history to form of the basis of nursing's contribution to collaborative patient care. However, the nursing staff faced "a lot of obstacles" in getting the nursing history to be part of the patient's permanent record.[50] Some physicians felt the nursing history "was cluttering up the chart,"[51] while others jealously guarded the contents of the patients' records.[52] The medical records department would also routinely remove the nursing history of the patient's record.[53] Nevertheless, the use of the nursing history codified the knowledge and practices that constituted professional nursing practice, and thus reflected the changing status of BSN education.

As the nature of nursing work expanded and patient care assumed greater complexity after the war (which, nurse educators argued, necessitated the curriculum reforms), much of the so-called traditional bed and body work of nursing was transferred to lesser-trained "technical nurses" (or bedside nurses), practical nurses, and nursing assistants. Practical nurses were typically trained in one-year programs that were principally located in hospital-based nursing schools or, increasingly, were offered by vocational educational systems.[54] Between 1950 and 1963, the number of practical nurse programs in the United States increased from 144 to 737.[55] In 1951, Mildred Montag introduced the concept of a new, specialized nursing worker, the technical nurse, whose training would be more than that of a practical nurse but less than that of the diploma or baccalaureate prepared professional nurses. Technical nurses were to assume responsibility for the hands-on bodywork of nursing. They would be trained in two-year associate degree programs based at community colleges, receiving general and nursing education and clinical instruction. The first three associate degree programs were established in 1952, and by 1960 there were more than one hundred associate degree programs throughout the U.S.[56]

The rapid expansion of associate degree programs in nursing reflected broader changes in American higher education, particularly the increasing commitment of education policymakers to significantly expand access to, and diversify institutions of, higher education.[57] In 1944, Congress passed the G.I. Bill of Rights, which included among its provisions tuition and monthly subsistence for veterans who wanted to attend college.[58] Three years later, President Harry Truman's Commission on Higher Education released its report, *Higher Education for American Democracy*.[59] The report called for the doubling of the number of students attending college in the U.S. by 1960, the elimination of financial barriers to higher education, and an end to racial, gender, and religious discrimination in higher education.[60]

At the center of the commission's plan for increasing access and equity in higher education was the massive expansion and reconceptualization of the nation's two-year colleges. In their redefined role, junior colleges would become community colleges and would provide students with general education and vocational education, leading to terminal degrees and providing support for students who would eventually transfer to four-year institutions. The commission expected that community colleges, as their new name reflected, would be fully integrated within and oriented toward the needs of the community. As part of this, community colleges would be responsible "for surveying and monitoring the educational needs of their communities so that their programs could be adapted to the needs of both general and vocational students at a local level." In turn, local communities, with additional support from the state, would be responsible for financing community colleges. States would undertake statewide planning to coordinate the location and educational offerings of community colleges within the state system, so as to avoid costly duplication and ensure that comprehensive education was being provided throughout the state. Ultimately, the postwar expansion of community colleges was intended to provide moderately priced and accessible education to all qualified students in communities across the country.[61]

The introduction and expansion of associate degree programs in nursing during the 1950s and 1960s contributed to the increasing number of nurses educated in institutions of higher education during these decades. It also created a new educational pathway into nursing—and higher education, in general— for women and men "without the material or social resources necessary to attend a traditional four-year college or university."[62] The introduction of associate degree programs in nursing, however, exacerbated already-existing hierarchies within the nursing workforce that stratified nurses by "education level, place of training (e.g., elite versus non-elite training schools), family income, and class."[63] These hierarchies were further compounded by race. By the late 1960s, the majority of nurses of color graduated from associate degree programs, reflecting broader trends in higher education in which students of color were overrepresented in community colleges and heavily underrepresented in four-year colleges and universities.[64]

In this new educational hierarchy, the baccalaureate (BSN)-prepared nurse assumed the status of the "professional nurse" and the responsibilities of the expert and independent clinical practitioner, while the AD-prepared nurse assumed the responsibilities of the "technical nurse." Professional nurses, typically after completing advanced graduate education, would go on to serve as clinical supervisors, educators, or administrators. In 1965, the National League for Nursing (NLN) passed a resolution that "recognized and strongly supported the trend toward collegiate nursing."[65] That same year, the American Nurses Association attempted to formalize this dual-level educational system and mandate the AD and BSN as the minimum educational requirement for entry into practice. While the effort failed, the debate over entry into practice has thrived since.[66] And as detailed in chapter 4, as the ANA and educational reformers worked to raise the educational preparation of nurses to the baccalaureate and graduate level, the graduates of diploma (and associate degree) programs were under pressure to upgrade their educational credentials but frequently encountered institutional and financial obstacles to their educational mobility.[67] The racial and class stratification of the differentially educated nursing workforce—and the obstacles to educational mobility—impacted which nurses were afforded opportunities for career advancement, leadership, and faculty positions.

But in the 1960s and 1970s, nursing leaders' claims of an educational hierarchy were largely rhetorical and aspirational. All nurses, regardless of whether they were educated in diploma, AD, or BSN programs, sat for the same licensing exams, and on completion, earned the title of registered nurse (RN). And despite efforts by educational reformers to distinguish the roles and responsibilities of AD- and BSN-prepared nurses, through the 1970s, the distinction between AD- and BSN-prepared nurses had become blurred in clinical practice.[68] Instead of establishing actual distinctions in practice, the differential educational pathways into nursing resulted in tensions between the differentially trained nurses working at the bedside, and bedside nurses and nurse educators.

The NLN and ANA resolutions also had implications for the status of hospital training schools. In 1960, more than 80 percent of nursing students were enrolled in hospital training schools.[69] However, by the late 1950s, hospital leaders were concerned about the rising costs of nursing education. As William K. Turner, director of Newport Hospital in Rhode Island, noted in 1959, the costs of nursing education were rising yearly and had become "a considerable surcharge on the bill for hospital service."[70] At Newport Hospital, for example, the net cost of nursing education had increased from $36,657 in 1954 to $71,747 in 1957. Although the number of student nurses had increased during those years with a concomitant increase in student service hours, the number of service hours per student had actually declined. This meant the hospital was spending more to educate each student, "result[ing] in a four-year rise of almost one-third in the net cost of education."[71] Turner reported similarly high costs of nursing education among hospitals in Connecticut and Illinois. While nursing education costs were often passed on to the patient through higher rates for hospital services, individual patients were increasingly unable to pay for their care, and there was a growing reluctance among private insurance companies to consider the cost of nursing education an allowable expense to be added to the patient's hospital bill.[72] According to Turner, the cost of educating the nation's nurses placed an "unfair burden" on hospitals.[73]

By the early 1960s, a growing coalition of nursing and hospital leaders were calling for the phasing out of hospital training schools.[74] Even so, throughout the decade there remained a lack of political will among nursing and hospital leaders to eliminate hospital training schools as they confronted ongoing nursing shortages and the need to quickly increase the number of nurses being educated. The NLN, which accredited nursing schools of all types, did not want to lose the significant income it received from hospital schools in the form of accreditation fees. So, too, the American Medical Association (AMA) continued to support—and lobby on behalf of—hospital schools through the mid-1970s, reflecting the reluctance of physician leaders to relinquish involvement in nursing education.[75] At the same time, advocates of hospital training programs, particularly the leadership, faculty, and alumni of those schools, pressured state and federal legislators to ensure hospital schools continued to receive legislative and financial support.[76] Nevertheless, the number of hospital-based nursing programs—along with the proportion of nurses educated at them—declined significantly over the next two decades. From 1960 to 1965, hospital training schools were closing at a rate of "approximately 18 a year, but from 1965 to 1970 the rate doubled to 36 a year."[77] In 1960, hospital training schools educated more than 80 percent of nurses. By 1980, hospital training schools educated less than 20 percent of the nursing workforce, and a decade later that number had fallen to 8 percent.[78]

Innovations in graduate nursing education also took place during these decades, which built upon Peplau's calls for specialized clinical training at the master's degree level. As early as 1952, the NLN had recommended that clinical specialty preparation should take place at the master's level. But through the 1950s, master's degrees in nursing were functional degrees: they prepared nurses for advanced education and practice in either administration, education, or clinical supervision.[79] There were a few exceptions to this functional focus, most notably in the emerging specialty of psychiatric nursing. During the 1950s, a handful of nursing schools, including Teachers College, Rutgers University, and New York University, with funding from the National Institute of Mental Health, established clinical master's programs in psychiatric nursing.[80]

By the 1960s, however, increasingly complex, specialized patient care had created new expert roles for nurses who had undergone advanced clinical training (at the master's degree level) in various other nursing specialties, including maternal-child health, oncology, nephrology, and critical care nursing. These expert clinical specialists were prepared in particular for leadership positions within service agencies and educational institutions (see chapter 5).[81] At the University of Colorado in 1965, public health nurse Loretta Ford, in collaboration with her physician colleague, Henry Silver, formalized the nurse practitioner role. In this expanded role, nurse practitioners were educated through a postbaccalaureate curriculum to provide total comprehensive care to children in outpatient settings.[82] As discussed in chapter 4, the nurse practitioner role was soon expanded to encompass the provision of primary health care services to adults. The establishment of the new nurse practitioner role took place amid persistent shortages of primary care physicians, particularly in rural and underserved urban areas of the country.[83]

Philanthropic foundations like the Russell Sage Foundation and the Kellogg Foundation, as well the Division of Nursing of the U.S. Public Health Service underwrote the planning and implementation of many of these educational reforms.[84] The Division of Nursing began funding nursing research projects in 1955, and in 1962 established the Nurse Scientist Graduate Training Program (NSGTP), which supported nurses pursuing research-based graduate degrees in university science departments (see chapter 2). Congress also responded to growing concerns about impending shortages of health care workers by passing a series of legislation intended to subsidize the education of health professionals, including nurses. The first of these, the Health Amendments Act of 1956, "allocated money to prepare nurses to become teachers, supervisors, and nursing service administrators."[85]

In 1961, at the behest of the Public Health Service's chief nursing officer, Lucile Petry Leone, the surgeon general convened a commission of health care professionals, administrators, and educators to investigate problems in the education, practice, and supply of nurses. In 1963, the surgeon general's Consultant Group on Nursing declared that the "nation's supply of nurses today has great inadequacies, both in numbers and in educational preparation." By 1970, the group concluded, the country would need 850,000 professional nurses, with 200,000 of them having at least a baccalaureate degree, and another 100,000 having graduate preparation to meet the critical need for nurses prepared for teaching and leadership positions. This translated into schools needing to graduate 53,000 new nurses each year by 1970.[86] That same year, Congress passed the Health Professions Educational Assistance (HPEA) Act of 1963, which provided construction grants for health professions teaching facilities and student loans to medical, dental, and nursing students.[87]

A year later, following the publication of the surgeon general's Consultant Group on Nursing's *Toward Quality in Nursing*, Congress passed the 1964 Nurse Training Act (NTA), Title VII of the Public Health Service Act. The act provided matching federal funds for the building of new nursing schools and the expansion of existing ones, as well as loans and traineeships to nursing students.[88] While the ANA lobbied for the NTA to prioritize the support of baccalaureate education and reduce support of hospital training programs, the American Hospital Association and AMA successfully lobbied for the inclusion of funding for diploma programs. The NTA thus reinforced the multiple educational pathways into nursing, which included three-year diploma programs, two-year associate degree programs, and four-year baccalaureate programs.[89]

Congressional support of health professions education continued through the mid-1970s through subsequent iterations of the HPEA and NTA.[90] However, as Lynaugh has documented, in the early 1970s, the Department of Health, Education, and Welfare under the leadership of Secretary Caspar Weinberger, "turned openly hostile toward nursing" and worked to severely limit Nurse Training Act funding.[91] In response, nurses throughout the country, led by the ANA and other nursing organizations, organized themselves politically and began lobbying Congress to preserve federal funding of nursing education. By the end of the 1970s, the NTA had provided more than $4 billion in federal funding for nursing education.[92]

To be sure, the efforts of nursing leaders and health policymakers to increase the number of nurses also included efforts to recruit greater numbers of foreign-trained nurses. As historian Catherine Ceniza Choy details in *Empire of Care*, by the late 1960s, Filipino nurses constituted the overwhelming majority of foreign nurses who entered the U.S. through the government's Exchange Visitor Program (EVP). Congress established the EVP in 1948, and "between 1956 and 1969, over eleven thousand Filipino nurses participated in the program."[93] Participants of the EVP came to the U.S. for up to two years to work and study in sponsoring institutions, which provided them with a monthly stipend. The ANA and individual hospitals were among the several thousand sponsoring U.S. agencies and institutions. While Filipino nurses had their own reasons for participating in the program, which were indelibly shaped by the history of U.S. colonialism in the Philippines, U.S. hospitals "used exchange nurses as an inexpensive labor supply to alleviate growing nursing shortages in the post–World War II period."[94] Congress's passage of the Immigration and Nationality Act in 1965 further encouraged the recruitment of foreign-trained nurses by American hospitals. With ongoing shortages of health care professionals, and concerns that those shortages would be exacerbated following the implementation of Medicare and Medicaid, foreign-trained nurses were in particularly high demand and large numbers of Filipino nurses immigrated to the U.S. in response. Indeed, as Choy notes, by 1967, "the Philippines became the world's top sending country of nurses to the United States."[95]

The Emergence of Academic Health Centers

The changes in nursing education occurred at the same time that many American academic health institutions were being conceptualized or reconfigured as academic health centers (AHCs). AHCs emerged as a new organizational form in the United States in the 1950s, replacing the traditional academic medical center model, which typically included an administrative alliance between the university's medical school, hospital, and medical staff. AHCs instead combined all of a university's health science schools, biomedical research institutes, and affiliated teaching hospitals and clinics under one centralized administration. Within an AHC, each health science school, in theory, was granted equal administrative status. AHCs were also intended to integrate the education and research that took place within nursing, medical, dental, pharmacy, public health, and allied health schools. This, administrators hoped, would not only help to dismantle the disciplinary silos that had previously characterized academic health institutions, but would also promote interdisciplinarity in research and education, and a team approach to clinical practice.[96]

The conceptualization or reconfiguration of health professional schools into AHCs presented nursing schools with new opportunities to assert their academic status and secure equal institutional standing among the health profession schools within their host institutions. Indeed, by establishing nursing's equal institutional status among the other health professions, nursing leaders hoped that AHCs would not only "protect" nursing "from medical dominance and authority" and assure nursing's academic standing, but also promote the concept of health rather than medicine or medical care.[97]

The development of AHCs also presented nursing schools with significant challenges. In all but a handful of AHCs across the country, physicians were appointed to lead the AHCs (usually given the title of vice president, provost, or chancellor). Thus, at the same time that nursing was moving out of hospitals (where it had been under medical control) into universities, universities were consolidating their health science schools into AHCs, typically headed by a physician with a direct line to the university president, while all deans within the AHC (who had previously had a direct line to the president) were now subordinate to the vice president of health sciences. For nursing leaders, this recreated an all-too-familiar institutional dynamic in which physicians had administrative authority over nursing education.[98]

UCLA's Center for the Health Sciences was one of the first AHCs to be organized in the 1950s. It was initially established as a traditional medical center when the regents of the University of California authorized a medical school at UCLA in 1945. However, it was quickly reconceived as an AHC following the establishment of a professional nursing school in 1949 and the initiation of plans to establish schools of dentistry and public health in 1960 and 1961. In 1970, the University of Minnesota reorganized its health science schools and hospitals into an academic health center. In contrast to UCLA's program, the development of Minnesota's AHC required administrative, intellectual, and physical reorganization of schools and colleges of the health sciences that dated back to the late nineteenth century, when the schools of medicine, dentistry, and pharmacy were founded. Minnesota's nursing school was established in 1909 as the first university-based school of nursing in the country, while the School of Public Health and College of Veterinary Medicine were established in the 1940s.

From the 1950s through the 1970s, individual nursing schools around the United States debated the merits of reformulating nursing education, experimenting with new curricula that eliminated dependence on a medical model of practice and emphasized instead nursing theory and patient-centered practice. The efforts of the nursing schools at UCLA and the University of Minnesota to reform the undergraduate nursing education amid these broader changes in health professional education reveal the highly contested nature of nursing education reform during these decades. They highlight the tensions that played out between bedside nurses, nurse administrators, physicians, and nurse educators in the university teaching hospitals when the nursing schools introduced educational reform. As nursing students now spent more time learning about the social and behavioral sciences and the nursing model of care, and less time working as student nurses in the hospital, learning less about the medical model and how to serve the physician, physicians and many staff nurses and nurse administrators were concerned that the new nursing students were not being appropriately educated to be effective bedside nurses.

The Gendered Politics of Health Education at UCLA

In 1949, Lulu Wolf Hassenplug was appointed founding dean of UCLA's School of Nursing. Hassenplug had graduated with a diploma from the Army School of Nursing at Walter Reed Hospital in 1924, and earned a baccalaureate degree from Columbia University Teachers College in 1927 and a Master of Public Health degree from Johns Hopkins University. She came to UCLA already a leader in nursing education, having played an instrumental role developing Vanderbilt University's baccalaureate nursing program.[99] At UCLA, Hassenplug oversaw the elimination of the hospital-based diploma program and the introduction of a four-year baccalaureate in nursing in 1950 and a Master of Science graduate program in 1951. In the late 1950s, the school began planning for a doctoral program in nursing.

UCLA's baccalaureate program was the first in the country to provide nursing students with the same preparation regardless of whether they wished to become clinicians, educators, or administrators. Students who wanted to pursue careers as educators, administrators, or clinical specialists would, after receiving their baccalaureate, enter the graduate program for advanced specialized education. All other nursing baccalaureate programs in this era tracked students into *either* education, clinical practice, *or* administration.[100]

From the late 1950s throughout the 1960s, however, the UCLA School of Nursing was under constant attack from the surgical faculty, medical school dean, and hospital director, all of whom lamented the loss of the traditionally trained bedside nurse. As Hassenplug recalled, "we got complaints" from physicians when the school revised the nursing curriculum because "the physicians thought our students were their own."[101] In February 1957, for example, UCLA neurosurgeon Eugene Stern wrote to the medical school dean lamenting the substandard education being received by UCLA's nursing students. The nursing students "are not learning adequate bedside care. . . . They appear to be more concerned with the psychological aspects of case studies to which they are assigned rather than being concerned with learning the rudiments of nursing care. . . . They likewise are taught minimal, if any, responsibility to the physician." For Stern, the decline in the quality of

UCLA's nursing education could be correlated with the elimination of the hospital-based diploma program and the now-minimal role of the physician in training nurses.[102]

Stern joined his colleagues in the Department of Surgery in calling for reform of nursing education at UCLA. Specifically, the surgeons wanted nursing students to return to the wards and operating rooms like the earlier diploma students, and for "nurse training" to be "implemented by a curriculum of which and in which the physician shares supervisions, consults, and participates."[103] As chair of UCLA's Department of Surgery William P. Longmire explained, the surgeons' hostility to the nursing reforms was because "many of us felt that our school was not graduating the type of nurse who would then become involved in patient care." Longmire took particular issue with the school's new philosophy, "that the student nurses were actually to have no ward assignments; they were to come on the wards as observers, to study the patient's case but not to actively participate in the patient's care."[104]

The surgeons had the support of the medical school dean, who drew up a proposal to reorganize the nursing school and transfer the nursing curriculum to the School of Medicine. In this plan, the nursing faculty would be appointed "to the appropriate department of the Medical School as a division of nursing with such titles as are appropriate, i.e., Professor of Nursing (Surgery), Professor of Nursing (Obstetrics), etc., as a division of the Department. Each Medical School department could sponsor the appropriate parts of the Nursing curriculum." A nursing faculty member would be assigned oversight of the curriculum and hold the position of associate dean within the medical school.[105]

This proposal circulated in the medical school and university administration for several years. But, as Dean Hassenplug recounted, in those years the nursing school had the "honest support" of the university chancellor and provost of health sciences.[106] In 1960, when physician Franklin D. Murphy was appointed chancellor and the position of provost for the health sciences was eliminated, the institutional politics at UCLA shifted. With the considerable power of his office, Murphy joined the assault on the nursing school. In February 1963, the dean of the medical school, Sherman Mellinkoff, wrote to Murphy that "it would be best to abandon a Nursing School at UCLA, except as a Hospital Diploma School . . . If a 'School of Nursing' is to be retained at UCLA it would require a great effort to reform it, and the 'School' should, in effect, become a Department of the School of Medicine."[107] In June 1968, in an attempt to "come to grips with the nursing question," the chancellor's office circulated a proposal that called for the termination of existing undergraduate and graduate nursing programs, the transfer of responsibility for undergraduate nursing education to an Office of Nursing Education located in the UCLA hospital, and the discontinuation of the nursing school. The department of surgery, the medical school dean, and the hospital director fully endorsed Murphy's proposal.[108]

Faculty throughout the university, however, including members of the departments of medicine, pediatrics, and psychiatry, submitted a position paper "in vigorous opposition" to the proposed closing of the school.[109] The University Committee on Educational Policy issued a report that concluded, "The administrative unit for the education of nurses at UCLA should be the School of Nursing."[110] Moreover, Dean Hassenplug mobilized a nationwide political campaign in support of the nursing school. On receiving the proposal on a Friday afternoon in late June, Hassenplug alerted "all the deans of university schools of nursing, the national nursing organizations, our friends in the federal government" about what was happening: "Our attack, I might say, was fast and furious, and it was supported at every step." By Tuesday morning, UCLA's president, chancellor, and regents were being bombarded with phone calls, newspaper coverage, and letters demanding continuation of the nursing school. Soon thereafter, the chancellor and his allies abandoned their efforts to close the school.[111]

Professional Conflict at the University of Minnesota

While UCLA's nursing faculty confronted criticism from physicians, the example of the University of Minnesota is emblematic of the resistance the new generation of nurse educators faced from their colleagues *within* nursing. Since 1919, the School of Nursing at the University of Minnesota had offered a five-year baccalaureate program that required nursing students to take two years of liberal arts education before beginning three years of hospital-based clinical education. In 1962, however, the school introduced a new "integrated" four-year baccalaureate degree that incorporated liberal arts and nursing courses throughout the four years, eliminated the thirty-hour-per-week clinical service requirement, and emphasized coursework in the behavioral and psychological aspects of nursing.[112]

Edna L. Fritz had been appointed director of the nursing school after the retirement of Katharine J. Densford in 1959 and oversaw the introduction of the new curriculum. Fritz had received her baccalaureate nursing degree from Russell Sage College in 1940 and her master's in nursing education from Columbia University Teachers College in 1942. When she arrived at Minnesota, she was completing a doctorate in education at Teachers College under the supervision of Mildred L. Montag; she received her doctorate in 1965.[113]

Prior to her arrival at Minnesota, Fritz had worked for NLN, first serving as director of a demonstration project integrating specialized clinical instruction into the curriculum, and then as assistant director of the NLN department of baccalaureate and higher degree programs.[114] Prior to her work with the NLN, Fritz had served as a nursing instructor at Cornell University, New York Hospital, and Massachusetts General Hospital School of Nursing. Fritz thus brought to Minnesota experience with, and a commitment to, curriculum development but little experience with university administration.

When Fritz arrived at Minnesota in 1959, the undergraduate nursing curriculum was already being developed by a small group of the faculty. According to retired faculty member Marilyn Sime, the reform group "had a new vision ... for delivering nursing education." The older five-year curriculum had been predicated on a "medical model" and the assumption that nursing care, at least within the hospital, would be delegated by the physician. In that curriculum, the emphasis had been on clinical instruction. The new curriculum considered nursing care something separate from delegated medical care. It taught students to "stud[y] patient behaviors, and arriv[e] at . . . a nursing diagnosis of the patient's needs and develop[e] a nursing care plan around those concepts rather than around the medical conditions."[115] In this way, the curriculum reforms drew explicitly on the work of Esther Lucile Brown, Hildegard Peplau, and Virginia Henderson, who called for nursing education to be grounded in the biomedical, behavioral, and social sciences to prepare nurses for independent practice that would be oriented to the individual needs—physical, psychological, and emotional—of patients.[116]

As Sime recalled, however, the new curriculum "wasn't loved by all. There were faculty that felt that too much had been lost and not enough gained by this new approach."[117] As Florence Marks, another former faculty member, elaborated, the faculty were no longer "teaching the didactic medical things, what you would do with this medical situation, this clinical situation. All those things were not there" anymore. Instead, the students "were supposed to know enough theory that they could figure these out for each patient. It was not something they learned, you know, as A, B, or C."[118]

In 1961, Marie Manthey was completing her baccalaureate degree while the curriculum was in transition. As she described it, "The faculty was divided. I don't think they really knew how to manage the transition without pretty much destroying each other." Manthey recounted taking a clinical course taught by three faculty members, two of whom were leading the reforms. The third had been on the faculty since the 1930s and was "an extremely brilliant clinician with a lot of understanding of the medical sciences." What Manthey "saw as a student was these teachers standing up in front of us, two of them humiliating the third one, and the third one was the only one talking about anything I was interested in, which had to do with dealing with patients who are sick."[119] Manthey went on to earn her master's in Nursing Administration from the university, and from 1964 to 1971 she served as associate director of nursing at Minnesota's University Hospital.

Reflecting on this period of educational reform, Manthey noted that "the curriculum swung so far over to a non-clinical side that it was *absolutely* frightening. People were coming out of the school with an RN, if they passed their boards . . . [they] came out not having ever given an injection, never having seen a delivery." As Manthey perceived it, nursing students were being "discouraged from doing physical care for the patients. So they were inter-viewing patients. They would come back and they would write down every single word that was said by the patient . . . analyze and, then, decide whether to admit [the patient] or not. People told me that if they so much as gave a pa-tient a drink of water, they would be marked down by the faculty for engaging in nursing care activity."[120] Students who graduated from the BSN program during those years shared similar reflections.[121] Collectively, their recollec-tions speak both to the speed with which the University of Minnesota School of Nursing implemented substantial curriculum reform and the faculty's dis-connect with hospital nursing. Indeed, the faculty replaced a curriculum that prepared students for functional practice with a curriculum that taught them to engage in the process of clinical thinking, but at a time when the majority of hospitals were still wedded to functional nursing practice.

In essence, the nursing curriculum reforms reflected a growing tension among nurse educators as to the fundamental principles of nursing and the appropriate balance between theory and practice in undergraduate nursing education. The difficulty of integrating theoretical and practical knowledge into the curriculum reflected an explicit tension built into the structure of nursing education. While in medical schools the teaching faculty held both faculty positions in the medical school and clinical positions in the teach-ing hospital, in nursing schools during this period—including the University of Minnesota's—they rarely held clinical positions in the teaching hospital's nursing service. Thus, faculty clinical practice was not integrated into the structure of academic nursing (this will be discussed at length in chapter 5). At the University of Minnesota, this led to conflict and division between the nursing faculty and members of the University Hospital nursing service. During those years, the faculty would hear from the nursing service, "You'll never make a good nurse. You don't get enough experience. Some things, you have to learn just by practice." In response, the faculty would say, "You get the foundational theory. Eventually, you get the practice."[122]

The University of Minnesota's nurse educators also faced resistance to the educational reforms from university administrators and regents. As part of the reforms, the nursing school eliminated its Practical Nursing Program in 1967. This program, launched twenty years earlier, had provided one year of technical training to prepare practical nurses for licensure (these were the category of nurses who now assumed responsibility for the lower skill bed and body work of the traditional diploma-trained nurse). When the school began the Practical Nursing Program in 1947, it was only one of four such programs in the state. By the mid-1960s, however, there were twenty-five practical nursing programs in Minnesota.[123] When the school revised the baccalaureate curriculum, it eliminated the Practical Nursing Program so as to better utilize the faculty's resources and delegated the preparation of practical nurses to the state's community colleges. School director Edna Fritz wrote to the university vice president for academic affairs in April 1966, "With the resources available to us, the greatest contribution the University can make to the nurse supply of the state and region is through efforts to expand enrollments in Masters programs that prepare faculty to serve the many schools that exist, thus permitting expanded enrollments in them."[124] Indeed, in 1966, 85 nursing schools in the upper Midwest reported 109 faculty vacancies and a need for 41 additional faculty positions.[125] As Fritz saw it, the university nursing school's priority was to train advanced degree nurse educators who could fill these positions.

The closing of the Practical Nursing Program, however, provoked "some very grave resistance by a few people," not least the university regents. Powerful regent Charles Mayo (of Mayo Clinic fame) was particularly upset because he viewed the university's Practical Nursing Program "as the one sound program" the nursing school had. Mayo was a physician wedded to the traditional diploma school model of nursing education.[126] The director of the university hospital and the director of its nursing service also worried that without the guaranteed supply of practical nurses graduating from the nursing school, the university hospital would be forced to compete with other local hospitals and clinics for the practical nurses trained by other, perhaps lower quality programs.[127]

The educational reformers at Minnesota, however, clashed most significantly with school director Edna Fritz. In 1967, the reformers wrote to Robert Howard, dean of the College of Medical Sciences (which had authority over the nursing school), demanding action to rectify "what we perceive to be the major problem in the school, namely administrative interference with faculty functioning. . . . We feel that the relationship between the faculty and the director of the School of Nursing must be examined objectively."[128] Howard disagreed with their assessment and put his full support behind Fritz, which ultimately led many of the faculty to resign from the school. Unfortunately, little archival or oral history evidence is available to support this group's contentions about Fritz's leadership style (sadly, they have all since passed away).

The tension seems to have centered on a fundamental disagreement about the degree of clinical instruction in the new curriculum. While Fritz supported curriculum reform in general, she wanted the faculty to be more engaged with clinical teaching. This approach followed from Fritz's earlier work on an NLN-funded demonstration project, which had integrated concepts associated with specialized clinical areas into the basic nursing curriculum at Cornell University-New York Hospital School of Nursing.[129] Fritz questioned the reformers' decision to replace "clinical laboratory practice" hours in the curriculum with "classroom laboratory" hours, noting, "It is this practice that has so minimized the opportunities of students to apply their learnings in reality situations."[130]

Fritz also advocated a faculty practice model, championed by Dorothy Smith at the University of Florida, in which responsibility for clinical education would be shared by the faculty and nursing service (discussed in chapter 5). This diverged significantly from the practice during Katharine Densford's tenure as director, when the hospital nursing service had primary responsibility for clinical instruction. By pushing the faculty "to doll up in a uniform and a white cap and go back into the clinical areas," Fritz ostracized some of the school's most senior faculty who had not worked on the wards since their training in the 1920s and 1930s. In doing so, Fritz contributed to a generational and philosophical divide that already existed among the faculty and between the faculty and nursing service.[131]

Building the State's Nursing Workforce

The efforts to reform nursing education coincided with growing regional and national concerns among health care leaders and policymakers about impending shortages of health care workers, including nurses. As mentioned earlier, several studies of the nursing shortage conducted in the early 1950s predicted that between 50,000 and 75,000 new graduate nurses were needed each year.[132] In 1963, the Surgeon General's Consultant Group on Nursing (on which Hassenplug served) declared that the "nation's supply of nurses today has great inadequacies, both in numbers and in educational preparation." By 1970, the group concluded, the country would need 850,000 professional nurses, with 200,000 of them having at least a baccalaureate degree, and another 100,000 having graduate preparation to meet the critical need for nurses prepared for teaching and leadership positions. This translated into schools needing to graduate 53,000 new nurses each year by 1970.[133]

The degree of nursing shortage varied across states and regions.[134] In January 1957, for example, the University of California issued a report that projected that unless enrollment in the UCLA and UCSF schools of nursing expanded, by 1965 the western United States would face a shortage of more than 18,000 nurses. Within that shortage, the committees predicted deficits of 8,000 baccalaureate-trained nurses and 5,980 nurses with master's degrees or higher.[135] Ten years later, the state's nursing shortage continued. In 1966, California's Coordinating Council for Higher Education (CCHE) identified "a critical shortage of nurses at all levels of preparation [that] exist[ed] in California," as well as "a serious need for qualified teachers in nursing." As a result of these findings, the California CCHE called on the California state colleges and the University of California system to expand all nursing programs, including graduate programs.[136] In Minnesota, by contrast, the nursing shortage was less severe. In 1966, the Upper Midwest Nursing Study reported that Minnesota's rate of nurse graduates from all nursing programs was nearly twice that of the rest of the country and, moreover, the upper Midwest region served as "an important source for nursing personnel."[137]

As a result of California's shortages, the authors of the University of California report proposed a statewide plan for nursing education in which the UCLA and UCSF schools of nursing would retain their undergraduate curricula but would also "put special emphasis on graduate education, particularly the preparation of nursing educators." Furthermore, "no other collegiate programs should be established on other campuses of the University of California." Because only UCLA and UCSF had adequate facilities in medical education, the report's authors contended that only these schools were equipped to provide nursing students "the quality of general and professional education now required for competence in the expanding fields of nursing."[138] Following the recommendations of the Brown and Ginzberg reports of 1948 and the Bridgman report of 1953, which provided detailed recommendations for establishing a collegiate nursing program, the University of California report called for the abandonment of hospital schools of nursing and for two-year curricula (leading to an associate degree) to be established at the state's community colleges, and four-year curricula (leading to baccalaureates) at the state's other four-year institutions.[139] Graduate nursing education should remain the province of UCLA and UCSF. The expectation, of course, was that many of these advanced graduate nurses would join the faculty at the community and state colleges to boost their undergraduate curricula. Ultimately, then, the report proposed a statewide division of educational labor in the university, state college, and community college systems.[140]

In response to these concerns, nurse educators framed their calls for educational reform as necessary for resolving the impending crisis in nursing supply and fulfilling the university's obligation to the state. Since the late 1940s, state legislators had looked increasingly to academic health institutions receiving state funds to expand educational opportunities and better coordinate the production and distribution of the state's health workforce. In March 1949, for example, at a meeting of the Finance Committee of the California Senate, Senator Bradford S. Crittenden offered his support for the budget of the University of California but warned "that he and other members of the committee and the Senate would be influenced in their enthusiasm by the present attitude and future planning of the University toward the problem of training enough professional people concerned with health and related problems to meet the needs of the State." Crittenden felt the committee's support was contingent, in particular, on the university addressing why the state had a shortage of doctors, dentists, nurses, pharmacists, and veterinarians.[141]

The nursing education reforms of the 1950s and 1960s were thus situated squarely within the politics of state health education and workforce policies. At UCLA and the University of Minnesota in particular, these politics indelibly shaped the outcome of educational reform. At UCLA, the nursing faculty warned administrators who wanted to shut down the school and reestablish nursing education as either a hospital-based program or a department within the medical school that they would violate the mandates set by the California Master Plan for Higher Education. In 1959, the California state legislature had asked the University of California and the California Board of Education to investigate the problems raised by exploding student population growth and mounting financial competition between the state's public universities and colleges, and develop a plan that would allow the state to continue to support higher education within its limited fiscal resources. The resulting Master Plan for Higher Education, codified in the Donahoe Higher Education Act of 1960, described a functional division of educational labor (consistent with the one already proposed for nursing education) between the University of California, the California state colleges, and the community colleges.[142]

In April 1962, UCLA's ad hoc committee on nursing, which had been appointed by Chancellor Murphy to review the organization of the nursing school in light of the medical school's complaints, concluded, "Clearly the University has an obligation . . . to continue a program in Nursing directed at alleviating" the shortages of nurses, nurse administrators, researchers, and educators, "at least until such a time as the State Colleges may take over some . . . of these functions." As such, the committee was thoroughly opposed to merging nursing into the medical school: "The prime function of nursing education at UCLA should not, in the long run, be an attempt to contribute significantly to the direct production of *practicing* nurses, but rather to provide nursing *faculty*, highly trained *nursing specialists*, and *scholars* in allied areas interested in applying this knowledge to problems of Nursing. Jurisdictionally, it would seem unwise and improper to incorporate a Department of Nursing in the School of Medicine" (emphasis added).[143]

Meanwhile, at the University of Minnesota, the nursing faculty addressed the concerns raised by the hospital's nursing service, regents, and administrators that the school's new academic orientation would lead to further decline in clinical nurses. As Director Fritz wrote to the Committee on Long Range Planning in the Health Sciences in September 1966, the school had "identified the most useful contributions that we might make to an augmented supply of nurses for our state and region." Based on data—including current and projected shortages—about the state of nursing in Minnesota, the Dakotas, and Montana, Fritz noted, "The greatest block to expanding student enrollments in nursing programs of all types is the serious shortage of qualified [that is, baccalaureate- and graduate-level-prepared] teachers." While there were a number of institutions in the region with practical nursing and basic professional programs, the University of Minnesota's nursing school was "the only institution in a four-state area presently able to provide preparatory programs for teachers of nursing to make possible improvement and expansion of the many other schools of nursing in this region." Fritz thus argued that the school's priority should be preparing the next generation of nursing educators and advanced clinical specialists.[144] The nursing school promised, however, to provide other nursing programs in the state, particularly at the community colleges, with "consultant services and continuing educational opportunities" to help them expand and establish practical nursing and associate degree programs.[145]

The nursing faculty at both UCLA and the University of Minnesota thus argued for the coordination of nursing educational hierarchies across their states to ensure a sufficient supply of nurses for the state and region, with university schools of nursing at the center. In this coordinated planning, the states' community colleges would be responsible for preparing associate degree nurses, the four-year universities and colleges would prepare baccalaureate nurses, and university programs would prepare advanced degree clinical specialists, researchers, and educators. As UCLA's nursing dean, Lulu Hassenplug, recalled, it was the nursing school's responsibility to set up a network of nursing education throughout the state: "The state university exists for that. We were in the community as much as we were in the university. . . . We thought we ought to be doing something like this to facilitate the growth of the baccalaureate and higher degree programs. We ought to be helping the whole region." As early as 1956, nursing leaders from the western states were working with the Western Interstate Commission for Higher Education to undertake regional planning for nursing.[146]

At the University of Minnesota, the nursing faculty became increasingly involved in regional planning in the mid-1960s after the initiation of the Upper Midwest Nursing Study. This project, funded by the Hill Family Foundation, described and analyzed the quantitative and qualitative supply of nurses and projected future demand for nurses in Minnesota, Montana, North Dakota, South Dakota, the Upper Peninsula of Michigan, and the northwestern portion of Wisconsin. With these data, the study group sought to tackle nursing shortages by better utilizing the region's existing supply of nurses.[147] Early in 1971, the School of Nursing joined the Minnesota Nurses Association (MNA) and other state nursing schools in the upper Midwest and applied for federal funding to initiate a regional planning project. They did so in response to the recommendations of the National Commission for the Study of Nursing and Nursing Education, which urged states to develop master plans for nursing and nursing education.[148] (This is discussed in more detail in chapter 4).

By placing their educational reforms in the context of state and regional health needs, nursing educators were able to secure their institutional objectives. Chancellor Murphy's efforts to discontinue UCLA's School of Nursing failed, and after several years of conflict, both schools regarded their educational reforms a success. Unfortunately for Fritz, however, by 1968 the practical implications of the nursing curriculum's shift away from clinical education were placed in stark relief. At the NLN evaluation team's site visit that March, the team noted the "serious imbalance" in the undergraduate program whereby the curriculum placed "disproportionate emphasis on the psychosocial dimensions of nursing, to the serious detriment of the biophysical aspects of nursing." Their findings confirmed reports that William Shepherd, vice president for academic affairs, had received in recent years from "students in the program about the adequacy of preparation in the biophysical aspects of nursing." Shepherd had also received reports from supervisors of the school's graduates who "regard[ed] them as poorly prepared for beginning nursing practice."[149] That fall, 25 percent of the graduating class failed their state licensing exams. While the curriculum's defenders, including Marilyn Sime, asserted that the state exams were not "measuring the new approach to nursing care" but "measuring knowledge from the old model," the failure provoked broad-based concern among the university administration and regents and led to Fritz being fired.[150]

The examples of the nursing schools at UCLA and the University of Minnesota reveal the ways state-supported academic health institutions have, since the 1950s, played an increasingly critical role in coordinating the supply and distribution of health care professionals in a region. And in so doing, academic health institutions have served as instruments of state health policymaking. We return to this topic, as it played out in the 1970s, in chapter 4.

New Politics, New Organizations

The educational reforms of the 1950s and 1960s also led to changes among the nursing organizations representing and advocating for nursing education programs. In 1952, the five extant nursing organizations voted to merge their organizations and membership in order to strengthen and unify the political voice of nursing. The Association of Collegiate Schools of Nursing, National Association of Public Health Nurses and the National League for Nursing Education merged to establish the National League for Nursing, while the National Association of Colored Graduate Nurses dissolved and its membership integrated—ostensibly at least—into the ANA.[151] Although only two decades later, in 1971, a group of Black nursing leaders established the National Black Nurses Association (NBNA), because of the failure of integration to eliminate racism and discrimination within nursing (discussed in later chapters).[152]

The NLN, which assumed responsibility for the accreditation of nursing schools in the U.S., established a Division of Nursing Education, which was divided into two departments. The Department (later Council) of Diploma and Associate Degree Programs represented hospital training schools and the newly established associate degree programs at community colleges, and as such represented the largest number of member schools. The Department (later Council) of Baccalaureate and Higher Degree Programs represented baccalaureate and graduate degree programs in nursing, which numbered far fewer—approximately 150 in 1952—than the hospital training schools.[153]

Both councils were charged with developing educational standards, implementing educational reforms, and providing guidance and resources to the deans and directors of nursing education programs. In this way, they provided leadership on issues related to nursing education and sought to represent and speak for the educational programs represented by their members. But the stakes of doing so were invariably different and often led to conflicting interests for the educational programs represented by the two departments—diploma and associate degree programs on the one hand, and baccalaureate and graduate degree programs on the other. As this chapter has detailed, as nursing leaders and educators at collegiate and university-based nursing schools reformulated baccalaureate programs and established new clinically oriented master's degree programs, many also called for the closure of diploma programs. This was typified by the push to establish the BSN as the entry degree into professional nursing practice. And yet the overwhelming majority of member programs within the NLN were hospital-based diploma programs and, increasingly—due to their exponential growth during the 1960s—associate degree nursing programs. By the late 1960s, the conflicting interests of diploma, AD, and BSN programs had led to many nursing school deans being dissatisfied and disillusioned with the NLN.[154]

The unique set of challenges that confronted university-based nursing schools, particularly those located within AHCs, led to an influential group of deans to call for the establishment of a separate organization.[155] By the late 1960s, the deans of nursing schools offering graduate programs had established themselves as a separate ad hoc committee of the NLN's Council of Baccalaureate and Higher Degree Programs (CBHDP) in order to focus on the "many issues now facing graduate nursing education."[156] Included among these issues were regional planning, comprehensive health planning and its implications for nursing, concerns about the proliferation of low-quality graduate programs, federal funding for graduate nursing education, and the need to ensure that nurse practitioner and clinical nurse specialty education was offered through master's degree programs in nursing schools.[157] For several deans, though, the ad hoc committee—tied as it was to the NLN—had neither the standing nor the capacity to sufficiently advance graduate nursing education. Among the limitations of the CBHDP was that its membership included faculty and deans of both undergraduate and graduate nursing education, and that because it was part of the NLN—which represented associate degree and diploma programs and whose board membership included nonnurses—its interests were often "diametrically opposed to," and thus undermined by, the interests of the larger organization.[158]

At the same time, as an ad hoc committee, it did not have standing to represent or speak for academic nursing's interests. Given the recent "health manpower" report by the American Medical Association's Commission on Graduate Education in Medicine, the forthcoming report by the National Commission for the Study of Nursing and Nursing Education (discussed in chapter 4), and threatened reductions in federal support to nursing programs, Rozella Schlotfeldt (dean of nursing at Case Western Reserve University) saw it as an imperative that deans of university-based nursing schools (those who by virtue of their position are "giving leadership to the field") organize politi-cally.[159] Schlotfeldt asserted that an organization of deans of nursing schools "under the aegis of higher institutions is an absolute necessity in the second half of the twentieth century!"[160]

In 1968, the CBHDP's ad hoc committee initiated plans to establish an independent organization of deans of graduate nursing programs. For Mary Kelly Mullane (dean of nursing at the University of Illinois Chicago), it was particularly critical to center the organization on deans of nursing schools af-filiated with AHCs. As Mullane explained, AHCs were sites in which "issues of both correlative and complementary roles, functions, and education" of medicine, nursing, pharmacy, and dentistry—that is, questions about inter-professional education and practice—came together and could be resolved. As such, Mullane saw it as essential that deans of nursing schools affiliated with AHCs "get together first and alone." Moreover, she reported, deans of medical schools "are searching for their counterparts in nursing to begin work with them on mutual problems."[161] AHC administrators were also keen to work with nursing school deans. In February 1968, Joseph Begando, chan-cellor of the University of Illinois Chicago's medical center, had alerted Mul-lane to that fact that the Organization of University Health Center Adminis-trators (which represented leaders of AHCs) wanted to meet with a group of deans of AHC-affiliated nursing schools at their next meeting in July.[162] But as one such dean had recently noted to Mullane, medical school deans find "nursing education to be such a large, amorphous group that they don't know where 'to put a handle in it to work with you.' "[163]

In the end, the ad hoc committee of graduate nursing deans voted in May 1969 to establish the American Association of Deans of College and Univer-sity Schools of Nursing.[164] Renamed the American Association of Colleges of Nursing (AACN) in 1972, the new organization represented the interests of AHC-affiliated nursing schools and all baccalaureate and graduate nursing degree programs. In the early 1970s, for example, the goals of the AACN were to "obtain broadened support (social and fiscal) for nursing education and research in universities," to "seek closer coordination with medical colleagues on increased responsibility for nurses and education for it," to "develop closer relationships between nursing education and nursing practice in teaching hos-pitals," and to enhance the role of nursing faculty in university-based nursing schools.[165] From the 1970s onward, the AACN became the voice of academic nursing, representing and promoting—on the national stage—the interests of academic nursing within health care, higher education, and health policy.

For its part, the NLN did not push back against the establishment of the AACN, its executive board having rejected (repeatedly) the ad hoc committee's proposals to establish an independent committee of graduate nursing deans within the framework of the NLN.[166] Instead, the NLN's CBDHP—whose functions, interests, and membership overlapped with those of the AACN— agreed to work cooperatively with the AACN, recognizing that the AACN's distinctive focus on legislative lobbying could complement rather than detract from the work of the NLN. By 1974, the AACN, NLN, and ANA had established an Interorganizational Committee for Implementation to provide "communication and interdigitation" among the three organizations and to ensure that cooperation remained a high priority among them.[167]

The lack of pushback from the NLN was also likely because the AACN was not interested in assuming responsibility for the accreditation of baccalaureate or graduate nursing programs in these early years. That responsibility, and the significant income it generated, remained in the hands of the NLN. This would come to have implications for nursing's academic project, however.

In the early 1980s, the AACN began developing educational standards for baccalaureate and graduate nursing programs—the "essential knowledge, practice competencies and values" that should "comprise the general and professional education of the professional nurse."[168] First published in 1986, these educational standards became codified as the AACN *Essentials*.[169] The AACN expected its member schools to ensure that the curricula of their baccalaureate and graduate nursing programs provided graduates with the knowledge base and clinical skills necessary for beginning or advanced practice, as codified in the AACN *Essentials*. But because the AACN had neither responsibility for, nor oversight over, accreditation, it had no direct mechanism for ensuring that the criteria by which programs were evaluated for accreditation were consistent with the educational standards it had set forth in the *Essentials*. Without control over both educational standards and accreditation standards, the AACN was hampered in its ability to implement across-the-board educational improvements. In turn, its member schools faced growing problems with the accreditation review process, as it involved not just the NLN but also state regulatory and credentialing agencies. The disconnect between educational standard-setting and accreditation—and the resulting accreditation "turmoil"—came to a head in the mid-1990s.[170] At that time, the AACN took the lead in resolving the issue, forming an alliance of regulatory and credentialing entities that worked to establish a new and autonomous credentialing agency for baccalaureate and graduate programs, the Commission on Collegiate Nursing Education. Although separate from the AACN, the new Commission helped to facilitate closer alignment between educational and accreditation standard-setting.[171]

Conclusions

The 1950s and 1960s were thus decades of change both for the American health care system and the nursing profession. A new generation of nurse educators sought to create greater professional autonomy for the nurse by introducing new models of education that emphasized science-based learning and clinical thinking over technical competence and functional practice. They also sought to create new clinical roles for the nurse, based on advanced graduate education. As they did so, these educators confronted generational conflicts in schools of nursing from older faculty and clinical instructors who feared becoming "second-class citizens" in increasingly *academic* nursing schools.[172] And they faced resistance from academic health care institutions comfortable with the gendered hierarchy of the health professions on which the traditional model of nursing education was predicted. The experiences of UCLA's School of Nursing during the 1960s were a stark reminder of the challenges that the gendered and hierarchical politics within academic health centers posed to nursing schools in this period.[173]

For nursing leaders, the lesson was clear: nursing's status as an academic discipline needed to be established and the role of nursing faculty secured within the university. As the next chapters detail, they did this by creating and demarcating the boundaries of a distinct science of nursing and establishing nursing PhD programs to prepare new generations of nurse scientists able to conduct the clinical research necessary to improve patient care. Along the way, however, nursing leaders continued to confront resistance from their colleagues in nursing who questioned the relevance of nursing's academic project. They also encountered opposition from university administrators, faculty in the biomedical sciences, and physicians who not only questioned the academic rigor of nursing but who also sought to protect the gendered hierarchical politics of academia and health care.

The Making of Nursing Science

In the decades after World War II, American nurses were engaged in an epistemological project to develop a science of nursing. They did so to formalize
the foundations of and legitimize nursing's professional work, and to prepare
nurses to better care for the changing health and illness needs of the population.[1] As the previous chapter details, through World War II, nursing's system
of knowledge was predicated upon the medical model, and as such, much of
nursing's work was dependent upon medicine's knowledge system, that of
the biomedical sciences. Beginning in the 1950s, however, academic nurses
worked to create nursing's own system of knowledge—nursing science—
and establish nursing as an academic discipline. Over the next two decades,
academic nurses developed the science of nursing, underpinned by nursing
theories that centered on the concepts of health, holism, and the environment, and by knowledge generated by nursing research, which focused on
the nurse-patient relationship and on improving individual and population
health and well-being.

There were two major factors that led nurses to advocate for the creation
of nursing science in the decades after World War II. The first was empirical and motivated by broadscale changes in the nature of patient care and,
therefore, nursing's work. In particular, as the previous chapter details, nurses
increasingly found themselves without the knowledge to provide appropriate
care to patients with more complex clinical needs.[2] They also did not understand how patients made decisions about their health care, or why patients
behaved in particular ways.[3] The second rationale was political: to establish
nursing as an academic discipline, which would secure the nursing profession's legitimacy and establish nurses as independent and expert practitioners. As the sociological literature of the 1950s and 1960s made clear, control

over an organized body of knowledge was an essential component of professional development; a point that Robert Merton made in a 1960 issue of the *American Journal of Nursing*.[4] To be sure, nursing was not the only practice profession engaged in an effort to establish its academic legitimacy. During these same decades, engineering, computing, clinical psychology, pharmacy, and social work were embroiled in similar empirical and political debates as they sought to establish their professions' disciplinary foundations.[5]

This chapter attends to the different and changing meanings that academic nurses ascribed to nursing science during these decades. In particular, academic nurses conceptualized the development of nursing science as a political process to justify nursing's positioning within universities and academic health centers, while also envisioning nursing science as a process of knowledge development and application to practice. While acknowledging the importance of academic nurses' own and shifting definitions of nursing science, the definition of nursing science that underpins my analysis is that which refers to the overall process of research, knowledge production, and application of knowledge into practice and policy.

Beginning in the 1950s, then, a small but growing number of academic nurses sought to build a science of nursing. They did so, on the one hand, by drawing upon the biomedical, social, and behavioral sciences. As chapter 1 notes, by utilizing the behavioral and social sciences, academic nurses sought to claim distinctive knowledge, skills, and expertise, rooted in an understanding of patient behavior and attitudes, which they—and not physicians—would contribute to the improvement of patient care.[6] On the other hand, academic nurses sought to establish nursing science as a theoretically oriented discipline. As part of this, nursing needed to develop its own theories rather than relying on those in the biomedical or behavioral sciences to guide nursing research and practice. As Myrtle Irene Brown asserted in 1964, "A clear mandate has been made to nurse researchers to build a body of scientifically tested nursing theory from which may be drawn facts, concepts, and principles on which to base the education of nurses and the nursing care and service of patients, families, and communities."[7] By asking research questions underpinned by *nursing* theories, nurse researchers would be able produce new knowledge that would be relevant specifically to nursing practice and would lead to the development of *nursing* science.

As nurse theorists and researchers worked to define nursing science and establish nursing as an academic discipline, they engaged in critical boundary and legitimation work—the process of selecting the requisite credentials of researchers, the types of research questions to be asked, and the methods and theoretical perspectives to be used for the purpose of drawing epistemic boundaries between nursing science and the existing biomedical and behavioral sciences.[8] As those requisite credentials included advanced degrees in nursing and, increasingly, doctorates in the biomedical or behavioral and social sciences, nursing's epistemological project was advanced primarily by white female nurses. Through these decades, Black, Indigenous, and other women of color faced significant barriers to accessing undergraduate and graduate nursing education and higher education in general.[9] And men, regardless of race, also encountered gender discrimination in their efforts to pursue undergraduate and graduate degrees in nursing.[10] The lack of diversity among the theorists and researchers engaged in constructing the science of nursing had implications for the types of research pursued and theories developed.

Through this boundary and legitimation work, nurse theorists and researchers demarcated nursing practice itself—particularly the nurse-patient relationship—as a site of knowledge production, and sought to demonstrate the ways in which application of nursing knowledge was integral to improving patient outcomes and health care delivery. In particular, nurse researchers conducted research to reduce hospital-based infections and adverse drug interactions, and to improve end-of-life care, pain management, and the management of chronic illness and debility. This was research that resonated with the broader quality assessment movement in health care, which aimed to systematically measure the outcome of patient care so as to determine which clinical interventions worked and which didn't and to hold physicians accountable for those outcomes.[11] At the same time though, nurse researchers opted *not* to pursue research on what today is referred to as the social determinants of health, despite calls from nurses of color and some public health nurses in the 1960s and 1970s to engage in this type of research. By exploring the choices nurse scientists made about the types of research they would pursue and the types of research methods they would use, this chapter highlights some of the limits of nursing's academic project and the consequences for that ongoing project today.

The efforts of academic nurses to develop a science of nursing occurred in parallel with the effort by academic physicians to establish a science of clinical medicine grounded in the new discipline of clinical epidemiology. It also took shape in the midst of a burgeoning feminist critique of science, which exposed the characteristics of scientific knowledge production—objectivity in particular—as distinctly masculine ways of relating to the world.[12] Yet, rather than seeking to question or transform the epistemological foundations of science, the overwhelming majority of nurse scientists were instead seeking access to doing science-as-it-was-currently-done—so-called normal science.[13]

But while academic physicians focused on constructing an empirical and statistically derived clinical science (applying the well-controlled experiment to the clinical setting), academic nurses worked instead to construct a science of nursing that was both empirical and theoretical. They did so because they saw the development of an abstract knowledge system underpinned by *theory* as key to achieving scientific legitimacy. Even as the majority of nurse scientists rejected engagement with feminist methodologies, they nevertheless created a system of abstract knowledge that emphasized nursing's distinctive perspective, rooted as it was in holism, caring, and an emphasis on environment—all qualities that some feminists have argued are distinctively feminist ways of knowing.[14] This chapter examines the difficulties this early generation of nurse scientists encountered as they sought to establish their scientific legitimacy and demonstrate the ways in which nursing science was integral to improving patient outcomes and health care delivery.

The Need for Nursing Science

As the previous chapter details, nurses were confronted with new clinical realities after World War II, particularly the increasing complexity of patient care. As the historian Julie Fairman argues, in this context, "Nurses increasingly realized they lacked the knowledge to provide safe and effective care to patients, especially because nurses were increasingly called on to make rapid, complex clinical decisions." These conditions prompted nurses to use "the knowledge they gained from experience" to "develop informal frameworks and theories to first describe and then to generate knowledge concerning their work and their patients." Early critical care nurses were pioneers in this type of knowledge development. In the 1950s, they began "to theorize that spatial location and the ability to observe their patients was critical to their survival," and identify "the different kinds of knowledge and skills they needed to critically evaluate patients' conditions and make nursing care decisions."[15] But as Rozella Schlotfeldt noted in 1960, the complexity of clinical nursing and the concomitant demands placed on nurses meant it was "unrealistic for nursing to continue to rely upon invention and intuition for its best practices."[16] Instead, there was now an "urgent" need for "systematic observation of effective nursing action with a view toward conceptualization of its rationale."[17]

The changing paradigm of health and illness from acute infectious diseases to complex, multifactorial chronic illness, together with an aging population, raised questions about the role of high-tech, interventionist, and predominantly hospital-based health care. It also drew increasing attention to the importance of patients' own health practices and decision-making. For example, the nursing care needs of acutely sick or dying hospitalized patients were quite different from those of aging and chronically ill ambulatory patients living at home and in their communities who were not subjected to the hierarchical structure of the hospital. Understanding patient behavior was especially important in this context because the prevention and treatment of acute episodes of chronic disease, as well as more effective management of chronic disease, relied on lifestyle changes as much as on pharmaceutical or surgical interventions. And as many clinicians realized, it was difficult to convince patients to make those lifestyle changes.[18] Ultimately, nurses needed to understand why a patient had particular problems and needs, why they behaved in particular ways, and how and why they made decisions about their health and health care.[19]

Several nurse researchers and educators joined Rozella Schlotfeldt in calling for the development of a "systematized nursing science."[20] In 1963, for example, the Surgeon General's Consultant Group on Nursing called for a greater focus on and support of nursing research directed toward the improvement of nursing practice, particularly "patient-oriented studies in line with the changing patterns of nursing care."[21] A year later, Virginia Henderson, in her definitional article "The Nature of Nursing," asserted that to improve patient care, nurses needed to "assume responsibility for validating and improving the methods" they used through the conduct of clinical nursing research.[22] Henderson had been arguing for the importance of clinical nursing research since the 1940s.[23]

To be sure, nurses had been engaged in research for decades. However, prior to the 1960s the majority of nursing research had focused on education and occupational studies aimed at improving preparation for nursing and the recruitment and retention of sufficient numbers of nurses to meet workforce needs.[24] One reason for this focus on "the workers rather than the work," Florence Wald and Robert Leonard asserted in 1964, was that nurses had "consulted with social scientists, asked social scientists to do research for them, and [had] undertaken doctoral study in the social sciences. As a result, nursing problems [were] being rephrased as social science questions rather than questions of practice."[25] It was time for nurses to direct research agendas, to ask questions underpinned by nursing theories, and produce a distinctive body of new knowledge—nursing science—that would be relevant specifically to nursing practice.

Leaders within nursing education and research also saw the development of nursing science as a political imperative, central to securing nursing's legitimacy as an independent and expert profession. As Dorothy Johnson explained in 1959, "The question of the existence of a body of substantive knowledge which can be called the science of nursing . . . is a question of considerable significance for nursing's continued development as a recognized professional discipline. Certainly, no profession can long exist without making explicit its theoretical bases for practice so that this knowledge can be communicated, tested, and expanded."[26]

For Wald and Leonard, by developing its own theories, "nursing would become an independent 'discipline' in its own right."[27] In this way, the effort to establish nursing science was, in part at least, a political project to establish nursing as an academic discipline. Doing so would increase nursing's professional status by achieving what Andrew Abbott has described as the three tasks of the academic knowledge system of a profession: "legitimation, research, and instruction."[28] But as Henderson asserted in 1956, "Whether or not nurses achieve full professional status is unimportant . . . unless this development results in, or is accompanied by, improvements in nursing care in all its physiological and psycho-social aspects."[29] Thus, the development of nursing science was at once a political and epistemological project, one motivated by a desire to improve both the status of the nursing profession and the quality of patient care.

The efforts to establish a science of nursing occurred alongside academic physicians' efforts to establish a science of clinical medicine. Since the late nineteenth century, knowledge generated by the laboratory sciences, including anatomy, physiology, biochemistry, pharmacology, and, from the 1950s, molecular biology, had underpinned medical practice. In this context, the development of new biomedical knowledge was typically generated through well-controlled experimental studies in the laboratory that were focused on increasing understanding of the cause, prevention, diagnosis, and treatment of disease.[30] As such, national medical research policy—and thus much biomedical research—was heavily oriented toward the elimination of disease. In the postwar decades, when the National Institutes of Health (NIH) became the primary patron of biomedical research, its research mandate was to "improve the health of the people of the United States through the conduct of researches, investigations, experiments, and demonstrations relating to cause, prevention, and method of diagnosis and treatment of diseases."[31] Throughout these decades, the NIH pursued its mission primarily through the funding of basic research in fields like genetics, biochemistry, molecular biology, biophysics, and immunology that would generate new knowledge about disease, and, when the knowledge base was sufficient to support it, targeted research aimed at finding solutions to specific health problems.[32]

Through the 1950s, physicians relied on the "integrity and expertise" of biomedical researchers to "produce reliable, untainted knowledge about the effects of medical treatment," which they could then apply in their own clinical practices. However, beginning in the 1950s and intensifying from the 1970s onward, physicians "abandoned their predecessors' trust in the judgment of experienced clinicians"[33] and sought instead "to make clinical care more scientific by developing a new clinical science, additional to the science of biomedicine."[34] This new clinical science centered on producing scientific evidence of therapeutic interventions—of what worked and what didn't work—and using that evidence (rather than subjective clinical judgment) to direct clinical decision-making.[35] This new clinical science was underpinned by the discipline of clinical epidemiology, which emerged in the 1960s and focused "on the application of quantitative methods to the empirical study of clinical practice."[36] The goal of this new clinical science was to make clinical medicine "every bit as scientific as the research laboratory" by applying the "scientific method"—typified by the well-controlled experiment—within the clinical setting.[37] As a research method for establishing the effectiveness of an intervention, the randomized controlled trial emerged as the gold standard.[38] It replaced observational studies and case reports, which centered on the authority of clinical experts, as the means by which interventions would be evaluated.[39] The randomized controlled trial, which was rooted in statistical analysis, reflected medicine's "trust in numbers," that is, the reliance "on quantification to produce objective knowledge and reduce uncertainty."[40]

But while academic physicians focused on constructing an empirical and statistically derived clinical science, academic nurses worked instead to construct a science of nursing that was not only empirical (utilizing both quantitative and qualitative methods) but also theoretical. Academic nurses did so in part because they believed theory offered the best path forward to demarcating the boundaries of nursing science and securing nursing's academic legitimacy.[41] But the privileging of theory also reflected the importance of the behavioral and social sciences to postwar nursing. Indeed, given the significance of both biomedical knowledge and the behavioral and social sciences to understanding and responding to the increasingly complex nursing care needs of patients in the postwar decades, academic nurses prioritized constructing nursing science as an interdisciplinary science that integrated components of the behavioral and social sciences as well as the biomedical sciences. In taking both a theoretical and interdisciplinary approach, nurse scientists were poised, ostensibly, to contribute to clinical research that which was missing from physicians' interventions-focused approach: evidence into the social and political context of patient care that could help explain why individuals made the choices they did about their own health and health care—including the prescribed interventions they would choose to use and those they would not.[42]

Enter the Nurse Scientists

As a first step in the construction of nursing science, nursing leaders sought to prepare the first generation of "nurse scientists" trained in the research methods, critical thinking skills, data analysis, conceptualization, and theory development necessary for building a science of nursing underpinned by both theory and research. As noted earlier, nurses had been doing research for decades. The emphasis on education and occupational studies, however, was in part explained by the educational preparation of nurses. Through the 1950s, most nurse researchers had received their graduate degrees in education.[43] By the mid-1950s, nursing leaders and the leadership of the U.S. Public Health Service Division of Nursing recognized that in order to promote a different type of research, nurses needed a new type of research training. In 1955, the Division of Nursing established the Nursing Research Grants and Fellowship Program, which supported research and research training in nursing particularly as it related to the "cause, diagnosis, treatment, control, and prevention of physical and mental diseases."[44] These extramural research grants and fellowships helped support nurses who would pursue research and research training, often in collaboration with biomedical and social scientists. That year, the Division of Nursing began awarding Special Nurse Research Fellowships to nurses pursuing research-based graduate degrees in the biomedical, behavioral, and social sciences. In 1964, the Division of Nursing began awarding research fellowships to doctorally prepared nurses undertaking postdoctoral research.[45] The Division of Nursing also provided institutional awards to nursing schools to promote research and research training. In 1962, it established the Nurse Scientist Graduate Training Program (NSGTP), which provided training grants to universities, which in turn awarded stipends to nurses pursuing PhD degrees in the university's biomedical, behavioral, and social science departments (discussed in more detail in chapter 3).[46]

Collectively, the Division of Nursing's support of research training through its Special Nurse Research Fellowship and Nurse Scientist Graduate Training (NSGT) programs led to a significant increase in the number of doctorally prepared nurses who could serve as researchers and faculty in nursing schools. Between 1955 and 1974, a total of 589 nurses received fellowships from the Division of Nursing, 330 of whom completed doctoral degrees in a range of disciplines, including 95 in education; 89 in the behavioral sciences of anthropology, psychology, and sociology; and 21 in the biological sciences of microbiology, biophysics, physiology, zoology, and biology.[47] The imbalance between the number of nurse fellows seeking doctoral preparation in the behavioral sciences and those enrolled in the biological sciences would

end up influencing the nature of nursing's subsequent boundary and legitimation work. It also reflected similar patterns in other post–World War II
sciences in which women flourished. As historian Margaret Rossiter documents, women tended to cluster in the life, behavioral, and social sciences—
disciplines more open to women and, not coincidentally, with less prestige
and less money. And such territorial segregation even occurred *within* scientific disciplines.[48] In primatology, for example, as Londa Schiebinger observes, "women are more likely to work in social behavior than in anatomy,
taxonomy, or physiology."[49]

There was also a significant lack of racial, ethnic, and gender diversity
among this new generation of nurse researchers, as practices of racial exclusion in nursing education continued even after civil rights legislation in
the 1960s dismantled the legal system of segregation and made racial discrimination in education and employment illegal.[50] Of the 589 nurses who
received fellowship support from the Division of Nursing between 1955 and
1974, only six men had participated in the program, one of whom was African American.[51] The fellowships were awarded to twenty African American
female nurses (fifteen of whom had completed doctoral degrees by 1975) and
eight Asian American female nurses (five of whom had completed doctoral
requirements by 1975).[52] This lack of diversity impacted the development of
nursing science, shaping what were and were not considered important areas
of research and theory development (discussed later this chapter).

As the federal government invested for the first time in nursing research,
so too did nursing's leadership work to establish the first journal of nursing
research, aptly titled *Nursing Research*. First published in June 1952 and ed-
ited by Helen Bunge, *Nursing Research* was the only peer-reviewed journal
dedicated to the publication of nursing research until the late 1970s. From
the early 1950s through the late 1970s, the journal was cosponsored by the
National League for Nursing and the American Nurses Association. In its
early years, as Ellen Baer observes, "*Nursing Research* represented a virtual
curriculum of how-to-do research," with "each column or department focused on a particular aspect of the research process." It also served as "a hub
around which much of nursing's research interest and effort coalesced," routinely including announcements of research funding opportunities, conferences, and research-focused education programs. Moreover, from the 1950s
through the 1980s, *Nursing Research*, led by its editor and editorial board,
was instrumental in establishing, contesting, and maintaining the boundaries
of what constituted nursing research.[53] By the end of the 1970s, several new
peer-reviewed journals had been introduced, including *Research in Nursing
and Health* and *Advances in Nursing Science,* both in 1978, and the *Western*

Journal of Nursing Research in 1979. Sigma Theta Tau's journal, *Image: The Journal of Nursing Scholarship*, had been published since 1967 but was not peer-reviewed until 1977.[54] The expanding number of peer-reviewed journals dedicated to the publication of nursing research signaled both the growth and growing importance of nursing research.

The decision by nurse leaders to educate a new generation of nurses in the existing biomedical, behavioral, and social science disciplines, however, presented problems for nursing's epistemological project. First, it led to identity issues for the nurses trained in these other disciplines. These identity issues centered on their status as nurses (now that they were no longer engaged in patient care), and their status as researchers, once they carried the research methods they had learned in their basic science disciplines out into the applied environment of the clinic. Second, it raised a series of critical epistemological questions: Would the creation of a corps of nurses trained in the established biomedical and behavioral disciplines simply lead to a shoring up of those already-existing disciplines or would it lead to a new type of disciplinary knowledge upon which the science of nursing could be built? If it were the latter and nurse scientists produced a new type of disciplinary knowledge—nursing knowledge—where would the boundaries of the already-existing disciplines end and the new discipline of nursing science begin? However, if instead these scientifically trained nurses contributed new knowledge to the already-existing disciplines, what then would be the value added of creating a new discipline of nursing science?

The premise of the NSGTP and the Special Nurse Research Fellowship program were that "the nurse scientist would then bring knowledge generated in these scientific disciplines into nursing."[55] In doing so, these nurse scientists would transform nursing's labor into a site of knowledge production. However, UCLA's Dorothy Johnson observed that despite the valuable scientific contributions made by nurse scientists, constrained as it was by the conceptual frameworks and research parameters of their scientific disciplines, the research being done by nurse scientists often had little to do with nursing practice.[56] And reports that tracked the careers of nurse scientists found that in many instances, nurse scientists who pursued doctorates in non-nursing fields never returned to nursing and instead remained in their field of doctoral study.[57]

In the end, nurses pursuing PhDs in the biological, social, and behavioral sciences were seen by most nursing leaders as a "stop-gap measure" to prepare a corps of nurse scientists trained in the research methods, critical thinking skills, data analysis, conceptualization, and theory development necessary for building a science of nursing. As Hildegard Peplau explained, the problem was "that we do not have nurses with PhDs who can act as graduate faculty." By earning PhDs in the basic sciences, the "nurse-scientists who have earned PhDs can bring their knowledge back to nursing and use it to chisel out a PhD in nursing."[58] Faye Abdellah, writing in 1966 shared Peplau's position. For Abdellah, the "PhD in nursing is still a dream to come true . . . When we can point to a scientific body of knowledge, a fully tested classification system, nurse theories, and patient care models," she continued, "we will be ready to consider a PhD in nursing."[59]

It was in this context that the movement to establish a science of nursing, underpinned by nursing theory, emerged in the 1960s. The pursuit of theory development, however, was not an inevitable path to securing nursing's academic legitimacy. As non-nurse supporters of academic nursing questioned in the 1970s, the majority of biomedical research was conducted without the guidance of explicit theories, so why was nursing so focused on looking to theory to guide nursing research and practice?[60] Moreover, during these same decades, academic physicians were looking to the laboratory, the new methods of clinical epidemiology, and the rigors of statistical analysis, not theory, to build the scientific base of clinical medicine.[61] Academic nurses, however, instead regarded theory development—in addition to clinical research—as integral to the making of nursing science.

Academic nurses looked to theory development for at least two reasons. First, while some of the nurses who received research training and doctorates during the 1950s and 1960s did so in the biomedical sciences, the majority did so in the social and behavioral sciences such as anthropology, sociology, and psychology, all of which had strong theoretical orientations.[62] As Ada Jacox, who had earned her PhD in sociology from Case Western Reserve University in 1969, explained, "We developed our notions of what science is in those disciplines and that's what we brought back to nursing in writing and teaching about theory construction."[63] Second, as sociologist Andrew Abbott explained in his seminal work on professionalization, *The Systems of Professions*, "only a knowledge system governed by abstraction can redefine its problems and tasks, defend them from interlopers, and seize new problems."[64] In this context, the establishment and mastery of esoteric theory reflected the highest level of abstraction. Academic nurses thus saw in theory development the most effective means to establishing nursing's scientific legitimacy and influence.

Constructing the Boundaries of Nursing Science

How should nurses create a science of nursing and what should constitute that nursing science? What theories should underpin nursing's research agendas and how should nurses go about developing those theories? What research would be necessary and what research methods should nurses use in order to produce a body of scientific knowledge unique to nursing? These were key questions that occupied academic nurses during the 1960s and 1970s. As they worked to address these questions and establish nursing science in these decades, nurse theorists and researchers engaged in critical boundary work. A series of conferences sponsored by the Division of Nursing's Nurse Scientist Graduate Training Program, held between 1966 and 1970, were important forums in which nurse theorists and researchers began the work of defining the boundaries of nursing science.[65] The discussions that took place at these conferences built upon and reflected the discussions that had been taking place in the pages of nursing's journals and at nursing research conferences since the late 1950s. Collectively, they captured the major elements of nursing's boundary work: 1) determining the degree to which nursing science would draw upon the theories, knowledge claims, and research methods of the biomedical and behavioral sciences, and 2) identifying what was unique to nursing and thus what nursing would do differently from the established disciplines, in order to clearly distinguish nursing science from related disciplines like biology, physiology, psychology, or sociology.

Some scholars, such as Dorothy Johnson and Virginia Cleland, saw this boundary work as drawing upon the theories and knowledge derived from the biomedical and behavioral sciences to develop either distinctive areas of nursing research or distinctive nursing theories. Nurse researchers, for example, could use "borrowed" theories from the biomedical, behavioral, or social sciences to address research questions of specific relevance to nursing—phenomena that researchers in these other fields had no interest in pursuing.[66] In borrowing from the existing sciences, however, it was critical for nurses to "be selective in [their] use of this knowledge and not automatically assume that knowledge from other areas is necessarily relevant."[67] For Rosemary Ellis, "Clinical practice must be the touchstone for determining what theories [from the biomedical and behavioral sciences] are significant, and what knowledge nurses must, and should, spend time pursuing." Theories that failed "in their usefulness for developing or guiding practice" were not significant for nursing.[68]

Ada Jacox, for example, who earned a PhD in sociology, pursued a research program focused on the subjective and psychosocial dimensions of the pain experience. Drawing upon biological and psychological theories of pain, Jacox examined the factors that influence how patients tolerate pain, whether and how they express pain, and how pain is related to other problems associated with their illness. In turn, she also examined the factors that influenced how effective nurses were at assessing and responding to pain in their patients.[69] Jean E. Johnson, who earned her PhD in social psychology from the University of Wisconsin–Madison in 1971, brought cognitive and behavioral theories into nursing. Johnson's early research interests focused on understanding people's reactions to threatening events. Johnson built upon the theory of cognitive dissonance to investigate the conditions that could decrease a patient's distress during a clinical procedure perceived as threatening.[70] In the late 1960s, Jeanne C. Quint Benoliel (then Jeanne C. Quint) was a doctoral student in nursing and sociology at the University of California, San Francisco, working with the sociologists Anselm Strauss and Barney Glaser. Strauss and Glaser had recently developed grounded theory, which was a new research methodology for generating theory from systematic collection and analysis of data.[71] Utilizing grounded theory, and drawing upon several theories from sociology and psychology, Benoliel undertook a series of studies that investigated care of the dying in hospitals and patients' experiences living with terminal illness, which proved foundational to the establishment of palliative and hospice care in the United States.[72]

But if nurse researchers borrowed theories from the biomedical, behavioral, and social sciences and applied them in the clinical setting, what would distinguish nursing science from the theory and knowledge of these other disciplines and from medicine? As Jacox explained in 1974, "It is difficult enough to define boundaries in these 'basic,' essentially academic areas [psychology, physiology, anthropology, and sociology] concerned with the *production* of knowledge. The difficulties are compounded when trying to specify clearly what part of the empirical world can be 'claimed' by disciplines in which the major concern is *use* of knowledge."[73] Another key aspect, then, of nursing's boundary work in this period was to identify the core concepts of nursing that distinguished it from the other health professions and demarcated the unique area of "empirical" focus for nurse researchers and theorists.[74]

The questions "What is nursing?" and "What is the nurse's unique area of responsibility?" had long been matters of debate within nursing. The increasing complexity of and demands for nursing after World War II served only to intensify the debate. As Ernestine Wiedenbach noted in 1970, given the "myriad and variety of activities in which nurses engage" and how quickly nurses' responsibilities were changing in response to rapid advances in biomedical science and technology, it would be difficult and unsatisfactory to characterize nursing—and thus nursing science—on the basis of what nurses do.[75] Instead, nurse theorists sought to identify the "essential components of nursing" that had served as "unifying focus" for nursing over time, and develop theories based on these core concepts.[76] These nursing theories would then serve as the foundation for nursing research and nursing education.[77]

Enter the Nurse Theorists

A number of nurses engaged in theory development during the 1950s, 1960s, and 1970s.[78] Collectively, they worked to conceptualize the role and scope of nursing's intervention in the health care system. Ultimately, the theorists sought to establish the theoretical frameworks by which nurses could better understand and influence the health behaviors of their patients, increase patients' roles in their own health care, and reduce patients' barriers to health and wellness.

The nurse theorists mobilized a variety of approaches to theory development. Some theorists borrowed theories and knowledge from the related disciplines to develop new and distinctive nursing theories. For example, Dorothy Johnson, who was a professor of pediatric nursing at UCLA and had earned a master's degree in public health in 1948, developed the "behavioral system model" for nursing, which she introduced in 1968. Johnson drew upon interdisciplinary scholarship in psychology, ethology, and sociology that "focused on the behavior of the individual as a whole—on what he does, why, and on the consequences of that behavior."[79] Johnson's theory derived, most notably, from the systems paradigm, first introduced by Talcott Parsons in 1951 and from general systems theory, which was introduced in the 1960s.[80] Johnson's theory conceptualized humans as being composed of two interrelated systems and their component subsystems: a biological system (the focus of medicine) and a behavioral system (the focus of nursing). According to Johnson, the behavioral system forms "an organized and integrated functional unit that determines and limits the interaction between the person and the environment and establishes the relationship of the person to the objects, events, and situations in his environment." While "for most individuals most of the time the behavioral system is at a level of balance that is functionally efficient and effective," during times of "psychological crisis or a physical illness" that balance could be disturbed and the person may "require external assistance" in order to restore the behavioral system's balance.[81] The role of nursing is to prevent occurrences of imbalance, and when they do occur, to "restore, maintain, or attain behavioral system balance and stability at the highest possible level for the individual."[82]

Another theorist who advocated the "borrowed theory" approach to nursing theory development was Sister Callista Roy, who was a master's degree student of Dorothy Johnson's at UCLA in the mid-1960s. Roy returned to UCLA in the 1970s, earning a PhD in sociology and continuing to work with Johnson, as well as the sociologist Ralph Turner, who was a prominent scholar of collective behavior and role theory.[83] Roy's theoretical work built upon and synthesized theories from the behavioral sciences and from sociology, particularly psychologist Abraham Maslow's hierarchy of needs, psychologist Harry Helson's adaptation level theory, and Turner's interactional role theory.[84] Roy's adaptation model of nursing, which she introduced in 1976, conceptualized of humans as "biopsychosocial being[s] in constant interaction with a changing environment." Humans, she asserted, cope with changes in their environment using "certain innate and acquired mechanisms" of adaptation that are "biologic, psychologic, and social in origin."[85] Roy also derived her theory from empirical work. After surveying five hundred samples of patient behavior, Roy identified four adaptive modes that she defined as constituting a person's mechanism for coping with a changing environment: physiologic needs, self-concept, role function, and interdependence. Collectively, these adaptive modes, which she conceived of as being both integrated and interrelated, are geared toward ensuring a person's *physiologic integrity, psychic integrity*, and *social integrity*."[86] In Roy's model, health and illness exist on a continuum, and as a person "moves along the continuum between maximum wellness and maximum illness" they "will encounter adaptation problems." The goal of nursing is to promote a person's "adaptation in each of the adaptive modes in situations of health and illness."[87]

Other academic nurses, particularly Florence Wald at Yale University, challenged the concept of borrowing theories from the basic and behavioral sciences and applying them to nursing. Instead, Wald, in collaboration with sociologist Robert Leonard, advocated an "empirical approach of building knowledge directly from systematic study of nursing experience."[88] Only by developing so-called practice theory, Wald and Leonard argued, would nurse researchers be able to identify and inform the ways in which nurses affect improvements in patients' health. In 1962, the Yale nursing faculty had begun a productive collaboration with Yale philosophers James Dickoff and Patricia James.[89] In 1968, when Dickoff and James presented their "theory of theories" at the Case Western Reserve University Symposium on Theory Development in Nursing, they extended Wald and Leonard's contention that nurses should develop practice theory. In particular, Dickoff and James called for nurses to develop "situation-producing theory" that would not only describe and predict but would also prescribe the activities of the practitioner.[90]

Prominent among the empirically oriented theorists was Ida Jean Orlando, who was a colleague of Wald and Leonard at Yale University during the late 1950s and early 1960s.[91] Orlando's educational background was in psychiatric and mental health nursing. Beginning in the mid-1950s, she led a five-year project at the Yale University School of Nursing, funded by the National Institute of Mental Health (NIMH), to "identify the factors which enhanced or impeded the integration of mental health principles in the basic nursing curriculum." Orlando's "theory of effective nursing practice," which she first published in 1961, resulted from this five-year study of "observing and participating in experiences with patients, students, nurses, service, and instructional personnel," collecting data, and formulating "the findings of the study, i.e., the content of instruction, the teaching process and the learning environment, needed by students for the development of a professional nursing role."[92] Orlando published an updated version of her theory in 1972 following the results of a second NIMH-funded research study, conducted at Mclean Hospital in Belmont, Massachusetts, in which she was able to test, validate, and refine the conceptualization she had introduced in 1961.[93] In her publications, Orlando made no reference to any other existing theories; instead she maintained her theory was entirely empirically derived.

Orlando's theory of effective nursing practice centered on the nurse-patient interaction, the goal of which is for the nurse to identify a patient's need and to help the patient meet that need. Patient agency—albeit mediated by the nurse—was integral to Orlando's theory. It is the patient themself who initiates the nursing intervention, first by perceiving that they have a need they cannot meet by themself, and second by signaling with their behavior—both verbal and nonverbal—that they have an unmet need. For Orlando, then, all patient behavior, no matter how insignificant the nurse might perceive it to be, "must be considered an expression of need until its meaning to that particular patient at that time is understood."[94] As such, it is the nurse's responsibility to identify and validate with the patient that the nurse's interpretation of the patient's behavior is in fact accurate, and if it is not, to correct that interpretation. Orlando's theory thus made clear "that patients have their own meanings and interpretations of situations, and, therefore, nurses must validate their inferences and analyses with patients before drawing conclusions about patients' experiences or needs."[95]

In Orlando's theory, the goal of nursing was to act deliberately rather than automatically, "guided by 'explicitness' of perceptions, thoughts, and feelings" in response to and directed toward resolving the patient's unmet need as identified by the patient.[96] Nurses were more likely to engage in automatic personal responses, Orlando argued, when they were taking actions "decided upon for reasons other than the patient's immediate need," such as when carrying out physician's orders or performing routines of patient care.[97] Orlando's theory thus advocated for nurses to no longer do things because a physician directed them to do so but rather to be deliberative and intentional about engaging in actions that were specifically in response to patient's own expression of their needs. In this way, Orlando's theory positioned the nurse as an advocate and mediator of patient agency and with a responsibility to center the patient as a key participant in their own health care.

Other theorists, such as Dorothea Orem, pursued neither an explicitly empirical nor "borrowed theory" approach to theory development. During the 1940s and 1950s, Orem held a series of positions in nursing education, working first as director of nursing service and director of nursing education at Providence Hospital in Detroit, and then serving in 1949 as a consultant to the Hospital Division of the Indiana State Board of Health, where she "had intensive involvement with nurses and their practice of nursing" in the state's general hospitals.[98] Orem then spent two years working in the federal government's Office of Education where she was involved in developing curricula for practical nursing programs. In 1959, she joined the nursing faculty at Catholic University of America.[99] Although Orem acknowledged being influenced by Talcott Parsons's systems theory and the work of several philosophers, she did not engage directly with Parson's or any other existing theories in her early theoretical writings.[100] Instead, she developed the "self-care deficit theory of nursing" from her own experiences of nursing. As Orem explained, "I didn't look at nursing references but I asked myself the question. I can still remember the situation in which I had the insight to answer the question "Why do people do nursing?" The knowledge was within me. I was able to use that knowledge in answering the question ... From that time onward, the knowledge I had about nursing began to structure itself. It wasn't anything I did deliberately, but the pieces started to come together."[101]

Orem's self-care deficit theory of nursing comprised three separate but related theories. Her first theory, the theory of self-care, defined self-care as the activities that "individuals personally initiate and perform on their own behalf to maintain life, health, and well-being."[102] It integrated biological, sociological, and psychological activities and demands, and included 1) universal self-care requisites, which include "all those demands and actions" that meet so-called basic human needs; 2) development-type self-care requisites, which "are associated with processes and conditions specific to human developmental stages," such as infancy, adolescence, pregnancy, and aging; and 3) health-deviation self-care requisites, which "are associated with regulation of the effects and results of disturbed functioning, of injury, of defects, and with the effects and results of medical care received from or prescribed by physicians."[103] As part of the self-care concept, Orem identified self-care agency as the capacity of individuals to develop self-care abilities as is influenced by age, developmental state, health, life experience, sociocultural context, and available resources.

Orem's second theory, self-care deficit theory, indicated the situations in which nursing is needed, namely when an individual is incapable of, or limited in their ability to provide, continuous and effective self-care. Critical to Orem's theory is the notion that the nurse works collaboratively with the person under her care to determine the characteristics and degree of both the person's self-care deficits and self-care agency, so as to determine the characteristics and degree of nursing care needed by the person, and that, ultimately, the person will be able meet their own self-care needs. This leads to Orem's third theory, that of nursing systems. She described three types of nursing systems in which the patient's self-care needs would be met by the nurse, patient, or both: wholly compensatory, partly compensatory, and supportive-educative. Ultimately, Orem's theory identified five methods the nurse could use, either individually or in some combination, to support the patient: 1) acting for or doing for the patient, 2) support, 3) guidance, 4) providing an environment that promotes self-care, and 5) teaching. In doing so, Orem's theory shifted the focus of nursing care away from those tasks delegated by physicians and centered on *doing for* patients (except in situations where a patient is completely incapacitated) toward nursing care that is centered on collaborating *with* patients and increasing the patient's agency in securing their own health and well-being.[104]

Another prominent nurse theorist during these decades was Martha Rogers. Rogers had earned a doctorate in public health from Johns Hopkins University, and from 1954 through 1975 she served as head of the Division of Nursing at New York University, where she was instrumental in advocating and implementing substantive changes in nursing education.[105] Like Johnson and Roy, Rogers drew upon knowledge and theories from other disciplines to develop a theory of nursing. However, in contrast to her fellow theorists, Rogers insisted that "principles drawn from the biologic, physical, and psychosocial sciences, no matter how excellent they may be in their own respective fields," were wholly inadequate for nursing because they were premised on a reductionist view of humans.[106] Instead, Rogers synthesized theories, "facts[,] and ideas" from other sciences, particularly physics (including general relativity theory and electrodynamics), biology (evolutionary theory), and sociology (general systems theory and adaptation theories) to create a completely novel and holistic basic science: the science of unitary man (which she later renamed the science of unitary human beings).[107] Rogers believed that unitary human beings cannot be divided into parts but must be understood as fully integrated wholes. The environment is also indivisible and in constant interaction with unitary human beings. Indeed, human beings cannot be understood separately from the environments in which they exist; they are "coextensive with the universe," and they "are integral with one another."[108]

Rogers' science of unitary human beings was based on four building blocks: energy fields, a universe of open systems, pattern and organization, and four-dimensionality (later, pan-dimensionality). The energy field is "the fundamental unit of both living and non-living."[109] Openness refers to the fact that the human and environmental energy fields are continuously open and continuously changing. Each energy field is characterized by a wave pattern and organization, the nature of which "is always novel, always emerging, always more diverse." Finally, energy fields are four-dimensional, thus they transcend time and space, and are "characterized by continuously fluctuating imaginary boundaries." Given their four-dimensionality, the present as a point in time is irrelevant. Rather, the human energy field "is the 'relative present' for any individual."[110] Given this relative present, a "unitary human being is always in the process of 'becoming' rather than 'being'; at any point, he is more than he has been because of all his previous actions, experiences, interactions, and being are incorporated into his present being."[111]

Rogers's theoretical contribution is distinctive among the early theorists because she did not formulate her theory explicitly around the concepts of health and illness.[112] Nevertheless, Rogers held that only the science of unitary human beings could be used to "evolve the descriptive, explanatory, and predictive principles basic to knowledgeable practice in nursing."[113] When the principles of this science were translated into practice, Rogers argued, the goal of nursing was "to promote symphonic interaction between man and environment, to strengthen the coherence and integrity of the human field, and to direct and redirect patterning of the human and environmental fields for realization of maximum health potential."[114] In particular, Rogers advocated a system of nursing centered on the human being–environment relationship, and in which the "human being is an integral participant in the intervention process" and nursing interventions "are predicated upon the wholeness of man [which] derives its safety and effectiveness from a unified concept of human functioning."[115] Rogers's theory, however, was highly abstract and esoteric, which made it difficult to both understand and operationalize.[116] As Rogers's supporters have remarked, her critics often labeled her as the "crazy nurse" and "crazy space nurse" (which refers to her later forays into explorations of space travel and intergalactic nursing).[117] In recalling the reaction of her peers to the publication of *An Introduction to the Theoretical Basis of Nursing*, Rogers explained "Well, there were those who said, 'She's crazier than a bedbug!' It was all so new and different. I was trying to get across an idea of life, change, and undirectionality. There were a lot of people who did much misinterpreting and a lot who said she doesn't know what she's talking about."[118]

The theories developed by Johnson, Roy, Orlando, Orem, and Rogers represent just a handful of the theories introduced by nurse theorists during the 1950s, 1960s, and 1970s.[119] However, they highlight the institutional diversity and varied educational and clinical backgrounds of this first generation of nurse theorists. They also reflect the collective efforts of the theorists to conceptualize the role and scope of nursing's intervention in the health care system and nursing's relationship to patients, premised, in particular, on understanding and then responding to the behavioral needs and actions of patients. These theories also capture some of the ways in which the theorists sought to demarcate nursing's empirical focus and thus distinguish nursing science from the biomedical and behavioral sciences. Indeed, by the late 1970s, the nursing theorists had identified four concepts that defined nursing's empirical focus: person, environment, health, and nursing. Nursing's focus is the whole person, not simply the locus of disease or disability. Persons are viewed as "biopsychosocial beings," constantly interacting with and being influenced by their social and physical environments.[120] As such, the environment is "a source of or an influence on the health or illness of a person."[121] Nursing's focus is health—its maintenance, restoration, and promotion—not disease or disability. Nursing actions (defined as what nurses do for and with the patient) enable and support patients as agents in the pursuit of their health goals. In this way, nursing "moved from doing *for* patients to working *with* patients, helping people to care for themselves and involving them in their care and decisions about their health."[122]

In important ways, the concepts of person, environment, and health reflected the efforts of nursing (and a handful of medical leaders) since the 1940s to move beyond "merely . . . treating disease entities" and to treat "patients as 'total persons'" (see chapter 1).[123] These were also concepts that had long been at the core of public health nursing.[124] As the historian Karen Buhler-Wilkerson has documented, when Lillian Wald invented the term "public health nurse" at the end of the nineteenth century, "she recognized that sickness should be considered within its social and economic context."[125] The charge of the public health nurse, then, "was not only to provide bedside care of the sick, but also to identify and correct the underlying causes of illness and misery," and "encompass an agenda of reform in health, industry, education, recreation, and housing."[126] And in the early twentieth century, the environment and other social determinants were increasingly understood by nurses engaging mental hygiene concepts to impact patients' mental health.[127] By the 1970s, though, the concepts of person, environment, and health had broader political significance. With an emphasis on a health perspective rather than a disease perspective, by considering the patient holistically, and by prioritizing the agency of the patient in shaping their health, the theorists constructed a system of abstract knowledge that emphasized nursing's distinctive perspective and distinguished it from the reductionist model of medicine that emphasized disease, diagnosis, and cure.[128] While wanting to make clear the boundaries of nursing science, the theorists were also responding to the growing criticisms being leveraged by civil rights health activists, the women's health movement, and a burgeoning patient-consumer movement against the medical profession and the reductionist, dehumanizing, and paternalist system of health care it lionized.[129]

Although the theorists were themselves removed from day-to-day interactions with patients and were largely uninvolved in the health activism of these years, they were, nevertheless, influenced by these events. Orlando, for example, wrote of being influenced by the "abundance of agreement from outside as well as within the nursing profession that the organization and delivery of care to the patient is inadequate." This included evidence from those outside of nursing who argued that the abundance of inadequate patient care was attributable "to the authoritarian, bureaucratic, power structure of treatment and care facilities and . . . that these 'restrictive' characteristics [should] be changed to allow more freedom and more democratic practices."[130] Among these critics was the sociologist Irving Kenneth Zola, who collaborated with Orlando in her theoretical work in the 1960s.[131] In 1972, the same year Orlando published an update of her theory of effective nursing practice, Zola introduced the concept of medicalization to explain the medical profession's expanding jurisdiction, authority, and practices over "an ever increasing part of human existence."[132] Zola went on to become a prominent disability rights activist and one of the founders of disability studies.[133]

Rogers was perhaps most explicit among the theorists in seeing the application of her theory as a means to move beyond the current model of health care and its attendant limitations. Rogers included among these limitations the "immorality of human experimentation without informed consent" and the health problems "stemming from social inequities" such as "poor and inadequate housing, ghetto areas, racial and occupational discrimination, economic and educational discrimination,"[134] and she emphasized the need to move beyond "the narrow, unimaginative, and inadequately conceived expansion of sick services"—premised on the medical model—to incorporate "the gamut of health and welfare services, whether directed toward habilitation or rehabilitation."[135] And by the 1970s, nursing journals—with which the theorists engaged—were publishing articles, editorials, and letters in which the nurse authors discussed the importance of acknowledging the rights of patients to have access to health care information so they could make informed decisions about their own health care; recognizing and valuing patients' experiential knowledge; and working with (instead of doing for) patients to secure the health care that patients chose for themselves.[136]

The potential political resonance of nursing's model of care and research was not lost on other nurse leaders. As Susan Gortner, former chief of the Nursing Research Branch of the Public Health Service's Division of Nursing and professor and associate dean for research at UCSF, observed, "nursing's deliberate concern with the whole human, with life styles, and with health behavior is attractive to those who find the disease orientation limiting and insufficient to explain response to therapy, spontaneous improvement in health status, and high-level wellness."[137] For Madeleine Leininger, dean of nursing at the University of Utah, the fact that physicians and their practices had come "under rather severe criticism" from American health consumers presented nurse scientists with an opportunity to stake their claim and assert their expertise to investigate and resolve the health care concerns that so troubled consumers. In particular, Leininger called on nurse scientists to conduct "research studies directed toward humanizing nursing and general health care services . . . especially in hospitals and clinics," identify the "ways that people are motivated and rewarded to stay well," and develop (and measure the efficacy of) "nursing care models of wellness and health maintenance."[138]

Nursing science, however, was not only to be constituted from nursing theory but also through transforming nursing practice into a site of research and thus knowledge production. How, then, did the boundary work of the nurse theorists shape the type of research being pursued by nurse researchers in the 1960s and 1970s? And how did nurse scientists transform nursing's practice into a site of valuable knowledge production and demonstrate the ways in which application of this knowledge was integral to improving patient outcomes and health care delivery?

Nursing Research, Health Outcomes, and the
Quality Assessment Movement in Health Care

Nursing's boundary work during the postwar decades shaped the type of research being pursued by nurse researchers in the 1960s and 1970s. Although nurses continued to conduct educational, occupational, and administrative research during these decades, increasing numbers of nurse researchers centered their research on "dealing with problems of how best we can take care of patients and what kinds of nursing will net us certain kinds of goals in patient care."[139] Reflecting this shift, between the mid-1950s and the mid-1970s, nursing leaders documented "a progressive increase in the investigation of clinical problems" by researchers.[140]

Nurse researchers, in particular, sought to understand the factors and conditions needed to maintain, restore, and promote individual health. As part of this, they were interested in understanding the processes that could bring about a change in health status, such as aging and reproduction, or "critical life events" like injury, trauma, or acute and chronic illnesses.[141] Once a change in health status had occurred, nurse researchers sought to understand how individuals adapted to and coped with such change. In all of these aspects, nurse scientists were interested in identifying the influences of the environment, both physical and sociocultural, on an individual's health status, and evaluating the influence of nursing interventions and nursing care on individual health outcomes.[142] A survey of more than 400 "nurse and nonnurse experts," published in 1975, identified nursing's clinical research priorities as determining the most effective interventions for reducing psychological stress of patients, enhancing the quality of life of the aged, promoting effective self-care education (particularly among patients with chronic diseases) reducing complications of surgical patients, performing crisis intervention, and managing pain.[143]

Despite the interventions of the nurse theorists, nurse researchers were ambivalent about the value of nursing theory to their research. Not all nurse researchers utilized theory in their research, and those that did more often relied on the theories of the social and behavioral sciences rather than specific nursing theories to guide their research. The types of research questions pursued, the research methods utilized, and the theories drawn upon were not inevitable. Rather, they reflected choices made by academic nurses regarding the types of knowledge they believed would not only contribute to improved patient care but also be both valuable and legible within the postwar research economy. In making the choice to conduct research to reduce hospital-based infections and adverse drug interactions, and to improve end-of-life care, pain management, and the management of chronic illness and debility, their research was shaped by an emergent quality assessment movement within health care, which sought to transform the ways in which biomedical research was conducted and health care delivered.[144]

The quality assessment movement, which had its roots in the early twentieth century, emerged in the 1960s and 1970s among researchers "attempting to develop a science of 'outcomes research' that would provide more objective assessments of medical care."[145] Through the 1960s and 1970s, a series of studies, including several by health services researchers, revealed that physicians "were treating patients with the same diagnoses in different ways" and that escalating health care costs were not being matched by comparable improvements in mortality and morbidity rates.[146] This raised concerns among health professionals, policymakers, and consumers alike about the efficiency, effectiveness, and safety of health care. The result was the emergence of outcomes research, which "promised a more scientific approach to evaluating procedure-based treatments than currently existed."[147] Outcomes research—of which both clinical epidemiology and health services research were a part—depended on the collection and statistical analysis of data about interventions and their outcomes.[148] Although physician researchers acknowledged the importance of bedside nurses to data collection, getting patients on board with the research, and ultimately operationalizing not only their outcomes research but also subsequent practice interventions, neither academic physicians at the time nor historians since have considered *nursing research* as part of the quality assessment movement. However, the nature of nurses' clinical research—focused as it was, on evaluating the impact of nursing interventions on patient outcomes and examining the ways in which patients' living environments shaped their health and health care actions—means it needs to be situated within the context of outcomes research and the quality assessment movement in health care.[149]

By the mid-1970s, for example, several nurse researchers were engaged in research to reduce patients' complications from surgery and hospitalization in order to improve patient outcomes. This included research to reduce the incidence of catheter-induced urinary infections and other forms of hospital-acquired postsurgical infections,[150] as well as research to reduce postoperative complications caused by mucus accumulation among tracheostomized patients.[151] Nurse researchers were also investigating ways to improve health outcomes for high-risk groups such as premature infants and the elderly. For example, several teams of nurse researchers, drawing upon developmental and psychological theories, determined the importance of environmental stimuli—particularly auditory, visual, and tactile stimuli—in the nursery to support premature infant development.[152] And Doris Schwartz, Barbara Henley, and Leonard Zeitz's study of elderly, ambulatory, chronically ill patients identified the psychosocial needs of this population of patients, which "served as a major description of the aged ill for the health professions."[153]

Nurse researchers also investigated factors that impacted patients' abilities to cope with chronic illness. For example, drawing on sociological and psychological theories of interactions and social networks, Patricia M. MacElveen investigated how patients on home kidney dialysis coped with treatment and the chronic illness of renal failure and found that the degree of cooperation among patient, spouse, and physician positively influenced patient outcomes.[154] As noted earlier, Jeanne Quint Benoliel undertook a series of studies that investigated care of the dying in hospitals and patients' experiences of living with chronic and terminal illness. Benoliel's work was informed by several different theories from sociology and psychology, including symbolic interactionism, theories of socialization and role identity, and social action theory.[155] Nurse researchers also engaged in efforts to develop and tests ways for hospitalized patients and "those living with health impairments" to manage anxiety, pain, and stress.[156] In the 1970s, for example, Linda Aiken researched the effect of relaxation exercises on the pain experienced by postsurgical patients, cancer patients, and patients with rheumatoid arthritis. Performing a randomized controlled trial, Aiken demonstrated that relaxation exercises carried out once or twice a day helped patients either to be "less aware of pain" or to "cope with the pain more effectively."[157] Drawing upon multidisciplinary theories of pain, Ada Jacox examined the factors that influenced how patients tolerated pain, whether and how they expressed pain, and how pain related to other problems associated with a patient's illness.[158] Several nurse researchers, some of whom utilized psychological theories of distress and fear, studied the effects of hospitalization on the behavior of children and adolescents with the goal of improving their behavior and, ultimately, their health outcomes.[159]

With few exceptions, the nursing research conducted during the 1960s, 1970s, and early 1980s were small-scale studies, ranging from as few as fifteen to as many as a few hundred research subjects. While some of these studies were controlled experimental studies and many utilized quantitative research methods, many were also based on qualitative research methods including ethnography, surveys, and grounded theory. In none of these studies did nurse researchers utilize nursing theories. Rather, those researchers that did use theory invariably drew from sociological and psychological theories to inform, analyze, and interpret their research.

Even as nurse researchers generated new insights about how patients adapted to and coped with such changes in health status, and even as they evaluated the influence of nursing interventions and nursing care on individual health outcomes, they struggled to secure recognition within the broader health research community. In part, this was because nurse researchers published their research primarily in nursing journals, which were rarely read by researchers outside of nursing. But more importantly, outcomes research and the broader quality assessment movement in health care shaped the ways in which research methods and the evidence they generated were evaluated and accorded status.

As historians and sociologists of medicine have documented, by the 1970s, the randomized controlled trial had emerged as the gold standard research method in clinical medicine.[160] It replaced observational studies and case reports, which centered on the authority of clinical experts, as the means by which interventions would be evaluated.[161] As the sociologist Jeanne Daly explains, advocates of this new evidence-based medicine shaped "the meaning of the word *evidence*, so that it [became] synonymous with that evidence produced by a randomized controlled trial or other method high in its hierarchy of evidence."[162] In turn, evidence obtained by research methods other than the randomized controlled trial, such as observational studies and case reports, came to occupy a lower rung on the hierarchy of evidence. Lower still was evidence generated by qualitative research methods. Such methods, including those often used by nurse scientists in the 1960s and 1970s—ethnography, grounded theory, and case studies—rely "on narrative arguments rather than statistical reasoning and [base] analysis on small samples generating a large quantity of narrative data. Researchers often explicitly draw on social theory for justification of their findings. Their scientific value is not assessed by tests for validity but by the convincing nature of the arguments presented."[163] In other words, the use of qualitative research methods and theory often went hand in hand: theory could help validate the evidence generated by qualitative research methods, while at the same time, that evidence could be used to further develop, refine, or modify the theory. But lacking the statistical inferences generated by quantitative research, qualitative research methods "have the lowest ranking in the hierarchy of evidence."[164]

In this context, nurse researchers' preference for descriptive quantitative studies, observational studies, and qualitative research methods (and the invocation of theory), undermined the effectiveness of their efforts to establish the scientific rigor of their research and secure research funding. Nevertheless, in taking this approach, nurse researchers were poised, potentially, to participate in multidisciplinary clinical research with physicians, offering to that research endeavor that which was missing from physicians' focus on the effectiveness of interventions. As critics of evidence-based medicine have observed, evidence-based medicine's reliance on the quantitative methods of the randomized controlled trial (and later, the meta-analysis of systematic reviews) excludes vital evidence for clinical practice, namely the social and political context of not only clinicians' decision-making but also patient decision-making. The observational studies and qualitative research methods favored by the early generation of nurse scientists had the potential to generate knowledge about how "patients actually live their lives and make sense of both illness and medication," which can help physicians and other clinicians understand "why interventions fail."[165] Nurse scientists also brought to their research an appreciation of and attention to the ways in which the environments in which patients live—including their family, community, and sociopolitical environments—"impinge on their health and their actions."[166]

Nurse scientists, however, faced a series of obstacles in conducting clinical research. First, they often confronted institutional barriers in their efforts to conduct patient-oriented research. Without an appointment in the hospital or clinic, nurse researchers did not have a population of patients on which to conduct their research (see chapter 5). In this situation, they usually had to secure permission from physicians to conduct patient research. Some nurse scientists expressed feelings of discomfort when they entered hospital settings to conduct their research. Because they were not on the units to provide patient care, they were "anxious not to disrupt" the unit's nursing service. They also reported becoming "more than usually compulsive about proving [their] nursing capabilities to the staff." In turn, nursing staff often viewed nurse scientists with suspicion, fearing that the researchers were actually engaged in "undercover work for hospital administration, spot-checking on nurses." In other cases, the nursing staff viewed their research as "irrelevant and academic." But as the researchers depended on the nursing staff to help them identify and recruit patients for their research, it was important that the nurse scientists cultivate good relationships with the staff.[167]

Second, nurse researchers struggled to secure adequate research funding. Throughout the 1960s and 1970s, there was, as Madeleine Leininger reported, "limited awareness about the value of nursing research and limited monies available for nursing research through State, Federal, and private sources."[168] It was also, as Florence Downs, then editor of *Nursing Research*, observed, that nurses' experimental "methodologies [left] much to be desired in terms of the clarity of the specifics involved." For Downs, though, this "methodological weakness" was simply a reflection of just of how recently nurses had begun to engage in clinical nursing research.[169]

Nurse researchers engaged in qualitative research found it particularly difficult to secure research support as federal funding agencies prioritized quantitative research, particularly research that utilized the randomized controlled trial.[170] Furthermore, as Susan Gortner lamented, the NIH, with its emphasis on "fundamental processes rather than trials of therapy or application," was not particularly interested in nursing research, which tended toward social scientific investigations of health and illness and problems in health care delivery.[171] The financial situation was even worse for theorists, who throughout the 1960s and 1970s struggled to justify the need for nursing theory to their nursing colleagues, let alone to funding agencies. For example, in 1980, the nurse theorist Imogene King reflected that "for the past ten years . . . any time a group (or an individual) has something going for theory development and testing, the obstacles begin to arise." In particular, she had struggled "to get funds to describe, explain, and predict events in nurse-patient interactions" because of "the rejections by peers who sit on the committees that give money." King noted, "I have had to use my own money and time for the past

10 years (and with $50,000 in grant money could have done it in 3–5 years) to move my own theoretical formulations forward."[172]

Even as nurse researchers made the choice to conduct research to reduce hospital-based infections and adverse drug interactions, and to improve end-of-life care, pain management, and the management of chronic illness and debility—research that resonated with the broader quality assessment movement in health care—they also chose *not* to pursue other types of research, including research that would have had resonance amid the health activism of the 1960s and 1970s. In particular, nurse researchers did not pursue community-based research into the effects of poverty or racism on health and health outcomes, despite calls from nurses of color and some public health nurses in the 1960s and 1970s to engage in this type of research—and despite decades of experience among public health nurses engaging in community-based demonstration projects that sought to reduce the effects of poverty, poor housing, and inadequate health care services in underserved communities.[173]

As noted earlier, these decades were a period of heightened health activism in which civil rights activists, the Black Panther Party prominent among them, called for an end to coercive and abusive medical practices—particularly those done in the name of medical research—and the systematic social and economic exclusion that contributed to disproportionately high rates of poverty, ill health, and poor medical care among Black Americans.[174] Among civil rights health activists were physicians, nurses, and other health care professionals—many of them members of the Medical Committee for Human Rights—who had seen firsthand the impact of racial inequities in health care access.[175] By the end of the decade, activist physicians and nurses were calling on their colleagues to focus their attention on the "problem of health care for the poor" and become agents of social change.[176] As nursing leader Rhetaugh Dumas asserted in 1969, the "social destructive force of poverty" is "one of the most serious hazards to the survival and health of man." For people of color, she continued, "the problems of poverty are precipitated and compounded by racism and other forms of prejudice and discrimination." For Dumas, nursing shared responsibility for effecting change in the health care system "to make health services more responsive to the needs of the poor."[177] Nurse and activist Marie Branch, who cofounded the Black Panther Party Free Clinic in Los Angeles in 1969 and served on the faculty of UCLA's School of Nursing, saw it as nursing's responsibility "to lead for other health professionals" in implementing radical change in the health care system so as to center on and improve the health and health care of people of color in the U.S.[178] In the early 1970s, members of the Committee on Nursing in a Society in Crisis also called on nurses, particularly those in academia, to reorient their priorities and focus their attention on the "interrelationship of sociopolitical issues and nursing."[179]

By the early 1970s, women's health activists also offered a critique of the health care system, challenging in particular the assumptions on which medical paternalism was premised.[180] They did so by emphasizing a woman-centered approach to reproductive health, promoting experiential knowledge as an alternative to biomedical knowledge, and establishing women as experts of their own bodies.[181]

The work of nurse researchers, like that of the theorists, however, remained largely isolated from these transformative health politics. Rather than engaging in community-based research, nurse scientists instead pursued research topics they hoped would be legible—and fundable—within the postwar biomedical research economy. They did so in order to gain access to doing science-as-it-was-currently-done—that is, so-called normal science. As noted earlier, the NIH's research mandate during these decades was overwhelmingly disease-focused and privileged basic research in the biomedical sciences.[182] In this context (and continuing through the early twenty-first century), community-based research occupied a marginal status within the research economy.[183] As such, even if nurse scientists had wanted to, they would have been unlikely to secure from the NIH (or other major research patrons) funding to support research aimed at addressing the social and cultural factors that impacted health and illness in low-income communities and communities of color. And yet, even in pursuing research that was ostensibly more legible to the NIH and other funding agencies, nurse scientists still encountered funding difficulties. There were also costs to their approach to do normal science, and these were laid bare in the criticisms lodged by feminist nurse scientists and nurse scientists of color in the 1980s and 1990s.

The Limits of Nursing's Boundary Work

Despite the work of nurse researchers to transform nursing's practice into a distinctive and valuable site of knowledge production, and despite the theorists' progress in demarcating the boundaries of nursing science, by the early 1980s the boundary work of creating a theoretically oriented nursing science was still incomplete. Nurse theorists varied in how they operationalized the four essential concepts of person, environment, health, and nursing; some theories were too vaguely articulated or inadequately developed to clearly signify directions for nursing research or practice, and many theories had yet to be empirically validated.[184]

Two major critiques of nursing theory in this period were that they were neither useful nor relevant to research or practice. Most notably, nurse theorists confronted resistance from their colleagues in practice who criticized them for being disconnected from practice concerns and failing to relate theory to clinical practice.[185] Although theorists had long stated a commitment to ensuring that nursing theory was relevant to and informed by practice, the theorists were primarily educators, not practitioners, and as such they were not engaged with the day-to-day realities of clinical nursing.[186] But as historians and sociologists well know, this type of critique is an inherent feature of disciplines and the academic knowledge system of a profession.[187] As the sociologist Andrew Abbott noted in 1988, the character of an abstract knowledge system is "dictated by its custodians, the academics, whose criteria are not practical clarity and efficacy, but logical consistency and rationality."[188] "In reality," Abbott continued, "this perfected abstract knowledge system exists only in the world of professional textbooks. By contrast, researchers operate within the disaggregated, rationalized system of single problems and aspects, while working professionals operate with the use-based diagnostic and therapeutic classification systems already discussed. It is only students and teachers who work in the arbitrarily complete classification system discussed."[189] It was wholly fitting, then, that the National League for Nursing, the organization responsible for setting accreditation standards in nursing, issued a requirement in 1972 that nursing curriculum should be framed by a nursing conceptual model for accreditation. Nevertheless, academic nurses saw—and still see—this educational requirement as having contributed to the schism between theorists and clinicians.[190]

Yet, according to Abbott, even as "the academic knowledge system of a profession generally accomplishes three tasks—legitimation, research, and instruction—and in each it shapes the vulnerability of professional jurisdiction to outside interference," nursing's knowledge system as it existed by the early 1980s was falling short.[191] As discussed above, not many nurse researchers during these decades utilized theory, and if they did, they tended to rely on the theories of the social and behavioral sciences rather than specific nursing theories to guide their research. For example, a survey of doctoral nursing dissertations completed between 1981 and 1984 found that only 10 percent engaged with a nurse theorist, while 12 percent engaged with theorists in psychology, sociology, or physiology. In other words, the overwhelming majority of doctoral nursing dissertations utilized neither theory in general nor nursing theory in particular.[192] Even as late as the 1990s, Florence Downs, the long-serving editor of *Nursing Research* (the leading research journal in nursing), lamented the ongoing failure of nurse researchers to utilize theory to power their research. As she wrote, "research without theory really does little to advance knowledge. I repeat this truism because failure to establish a working rationale for a study has become one of the most frequent reasons for rejection of manuscripts. The study that lacks a theoretical rationale lacks substance and fails to answer the 'so what' question."[193]

Nursing's efforts to develop a theoretically oriented nursing science were also criticized by other scientists who viewed their efforts at theory development and science-making as naive and romanticized. For example, Joseph Matarazzo, a medical psychologist from the University of Oregon, explained to a conference of academic nurses in 1971 that "science . . . has little relationship to practice. This is true of all fields and all disciplines. . . . There is simply little relationship between what textbook writers say nursing is all about and what, in fact, scientists really do." Matarazzo criticized the "agonizing soulsearching and stock taking about practice derived from principle and scientific theory in relation to practice" that nurses engaged in at conferences and in published articles. As he noted, "these articles read like sophomore level textbooks . . . they are nonsense and a wasteful exercise," and they reflected the fact that "nurses talk and talk and talk about science instead of doing it."[194] A biologist attending the same conference similarly lamented nursing's efforts at constructing a science of nursing. As was reported in a summary of the biologist's remarks, he had "difficulty relating to nursing, particularly when nurses talk so much about methodology and the science of nursing. No matter how long he listens, he is still not sure what they are saying; but it appears that they are going to talk themselves to death in meetings."[195] For this biologist, it was "difficult to conceive of a science of nursing because . . . he cannot even define a science of biology."[196] He further explained, "every discipline 'steals' from every other; there is little that is absolutely unique to a single discipline." From his perspective, nursing should "grow as any other field does by appropriating what it needs from other disciplines."[197]

Additional critiques came from the small corps of feminist nurse scientists and nurse scientists of color. Despite the confidence of nursing leaders that nursing science offered a much-needed corrective to the paternalism, reductionism, and disease orientation of medicine, feminist nurses challenged that assessment. As Peggy Chinn and Charlene Wheeler reflected in 1985, "with few exceptions, nursing literature has not incorporated feminist thinking and feminist theory."[198] Furthermore, they argued, "Nursing theories embody many underlying patriarchal assumptions about human experience." For example, they continued, while feminist theory "has questioned and challenged the social imperatives perpetuated in the patriarchal family that create and sustain the oppression of women," in nursing theory "the ideal of the patriarchal family is unquestioned." Nevertheless, Chinn and Wheeler maintained that nursing theory and feminist theory had much in common. In particular, the central concepts of all nursing theories—"reverence for life, reverence for the environment, and respect for each individual's uniqueness"—were, they argued, "also central to feminist theories."[199] Indeed, although nurse theorists were not, in general, interested in claiming for nursing science a distinctively *feminist* way of knowing, by rooting their abstract knowledge system in holism, caring, and an emphasis on environment, they centered on qualities that some feminists have argued *are* distinctively feminist ways of knowing.[200]

Chinn and Wheeler were founding members of the radical feminist nursing group, Cassandra.[201] Frustrated both by the demise of the Equal Rights Amendment and with the American Nurses Association's apparent disinterest in feminist issues, a group of twelve nurses established Cassandra in the summer of 1982 with the goal of transforming the health care system and empowering nurses. From the beginning, Cassandra members identified strong support of "nursing research employing a feminist approach and exploring new dimensions of women's health" as a key issue.[202] As Ann Voda wrote in the first issue of the group's newsletter, nurse theorists and researchers had "borrowed heavily" from so-called masculine disciplines like medicine and psychiatry "in order to be 'respectable' and achieve some semblance of having a legitimate body of knowledge." The result was that nursing was not being practiced using a "truly" nursing perspective. For Voda, this meant that nursing was not utilizing a " 'woman-centered' perspective." To do so, Voda argued, nurse researchers would have to challenge the pathologization of women's reproductive lives by physicians and scientists. But doing so would put the nurse researcher "at risk . . . since such perspective[s] raise questions and ideas that are inconsistent with the way in which our universe has been defined through patriarchal eyes. So rather than question," Voda reflected, "nurses as women and women scientists generally work terribly hard to apply male generated theories and to make science as male scientists do."[203] As historians of gender and science have shown, this was indeed a common strategy of women scientists throughout the twentieth century.[204] It was time, Voda argued, for "nurses to believe that there might be a different way of thinking and being" than that prescribed by the "patriarchal framework" of biomedical science.[205]

Feminist nurses also noted that the preference among research funding agencies for quantitative research was gendered. As Kathleen MacPherson argued, qualitative research methods were central to a feminist nursing research agenda.[206] For MacPherson, a feminist research agenda would focus

on "women-related research questions," including research on topics long ignored such as "rape, incest, and hormonal and surgical abuse."[207] It would also
prioritize "analyzing the conditions of women's lives, in understanding them,
and in delineating the causes and consequences of women's oppression and a
concern for improving their state."[208] To this end, feminist nurse researchers
would rely on qualitative research methods such as participant-observation,
small sampling, and in-depth interviewing in order to privilege women's
"self-reports" of their "own experiences of health/illness, family life, work in
and outside the home, sexuality, friendship, and aging."[209] In this way, feminist nursing research would be "grounded in women's actual experiences."[210]
But, as Voda warned, the danger for nurse scientists who "do not 'do' our
science like well established disciplines do with their worship of 'methodo-
lotry'" (that is, their emphasis on quantitative research methods) was that
"we pay the price not only in procuring funds for research but in the publication of our findings. We pay the price in terms of refusal of an article because
we have not used the correct patriarchal framework. Or we pay the price in
terms of refusal if we dare to interpret our findings from a woman-centered
perspective which contradicts the patriarchal view of the world."[211] Indeed,
in the spring 1983 issue of Cassandra's newsletter, a nursing faculty member
wrote that she had been denied research funding for her feminist research
agenda and instead "was told to learn to 'play the game'" of academia.[212]

This critique of nursing science by feminist nurse scientists was part of the
broader feminist critique of science in general, which held that the "exclusion
of values culturally relegated to the female domain has led to an effective
'masculinization' of science."[213] In its place, some feminist scholars—including
feminist scientists—called for the establishment of a feminist science that
privileged supposedly distinctive feminist ways of knowing and utilized alternative methods of research, particularly qualitative methods, that would
"bring together subjective and objective ways of knowing the world."[214] But
for the majority of nurse scientists in the late 1970s and early 1980s, the goal
was to gain access "to normal science, leaving the latter unperturbed."[215]

Yet, even as feminist nurse scientists criticized nurse researchers for being
too wedded to the methods and epistemology of the "masculine" biomedical
sciences, by the late 1980s, Florence Downs was warning that nurse scientists
had in fact become overly focused on the psychosocial aspects of nursing
at the *expense of* the biophysical.[216] For Downs, the lack of nursing research
"that deals with physiological and biological aspects of patient care [was]
striking" and reflected an unhealthy emphasis among some within academic
nursing on eschewing anything biomedical.[217] As she wrote, "What comprises
a 'nursing context' has obviously troubled many manuscript reviewers during

the past decade. Animal studies and physiological variables have raised their hackles. Reviewers have asked, 'What is the significance of this study for nursing?' Others have gone further and recommended that the work be rejected for publication in Nursing Research. 'We can read about it in 'their' journals. We should be publishing nursing science.'" Even though, in many cases, the studies had been carried out by nurses and funded from nursing sources, this resistance to biological research indicated to Downs that "there is a difference of opinion about what kind of research is significant for either the discipline or practice."[218] The result, in many instances, was that nurse researchers interested in physiological variables "[felt] alienated by the eminent position accorded psychosocial variables."[219] Downs asked whether the dominance of psychological variables in nursing research meant that "psychosocial variables [were] considered more theoretical or holistic than physiological variables."[220] She was "unclear" as to how biophysiological research had become so unacceptable within nursing science. But no matter the process, she explained, "if physiological phenomena are dismissed, it hardly seems as though we have more than half a grasp on what needs to be known to understand behavior." After all, she reminded nurse researchers, "A lot of activity takes place in the unseen region beneath the skin that affects what we do and think." Moreover, nurses practicing "in arenas as disparate as primary care and the high technology intensive care units where patients are physiologically fragile" are themselves "acutely aware of their need for more substantive [biophysiological] knowledge to provide effective care."[221]

Downs's critique of nurse scientists' reticence at best—and outright rejection at worst—of biological and physiological variables resonates with recent scholarship in feminist science studies. In particular, Elizabeth Wilson draws attention to the limits of feminist theory that was, for decades, "instinctively antibiological."[222] For Wilson, the long-standing and widespread "aversion to biological data" within feminist theories "bespeaks an ongoing discomfort with how to manage biological claims—as if biological data will overwhelm the ability of feminist theory to make cogent conceptual and political interventions."[223] Read in such a feminist register, nursing science looks to have conformed with the antibiological impulse within feminism. That even as the first generation of nurse scientists sought to establish nursing science within the parameters of normal science, hewing to its epistemologies and methodologies, they at the same time worked to reject that within normal science that was explicitly biological. Indeed, for many nurse scientists, rejecting the biological was integral to their work of creating boundaries around nursing and distinguishing it clearly from the biomedicine of physicians. In this regard, even if the majority of these nurse scientists were not engaged in feminist *science*, they were nevertheless engaging in feminist work—most importantly, establishing the gendered domain of nursing as a legitimate site of knowledge production. Thus, nursing science offers an interesting and complex site for feminist analysis.

The lack of racial and ethnic diversity among doctorally prepared nurses in these decades also influenced the development of nursing science. As noted earlier, only twenty African American female nurses, one African American male nurse, and eight Asian American female nurses were among the 589 nurses who received fellowship support from the Division of Nursing between 1955 and 1974.[224] Data published by the American Nurses Foundation in 1972 indicated that of the 964 doctorally prepared nurses in the United States, only fifty-eight self-identified as nurses of color. Among them were nine African American nurses who had since left nursing to pursue careers in medicine.[225]

This lack of diversity shaped what were and were not considered important areas of research and theory development. As Lucille Davis, a faculty member at Rush University, asserted in 1974, nurse researchers from minority groups "bring a unique perspective . . . to the research process." Davis saw it as "absolutely essential that we have more nurses from minority groups" trained as researchers if nursing is to develop "research models relevant to the health care needs of minorities."[226] When the National Black Nurses Association was founded late in 1971, one of its ten published objectives was to "Conduct, analyze, and publish research to increase the body of knowledge about health care and health needs of blacks [*sic*]." Two more of the NBNA's objectives called on Black nurses to "Define and determine nursing care for black consumers by acting as their advocates" and to "act as change agent in restructuring existing institutions and/or helping to establish institutions to suit the needs of black people." The NBNA recognized that such research and advocacy—led by Black nurses—was integral to improving the health and health care of Black Americans.[227] For Gloria Smith, dean of nursing at the University of Oklahoma, the presence of "minority group faculty is an ongoing reminder for the faculty of its responsibilities for educating nurses and for developing research to meet the needs of many cultural groups."[228] Throughout these decades, however, nursing schools struggled to recruit and retain doctoral students and faculty of color because of persistent structural racism.[229]

In the western U.S., nursing leaders were engaged in efforts to increase the number of nurses of color participating in research and the number of research studies addressing issues of concern to patients of color. In 1971, the Western Council of Higher Education for Nursing (WCHEN) had established a regional development program (with funding from the Division of Nursing) to increase "the quantity and quality of clinical nursing research and the use of research findings to improve patient care."[230] In 1974, when WCHEN renewed the program, it did so with the express aim of increasing the number of participants in sponsored research projects "from ethnic minority backgrounds."[231] Despite "a concerted outreach effort . . . the proportion of ethnic nurses recruited was not as a high as had been hoped." Although 6 percent of nurses who participated in the program between 1971 and 1974 were nurses of color, between 1974 and 1977, the number of nurses of color who participated increased only to 10 percent.[232]

During the same period, the Western Interstate Commission for Higher Education—of which WCHEN was a part—sponsored "Faculty Development to Meet Minority Group Needs" with funding from the W. K. Kellogg Foundation.[233] The project was led by Marie Branch, who in 1969 cofounded the Black Panther Free Clinic in Los Angeles while also serving on the faculty of UCLA's School of Nursing.[234] The goal of the project, which ran from 1971 through 1974, was to assist nursing faculty in developing strategies to recruit and retain nursing students of color and revise nursing curricula in order to prepare nursing students to better meet the health care needs of communities of color. It led to the publication of Branch and Phyllis Paxton's *Providing Safe Nursing Care for Ethnic People of Color* in 1976, which was intended as a primer for educating nurses and nursing students to provide inclusive nursing care.[235] Then in 1978, building on these and WCHEN's earlier initiatives, the Western Interstate Commission for Higher Education brought together a group of nurses of color from the western states to further develop strategies for increasing the number of nurse researchers of color and to define research priorities centered on addressing the nursing problems of patients of color. This culminated in the establishment of the Ethnic Nurses for the Advancement of Health Care, an organization committed to fostering research into the health care of people of color. The organization held its first annual research conference in Los Angeles the following year, where the majority of the research papers addressed "clinical problems of ethnic patients of color."[236]

However, by the early 1990s, there remained a dearth of nursing research on the experiences and nursing care needs of patients of color. Indeed, of the 8,261 clinical studies published in U.S. nursing journals between 1983 and 1991, nurse and anthropologist Eileen Jackson, found that only fifty-nine (0.7 percent) included African Americans in the study sample. The majority of these fifty-nine studies did not focus on "the eight major health problems identified among African Americans."[237] In particular, they failed to address the reasons for or propose solutions to disproportionately high morbidity and mortality

rates in Black communities. As Jackson concluded, "simply including marginalized groups in a study sample does not make the research relevant to the
health of those being studied."[238]

The ongoing shortage of nurse scientists of color and the lack of nursing research on patients and communities of color reflected and reinforced
what Jackson termed "whiting-out difference" and nurse and anthropologist
Evelyn Barbee characterized, simply, as "racism in U.S. nursing."[239] As Barbee
argued, by the early 1990s, "nursing's theoretical models," along with "the curricular emphases" in nursing schools, had led to the "lack of awareness of the
influence of structural variables on the work of nursing" and of the influence
of race and racism on health outcomes.[240] In particular, Jackson explained,
nursing theorists' focus on the environment—rather than on society—"as a
fundamental factor affecting the patient" had "had the effect of both increasing the holistic perspective of nursing and de-emphasizing social structure
and socioeconomic differentiation."[241] This had led to both a class and race
bias in nursing research in which the influence of racism or socioeconomic
or cultural factors on the health outcomes of individuals and communities of
color, particularly the causes of and potential solutions to health disparities,
had been ignored.

For both Jackson and Barbee, the very nature of nursing's academic project had led to this situation. "The desire to gain acceptance for nursing as a
scientific discipline," Jackson asserted, had led "nursing's ideology" to mirror
"the funding priorities of the major funding agencies that support nursing research." These were an emphasis on "individual responsibility for health" and
a preference for "high-technology, revenue-generating treatment localized in
hospitals and translated into home care." The result was nursing's "focus on
individual-level variables in isolation from the broad social context of patients."[242] Given the imbrication of racism within nursing's academic project,
Barbee asserted, "a question that need[ed] to be voiced [was]: What is the cost
of our striving for legitimacy?"[243]

The limits of nursing's boundary work were also reflected in the efforts
of nurse educators to secure academic legitimacy for their new discipline
and establish nursing PhD programs during these decades. Indeed, the move
to establish nursing as an academic discipline held particular significance
as the primary sites of nursing education shifted to colleges and universities and nursing schools worked to secure their status on university campuses. By contributing to the production of new nursing knowledge, nurse
researchers and theorists would not only hope to help advance patient care,
but they would also secure membership in the "community of scholars."[244] In
this way, nursing faculty would no longer be just teachers but would become

full-fledged members of academe. But as the next chapters show, as nurse theorists grappled with the definitional and conceptual questions of nursing science, nursing faculty struggled to convince university administrators of the strong conceptual underpinnings of the nursing PhD, the disciplinary parameters of nursing science, and the academic rigor of nurse scientists. Thus, even as many among this early generation of nurse scientists saw the creation of an abstract knowledge system underpinned by nursing theory as key to gaining entry to "masculine" science, their efforts were not always valued or taken seriously by the broader culture of science and medicine. While there was gender at work here, it was also, as the next chapter documents, about the ways in which nurse scientists were choosing to do science.

Nursing in the Postwar Research University

Writing in 1965, Dean Rozella Schlotfeldt of the Frances Payne Bolton School of Nursing at Case Western Reserve University (then called Western Reserve University), noted that nursing faculties had yet to achieve "two major accomplishments" which would signal nursing's arrival as an academic discipline: "First is that each [nursing] school must make its contribution toward developing and testing the theoretical constructs which represent nursing knowledge. The second is that all faculties in nursing schools must exemplify the characteristics appropriately expected of professionals and scholars who hold university appointments." As part of this, nursing faculty should be engaged in "developing and refining nursing knowledge . . . preparing generalist and specialist nursing practitioners of the future, [and] finding answers to significant questions concerning nursing practice." To this end, another core component of nursing's academic project was the establishment of PhD programs in nursing. While many nurses had earned doctorates in schools or departments of education and, increasingly from the early 1960s, in the basic or behavioral sciences, the development of the *nursing* research doctorate, the PhD, would for the first time prepare nurses *within* nursing schools to conduct research—grounded in nursing theory—aimed at producing new nursing knowledge (nursing science) that would, ultimately, advance nursing practice. By contributing to the production of new nursing knowledge, nurse scientists would not only help advance patient care (as discussed in chapter 2), but they would also secure membership in the "community of scholars." In this way, nursing faculty would no longer be just teachers but would become full-fledged members of academe, and as such should be accorded equal intellectual and institutional status as their university peers.[1]

Nursing's academic project took place in the context of the changing political economy of American universities. As the federal government became the primary patron of basic research after the war, universities increasingly prioritized research—and the acquisition of federal research funding—over teaching and service.[2] At the same time, the federal government and its policymakers ensured that graduate education (particularly at the doctoral level) became an integral component of the research enterprise.[3] In response, nursing leaders sought to establish the legitimacy of nursing as a scientific discipline so as to capitalize on new federal funding opportunities and secure the academic status of nursing schools. Just as engineering and the physical, biological, and social sciences were transformed by the institutional context and patronage relationships of the postwar research university, so, too, was nursing.[4]

During the postwar decades, as the previous chapter documented, nurse scientists transformed nursing's practice into a site of knowledge production and demonstrated the ways in which application of this knowledge was integral to improving patient outcomes and health care delivery. As a predominantly female profession, however, nursing's transformation within the postwar university was indelibly shaped by the politics of gender. As historians of gender and science have documented, while women scientists made academic gains during World War II, they were pushed aside after the war as male faculty and students—supported by G.I. Bill funding—returned to campuses.[5] The result was the "remasculinization of the sciences."[6] But while the discriminatory gender politics of postwar science led to the demise of predominantly female disciplines like home economics, nursing was able to secure a footing, however tenuous, within the research economy.

To be sure, the efforts of nursing researchers to secure their academic standing within the postwar university were impacted by gender discrimination. But their struggle for status was also shaped by the limits of their academic project—by the way they chose to *do* science. As the previous chapter describes, nurse scientists primarily utilized observational studies and qualitative research methods, particularly ethnography, case studies, or grounded theory, to generate evidence. They did so, however, as the broader culture of biomedicine regarded large-scale randomized controlled trials as the gold standard of biomedical research. That nurses were not using the research methods that were most highly valorized in the biomedical culture thus impacted the effectiveness of their efforts. As a consequence of this, nurses struggled to demonstrate to university administrators that as an academic discipline, nursing science added value in ways that mattered, such as securing federal research funding and generating new knowledge not attainable by the other disciplines.

Ultimately, this chapter explores how this early generation of academic nurses understood their roles as nurses and as academics, and how their roles within the university (as opposed to in clinical settings), shaped the kinds of knowledge they produced and the types of knowledge workers they educated. By emphasizing the conflicts that occurred as nurses worked to establish themselves in the postwar research university, this chapter reveals what those at the time believed was at stake and what would be lost as well as gained in the academization of nursing.

The Postwar University

Nursing's academic project took place in the context of the changing political economy of American universities in the decades after World War II. As the federal government assumed primary responsibility for the support of basic research, federal research funding flowed to university and college campuses. The 1960s, in particular, were "the golden decade" for academic science in the United States.[7] By the early 1960s, the federal government was spending more than $1 billion on research and development conducted on university campuses, with 36 percent of that funding coming from the National Institutes of Health and 26 percent from the Department of Defense.[8] Although never as substantial as the federal government's investment in research and development, industry spending also increased in the postwar years. The defense industry, in particular, invested heavily in the physical sciences and engineering, while the pharmaceutical industry became an increasingly important patron of biomedical science. In turn, universities provided most of the basic research and trained all of the scientific labor for the defense and pharmaceutical industries.[9]

As universities competed for federal and industry dollars during and after the war, they became service institutions, offering services such as targeted research and innovation or policy advice to their patrons in exchange for research funding.[10] In this context, the research university became a "multiversity," responsive to the needs and interests of multiple constituencies.[11] This had a transformative effect on the academic disciplines as federal and industry funding influenced the kinds of research pursued and the types of technologies developed.[12] It also led to changes in the role of faculty members, who were no longer valued for their teaching but for their ability to secure research money and generate patents and publications. In this context, academic entrepreneurship—with emphasis on attracting patronage and building research empires, often at the expense of undergraduate teaching—became the norm. Patronage often parlayed into institutional power. For individual faculty members, "access to outside funds rather than seniority conveyed power and authority within departments."[13] In turn, the total amount of external funding secured by departments, centers, or schools often determined the degree of institutional power accorded that unit and its administrator within the university.

Medical schools were particularly effective at capitalizing on the postwar research economy.[14] In the postwar decades, the NIH became the primary patron of biomedical research.[15] At the same time, though, the costs of medical education increased significantly. Medical schools responded by accommodating themselves to the priorities of medical research, placing increasing emphasis on the research capacity of its faculty. This included hiring more research-engaged faculty and postdoctoral research fellows and enlarging PhD programs in the basic biomedical sciences.[16] As a result, the number of scientists employed by medical schools increased from 15,600 in 1958 to 50,000 in 1965. In turn, the number of full-time faculty—typically faculty engaged in research in the basic sciences—grew from 9,600 in 1958 to 23,000 in 1968. During these same years, the number of medical students grew only 20 percent, from 30,000 to 36,000, while the "contingent of graduate students grew far more rapidly, reaching 10,000."[17]

Medical schools also significantly expanded their clinical services during the postwar decades, as they hired increasing numbers of faculty engaged in clinical practice (typically designated as clinical faculty). This was largely due to changes in the economic structure of medical education and patient care, such as the growing number of patients with health insurance.[18] The passage of Medicare and Medicaid in 1965 greatly increased the availability of clinical income, which not only led medical schools to hire greater numbers of clinical faculty, but also helped to underwrite the expansion of clinical research in medical schools. These developments, as Roger Geiger argues, "gave medical research a structure and dynamic all its own."[19] By the end of the 1960s, medical schools were the largest performers of academic research on their campuses, and their deans, as a result, "enjoyed far more budgetary flexibility" than did the deans of other schools and colleges in the university.[20] Even within newly emergent academic health centers, which were intended—ostensibly, at least—to promote parity among constituent health science schools, the political and economic interests of medical schools tended to dominate.

During the postwar decades, the government's science advisors, along with federal policymakers, made clear that graduate education would be an integral component of the research enterprise. Most notably, in 1960, the President's Science Advisory Committee published its report, "Scientific Progress, the Universities, and the Federal Government." The report argued that basic research and graduate education "*belong together* at every possible level" and called for the federal government to support the significant expansion of graduate education.[21] Two years earlier, in 1958, Congress had passed the National Defense Education Act, which "created a new program of graduate fellowships, most of them in science and engineering."[22] This, together with President Kennedy's signing of the Higher Education Facilities Act of 1963, which established "an expansive program of grants and loans to universities and colleges for building and equipping classrooms, laboratories, and libraries," underwrote the expansion of graduate education on university campuses in the 1960s.[23]

On a national scale, the postwar expansion of graduate education was intended to provide the highly trained scientific and engineering labor needed to ensure the U.S.'s scientific and technological leadership during the Cold War. Within individual institutions, graduate students facilitated faculty research by serving as research assistants, and "as future researchers they enhanced the reputation of the department and their mentors."[24] The establishment and expansion of doctoral programs, in particular, Geiger explains, "raised the prestige of an institution, allowed it to recruit and retain better faculty, encouraged research, qualified it for special forms of federal aid, and, especially for state schools, justified appeals for increased resources."[25]

Despite the characterization of the postwar decades as a golden age for American scientists, not all scientists (and not all scientific disciplines) benefited equally from the research boom. Women scientists faired especially poorly in the postwar research economy. As Margaret Rossiter has documented, women scientists were marginalized and underutilized in the postwar decades. Even as some government officials encouraged young women to pursue scientific careers, "previously trained women scientists were finding it hard to get hired or promoted or even to be taken seriously."[26] Because of prevailing discriminatory assumptions about women's societal roles, women scientists were "defined as obstacles to progress, and their removal" from academic institutions was "a desired goal."[27] The decline of home economics is particularly revealing of the struggles facing women scientists in the postwar decades.[28]

In the 1950s and 1960s, Rossiter describes, "the most numerous and the highest-ranking women scientists employed on the faculties of the nation's top universities . . . were those concentrated in the highly but not totally feminized area of home economics." But during these decades, university administrators (who were uniformly male at the time), "held skeptical and hostile attitudes about home economics while at the same time admitting unabashed ignorance about what the field was and what it was trying to do." Administrators were especially troubled by the "field's strong vocationalism or explicit links to teacher education . . . and the low proportion of doctorates among its faculty." As Rossiter argues, however, it was primarily "the field's high proportion of women (usually 90–100 percent)," that administrators held up "as further evidence that the field was out-of-date."[29] Home economics also struggled to secure much-needed research support in these decades, as the major federal patrons of postwar science, the National Science Foundation (NSF) and the NIH, "did not recognize 'home economics' as a field of science."[30] Although the U.S. Department of Agriculture supported research in home economics, the amounts were "never enough . . . to satisfy the relentless demand" for more research.[31] As Rossiter shows, by the mid-1960s, as the field had become "less attractive to women students and intolerable to many of the male faculty and administrators," university administrators at "several major campuses seized upon the opportunity to reshape this formerly female bastion into the somewhat more gender-neutral subjects of 'nutritional sciences,' 'human development,' or 'human ecology.'"[32]

While nursing leaders did not comment (at least not publicly) on what their colleagues in home economics were dealing with in these years, it is hard to imagine that they failed to notice given the similarities between the two fields. As with home economics, nursing had strong vocational ties with roots in education, the faculty were overwhelmingly female, and there were very few doctorally prepared faculty. To be sure, nursing faculty were all too aware of their potential vulnerability within the gendered environment of the postwar research university. The reconfiguration of American academic health institutions into academic health centers (AHCs) in the postwar decades (discussed in chapter 1) had theoretically granted equal administrative status to each health science school. But as the operational budget and revenue generation of medical schools significantly outpaced the fiscal capacity of the other health science schools, university presidents consistently called upon physicians who had proven their administrative mettle in medical school administration to lead the AHCs.

For nursing leaders, this created an all-too-familiar institutional dynamic, one they thought they had left behind in hospital training schools: physician oversight of nursing education. As Madeleine Leininger, who had held leadership positions in three academic health centers and surveyed several others, noted in 1974, this realignment of institutional relationships within universities had led to "conflicts and serious problems." In particular, there "[had] been open confrontations by astute nursing deans and faculty with the structure as nursing schools were most reluctant to be placed under medicine again after only being liberated from them." The appointment of physicians as leaders of AHCs had, Leininger asserted, "aggravated and increased the fears and distrust of medicine as further evidence of a solid power-base of medicine over other disciplines."[33]

The gendered hierarchies within AHCs could also lead to discrimination. At the University of Florida, for example, the dean of nursing, Dorothy Smith, had excellent relations with both the dean of the medical school and the AHC's provost (also a physician). But the other health science leaders considered her expertise and status "suspect" because she was both a woman and a nurse. Writing to the provost in 1965, Smith reflected on a series of power struggles within the Health Center Council, which was composed of the deans of medicine, nursing, and dentistry, the hospital administrator, and the provost. "The ironic thing," Smith wrote, "is that with the exception of you—and I don't know what your experiences have been—I have had more experience within group development and group process than probably anyone else in the group. I suspect that I have studied more about it—in fact, I know I have—and yet, because I am a woman and because I am a nurse to some extent everything I say is colored by the group's concepts of women, nurses, and . . . the importance of process in terms of reaching a goal. The University says that we are peers but saying this does not make it so."[34]

The experiences of UCLA's School of Nursing during the 1960s reflected in the extreme the challenges that the gendered and hierarchical politics within academic health centers posed to nursing schools in this period. As discussed in chapter 1, throughout the decade, the dean of UCLA's medical school (along with faculty in the department of surgery) lobbied UCLA's chancellor (a physician) to dismantle the School of Nursing and reestablish it as a department of nursing within the medical school. For nursing deans looking to institute educational reform, transform the culture of their schools, and establish their school's academic standing, the experiences at UCLA offered a chilling warning. As Mary Kelly Mullane, dean of University of Illinois Chicago's College of Nursing, warned, "recent events at UCLA" had made clear that the "inauguration of a nursing program in a university is no guarantee of its continuance." The lesson, for Mullane, was that university-based nursing schools "will remain and prosper there [in universities] only if the next generation of nurses in sufficient numbers produce the scholarship and research which underlie university teaching and typify the university professor in any field."[35] In other words, nursing schools needed to become part of the postwar research economy. For nursing leaders then, this meant that nursing faculty should be doctorally prepared and engaged in externally funded research. And given the imbrication of the academic research enterprise and doctoral education, nursing schools would need to establish PhD programs to underpin their research enterprise and secure their standing within the postwar research university.

Establishing Nursing Schools in the Postwar Research Economy

In the transition from service-based to university-based education, nursing schools were slow to adopt an academic culture that supported and rewarded research. Nursing faculty in this period typically focused on teaching, curriculum development, and educational administration. In the 1950s at the University of Washington School of Nursing, for example, individual faculty members typically taught thirty hours or more of clinical teaching per week. And faculty efforts, explained Mary Tschudin and Lawrence Sharp, "were directed almost exclusively to discovering ways of improving undergraduate education."[36] In turn, pedagogical contributions and effective teaching were the primary measures by which faculty were evaluated for promotion. Research was neither envisioned nor rewarded as an essential faculty role.

This emphasis reflected the educational preparation of nursing faculty in the 1950s. Through the 1950s, most nursing faculty had received their graduate degrees in education, the majority at the master's degree level. Of the small number of doctorally prepared nurses, most were graduates of either Teachers College, Columbia University, or New York University School of Nursing—the only doctoral nursing programs at the time.[37] Teachers College launched the first doctoral program in nursing in 1924. As an education doctoral program, the emphasis was on preparing nurse educators rather than nurse researchers. In 1934, New York University's School of Nursing established the first nursing PhD program. Although the program emphasized the teaching of theory development, it was still largely modeled on an educational degree with half of the required courses being in nursing education.

In many ways, university-based nursing schools' emphasis on undergraduate teaching typified the prewar university in which undergraduate education was a clear priority. But in the changed political economy of the postwar university, in which faculty's professional advancement "depended wholly on research and publication, which in turn depended on development of patronage,"[38] nursing schools' emphasis on teaching and a lack of focus on research stood to isolate them from the rest of the university. As Mary Tschudin, dean of the University of Washington School of Nursing argued in 1965, "For too long we have been remiss in not accepting our full responsibilities as members of the university family." While university faculty were expected to fulfill the tripartite roles of research, teaching, and service, nursing faculty were traditionally focused only on teaching and service. As such, Tschudin continued, "we have been 'in' but not 'of' the university because we have not been prepared to participate in carrying out the full range of university functions."[39]

By the late 1950s, the deans of the leading university-based nursing schools recognized that nursing had not yet adapted to the postwar political economy and would need to if nursing was to be taken seriously as an academic discipline. Integral to this adaptation was that nursing faculty needed to be doctorally prepared and engaged in externally supported research to become full-fledged members of the university. Thus, research needed to become, and be rewarded as, an essential faculty role.[40] In this way, nursing schools had to incorporate the research ethos of the postwar university in order to secure their status on university campuses. At Yale University School of Nursing in the 1950s, for example, "the faculty felt pressure from the [Yale] Corporation to justify the school's place in the university. Increasing competence in research," Donna Diers explained, "was one way to provide evidence that the School of Nursing could attain the levels of quality apparent in other departments."[41]

During the 1960s, the deans of several of the country's leading nursing schools worked to transform nursing schools into sites of knowledge production. They did so by prioritizing the recruitment of faculty with doctorates, particularly those who had earned PhDs in the biomedical, behavioral, and social sciences (often through the Nurse Scientist Graduate Training Program discussed below) who were committed to engaging in nursing research.[42] They also encouraged their master's-prepared faculty and students to pursue full-time doctoral study, and provided the faculty with time for research and rewarded that research effort in their school's workload and promotion and tenure policies.[43] These efforts were largely underwritten by the U.S. Public Health Service Division of Nursing, with additional support provided by philanthropic foundations like the American Nurses Foundation, the W. K. Kellogg Foundation, the Commonwealth Fund, and the Russell Sage Foundation. For example, in 1959, the Division of Nursing had established the Faculty Research Development Grant (FRDG) program to develop the research competence of nursing faculty and transform participating nursing schools into sites, not only of education, but also of research.[44]

Between 1959 and 1966 (when the final award was made), the Division of Nursing awarded FRDGs to eighteen nursing schools to enhance their research capacity.[45] The FRDG program was similar in many respects to the National Science Foundation's University Science Development Program, which was launched in 1965 to raise the "research capacities of second-tier institutions so that they might merit greater research support through regular channels."[46] Both programs reflected the federal government's interest not only in supporting institutions already doing research, but also, as Roger Geiger explains, "supporting the aspirations of institutions wishing to do more research."[47]

A key element of the FRDG program was that it enabled participating nursing schools to hire full-time research consultants to provide research training, hands-on guidance, and encouragement to faculty interested in initiating research projects. The research consultants were typically doctorally prepared researchers in the behavioral or social sciences. The UCLA School of Nursing, for example, hired a series of full-time research consultants (including two psychologists and one physicist-turned-sociologist) who assisted the nursing faculty as they embarked on research projects. The University of Washington School of Nursing hired a series of four research consultants who were trained either as sociologists or psychologists.[48] At Yale University, the nursing school used the grant to establish dual appointments for several faculty in sociology, psychology, and philosophy, and hospital administration and public health.[49] At all three schools, the research consultants conducted seminars, classes, and workshops in research methodology that faculty were encouraged to attend.

In many of the nursing schools that received FRDG funding, the research training provided faculty with both the stimulus and the context for revising the schools' undergraduate and graduate curricula in order to incorporate research as an integral part of coursework. This included adding a new research course as a requirement, making a pilot study or senior project as a requirement for graduation, or adding new courses in statistics or research methodology.[50] At Yale University, the School of Nursing increased the number of research courses it offered from one elective course in 1962 to two required and three elective courses by the end of the grant period in 1968. Over the duration of the grant, the faculty also observed "an increase in comfort with which [master's] students approach research, an increase in their competence to design and conduct meaningful research, and a decrease in the conflict of loyalties students used to have between research and clinical practice."[51] At the Frances Payne Bolton School of Nursing at Case Western Reserve University, every student in the master's program was "required to design, carryout, and report an independent investigation. Several who demonstrated research potential were encouraged to enroll in doctoral study."[52] Similarly, at UCLA, over the course of the FRDG project, the number of master's students writing theses increased, and the quality of those theses (in terms of the caliber of research), improved. At several of the participating nursing schools, under-graduate and graduate students served as research assistants on the faculty's research projects. The intent of incorporating research training and research experiences into the student experience was to stimulate "the next generation of nurses increasingly to value research"[53] and "to think of research as a part of the basic triad of the profession's responsibilities."[54]

Much of the research carried out under the auspices of the FRDG pro-gram centered on studies of patient care and the influence of nursing inter-ventions on patient outcomes.[55] This reflected the Division of Nursing's stated priority of supporting research focused on nursing care and patient care problems rather than educational or administrative research on nurses.[56] It also reflected, however, broader changes taking place in health care research in the second half of the twentieth century, particularly the emergence of the field of outcomes research and the related quality assessment movement in health care (see chapter 2).

The efforts of deans and their research-oriented faculty to transform nurs-ing schools into sites of knowledge production in the 1960s and 1970s were circumscribed, however, by generational politics. An older generation of nursing faculty were socialized to a reward structure that used "teaching ef-fectiveness for faculty evaluations and salary merits and only very limitedly on research and research productivity."[57] As Madeleine Leininger noted in 1977, "highly conservative and traditionally-oriented faculty who have been limitedly prepared in research (and who are often tenured through time rather than by academic criteria) often pose serious problems in schools and thwart research climate and direction."[58] Leininger had encountered such resistance in her efforts to establish a research culture and raise academic standards first at the University of Washington School of Nursing, where she served as dean from 1969 to 1974, and then at the University of Utah College of Nursing from 1974 through 1980.[59] At Utah, for example, a small group of dissenting faculty who were threatened by the changes introduced by Leininger "con-tinually utilized harassment techniques" aimed both at Leininger and at the faculty who openly supported her. Although their efforts to block Leininger's changes failed, "the faculty time, effort, and energy needed to neutralize them [were] prodigious" and distracted from the work of the College of Nursing.[60]

In this context, deans and their research-oriented faculty often had to do "considerable work to change the dominant teaching emphasis and give pro-portional emphasis to research."[61] As part of this, Leininger recommended including research productivity—publishing and presenting research papers and applying for and securing external research funding—as criteria for pro-motion and retention.[62] At the Frances Payne Bolton School of Nursing at

Case Western Reserve University, for example, Dean Rozella Schlotfeldt and the research faculty revised the faculty workload policy and the school's reward system "to reflect the extent to which research would be valued."[63] The new workload policy enabled faculty to program "time for research as well as for teaching and practice" and held them accountable for "their research involvement and productivity." The criteria for faculty promotions and tenure were also designed to reflect faculty contributions "to research and scholarly endeavors as well as to give recognition of their competence in teaching and in specialty practice." In this way, the school's promotion and tenure policies were for the first time closely aligned with promotion and tenure policies of other university faculty.[64] At Wayne State University, in contrast, the College of Nursing made minimal adjustments to its workload and tenure policies, holding the research faculty accountable for their research productivity but doing little to encourage or reward research among faculty who felt their primary function was to teach.[65]

The efforts of deans and faculty to transform nursing schools into research enterprises also faced institutional and financial difficulties. The experiences of the nursing faculty and dean at Wayne State University as they worked to transform its College of Nursing into a site of innovative research are particularly instructive. In 1965, the College of Nursing was awarded a five-year FRDG from the Division of Nursing. The nursing faculty undertook a series of research studies on the nursing care problems of medical-surgical patients, including the incidence and prevention of catheter-induced infections and hospital-induced infections among tracheostomized patients.[66] Two-and-a-half years into the FRDG, however, the nursing faculty realized "something more was needed if research in the College of Nursing was to flourish."[67] In particular, the dean, Margaret Shetland, and her faculty believed that a research center would enable them to bring together scientists of different disciplines and "pool their expertise, as it were, and work together toward developing several programs of research in the area of health."[68] A research center would also allow the faculty to share equipment, support staff, and other resources, which they hoped would help control the costs of research. To this end, in 1969, the College of Nursing established the Center for Nursing Research.[69] Shetland recruited Harriet Werley to serve as the center's first director. Werley had begun her career in the U.S. Army, serving in the Mediterranean theater during World War II, and by the time she was hired by Wayne State University, she was an accomplished and highly regarded nurse researcher.[70]

By the mid-1970s, according to typical measures of research productivity—such as degree of external research funding—the College of Nursing had established itself as a research school. In 1969, for example, the college established the first research center in the country dedicated to nursing research with funding primarily from the NIH, as well as research grants from private foundations and institutional funding from Wayne State University. By 1972, the center had secured more than $100,000 of annual research support. As such, it was eligible for and received an NIH General Research Support Grant (as of 1972, one of only four nursing schools to receive such funding).[71]

Much of the Center for Nursing Research's focus during its first decade focused on evaluating and improving patient outcomes, and on improving patients' access to and experience of health care. In this way, the center's research aligned with the growing focus on outcomes research and quality assessment in health care (see chapter 2).[72] This included controlled experimental research studies that investigated ways to reduce patients' complications from surgery and hospitalization, such as hospital-acquired infections and elevated stress and anxiety; the latter studies being guided by psychological theories.[73] The center's research also focused on evaluating the effects of nursing interventions on the outcomes of acutely ill and terminally ill patients.[74] Another series of studies investigated the impact of health problems on the family, the eventual goal of which was to promote family-centered care.[75] Another major area of the center's research program—primarily descriptive quantitative research utilizing questionnaires—focused on family planning. Werley and her colleagues, for example, investigated how the attitudes of nurses, physicians, and social workers toward population growth and family planning (birth control, sterilization, and abortion) influenced clients' use of family planning services.[76] In related research, Werley and her team assessed nurses' attitudes toward abortion and evaluated their experiences providing abortion care prior to the legalization of abortion in order to facilitate the implementation of abortion reform and improve the abortion care provided by nurses.[77] Some of their other research sought to improve the health care of sexually active teenagers, including increasing teenagers' knowledge of, access to, and use of contraceptives and sex education programs.[78] The researchers hoped to use their findings to improve access to family planning services, including sterilization and abortion services, and reduce the incidence of unplanned pregnancies (especially among teenagers).[79] Despite these markers of success, however, the school and its research center struggled to secure support from the university administration and from external funding agencies, each of whom weighed nursing's utility as a research discipline against budget cuts and shifting funding priorities.[80]

The difficulties encountered by nurse scientists seeking to secure external research funding during the late 1960s and 1970s reflected, in part, changes in the political economy of the research university in the early 1970s. The escalation of the Vietnam War during the late 1960s had increased the cost of the war, which led the federal government to significantly and abruptly reduce the amount it was spending on research and development. Restrictions in federal funding, together with declining university enrollments, persistently high inflation, and diminishing state support for higher education, "created far less favorable circumstances for universities and colleges" in the 1970s than they had experienced during the previous decade.[81] The 1970s have accordingly been termed "the stagnant decade."[82] Between 1968 and 1971, for example, the "federal research budget fell more than 10 percent in real terms." And from 1968 to 1984, total federal awards to universities declined from $4.2 billion "to $3.9 billion in 1984 (in 1982 dollars), while academic research costs increased 50 percent between 1967 and 1975."[83]

This context of declining federal research support undermined the efforts of nurse researchers like Werley and her colleagues at the Center for Nursing Research. Throughout its first five years, the work of the center was as much about "survival" as it was about developing and conducting research. Werley and her staff continually wrote research proposals and pursued opportunities for securing "hard money" so that the school could retain the "tried and proven" qualified researchers once their current grants expired.[84] But Werley struggled to secure stable institutional financial support for the center. She made repeated requests to the dean and to the university administration to secure ongoing support for the center once the term of the NIH Research Development Grant ended, but such support was not forthcoming.[85]

The funding difficulties encountered by nursing schools like Wayne State University also reflected, in part, the type of research they were pursuing and, particularly, the research methods they were using. Although some of those methods included controlled experiments, like the majority of nurse scientists in these years (as detailed in chapter 2), the center's researchers primarily utilized descriptive quantitative research, observational studies, and qualitative research methods to generate evidence. They did so, however, as the broader culture of biomedicine regarded large-scale randomized controlled trials as the gold standard of clinical research.

But for Werley, the center's difficulties securing research funding were less about the research methods being utilized and more about nursing's low standing as a scientific discipline and what Werley perceived as gender discrimination. The staff's research proposals were often rejected on the grounds that they were not published in the particular content area for which proposals were submitted, even when they collaborated with researchers in allied fields (such as psychology, sociology, and medicine) who were already published in their respective field of study. The center staff also felt that research "funds were denied because nursing was not viewed as a legitimate research discipline." Some "individuals declined program participation in a *nursing* research center, although before knowing the name of the Center, they had expressed interest and enthusiasm about the request to participate" in the center's research program.[86] In an effort to overcome "the misunderstanding of people in the scientific community about the nature of nursing research," the College of Nursing renamed the center the Center for Health Research in 1972.[87] The name change, however, failed to solve all the problems, particularly those caused by sexism. After all, as Werley reflected, "the Center [still] stems from a nursing situation and from a predominantly female group."[88] Werley's efforts were also undermined by the generational conflicts described above, which culminated in a lack of understanding among many of the nursing faculty about the nature of research and the importance of building the college's research capacities.

In spite of the challenges encountered by Werley and her colleagues in transforming the academic culture at Wayne State University College of Nursing and establishing research as an essential component of the nursing faculty role, by the mid-1970s there were clear signs of progress. The research productivity of the college's faculty had increased. Between 1970 and 1975, the nursing faculty had submitted twenty-one research proposals for internal university funding and thirty-eight research proposals for external funding (including from the NIH, the National Institute of Mental Health, the NSF, the American Nurses Foundation, Sigma Theta Tau, the Robert Wood Johnson Foundation, Blue Cross Blue Shield, the March of Dimes, and the Population Council). Nineteen of the proposals were funded, with three still under review. The faculty also published thirty research-based articles. Research was better integrated into the nursing curriculum, particularly at the graduate level, with all master's students being required to conduct an empirical research project as part of their degree. A research elective was also offered to senior undergraduate students, with more and more students electing to take the course each year. The center also hired students as research assistants. The Center for Health Research had also established a regular research seminar, "Frontiers of Knowledge," and six research report sessions each year, which were open to the college's faculty and students.[89] Thus, according to the academic measures that were legible within the postwar research university, Wayne State University College of Nursing had successfully established itself within the research enterprise.

The deans and faculty at several other nursing schools across the country—many supported by Division of Nursing funding—reported similar conflict and some success as they worked to establish their nursing schools within the research economy.[90] As a result, by the 1970s, an increasing number of nurses were engaged in externally funded research, much of it focused on problems in clinical nursing.[91] And as the previous chapter notes, by the end of the 1970s, the growth of nursing research had led to an expanding number of journals dedicated to publishing peer-reviewed nursing research.[92] At the same time, the Division of Nursing's Nurse Scientist Graduate Training Program (NSGTP) was producing a growing corps of PhD-prepared nurses educated in the biomedical, behavioral, and social sciences.

The Division of Nursing established the NSGTP in 1962, providing institutional training grants to universities, which in turn awarded stipends to nurses pursuing PhD degrees in the university's biomedical, behavioral, and social science departments.[93] Between 1962 and 1974, ten universities in the U.S. established nurse scientist PhD programs with support from the NSGTP.[94] The first NSGTP was established in 1962 at Boston University, with PhD preparation supported in anthropology, biology, psychology, and sociology. That same year, the University of California, San Francisco (UCSF) established an NSGTP with the sociology department on the University of California, Berkeley campus. The following year, in 1963, the University of California, Los Angeles (UCLA), the University of Washington, and the Frances Payne Bolton School of Nursing at Case Western Reserve University (then known as Western Reserve University) established NSGTPs. At UCLA, nurses could pursue a PhD in psychology, while at the University of Washington, nurses could pursue PhDs in anthropology, microbiology, physiology, and sociology. At Case Western Reserve University, the NSGTP supported nurses pursuing PhDs in anthropology, biology, psychology, physiology, and sociology.[95] For Schlotfeldt, who was dean of Case Western's Frances Payne Bolton School of Nursing, nurses with PhDs "in the basic disciplines" were needed so that nursing could "begin to inquire systematically and with proper rigor into the questions that are nursing questions."[96]

The timing of the NSGTP was critical, Wayne State University's Virginia Cleland noted, because it provided "heavy subsidization of the teaching program in the related discipline," which "was necessary at that time because of the prejudicial treatment of women, including nurses in those disciplines."[97] As Katherine Hoffman, who was professor and assistant dean at the University of Washington's School of Nursing in the late 1960s, explained, while the faculty and administrators of departments in the biomedical, social, and behavioral sciences were supportive of nursing's needs, "when faculty time and physical facilities are limited and a choice must be made between a candidate [to the PhD program] who plans to remain in the field after graduation and a second candidate who plans to return to nursing, the choice" of those departments was "to use the limited faculty and facilities for the student whose primary goal [was] to remain in that discipline as their career." The NSGTP included a provision, however, that enabled the departments in which nurse scientists were pursuing a PhD to hire an additional full-time faculty member to teach and conduct research in that department and serve as the liaison to the nurse scientists pursuing their PhD in that discipline. The faculty hired as part of the NSGTP would be granted a joint appointment in the nursing school, but the expectation was that they would be "citizens first in their own fields and ambassadors to nursing secondly."[98] In essence, the NSGT programs "were a means of 'buying a way in' to the basic science programs that previously had been closed to nurses."[99]

The interdisciplinary potential of the NSGTP was perhaps best typified at UCSF. In 1960 (two years before receiving an NSGTP), the dean of nursing, Helen Nahm, had already begun recruiting sociologists to teach research methodology to students in the master's program, as well as courses in the sociology of health and illness. Among the first sociologists she recruited was Anselm Strauss, who subsequently developed, with fellow sociologist Barney Glaser, a new qualitative research method: grounded theory. Strauss would also go on to become a leading figure in medical sociology. With additional support from the NSGTP, the role of sociologists within the nursing school increased, and in 1972 the School of Nursing established the Department of Social and Behavioral Sciences with Strauss as the founding chairperson.[100]

The nurses who earned their doctorates in the biomedical, behavioral, and social sciences, however, experienced several challenges that extended beyond the typical demands of graduate education. As nurses and women in male-dominated sciences, they challenged gendered assumptions both about women's intellectual worth and nurses as mere handmaidens to medicine, and proved to the faculty and their student peers that they were intellectually capable of doctoral-level work.[101] But in doing so, these nurses also experienced "an 'identity' problem when they ['left'] the field of nursing and [took] on another."[102] "In moving into related science fields," Helen Grace (associate dean at the University of Illinois Chicago) explained, "nurses have had to, in a sense, 'put aside nursing' while pursuing other academic lines of study. The pressures to become 'real scientists' have often necessitated a type of disjunctive learning experience within their doctoral programs." In their push to become physiologists, anatomists, psychologists, or sociologists, for example, and "gain recognition as a 'scholar,'" these nurses found it "difficult, if not impossible" to link "their nursing identities to these scientific disciplines." Grace wrote, "Most nurses, in this process, become intent on being as good a scientist, whatever the discipline, as their classmates, and rightfully so but within the particular culture of these scientific fields have had to mask their nursing identity to achieve scholarly recognition."[103] Marian E. Olson, for example, who completed a PhD in social psychology at UCLA in 1966 explained that "in order to 'make' the social psychology program, I had to *be* a social psychologist for a while."[104]

For those nurses who "re-entered academic nursing" after completing their doctoral degrees, the process was then reversed; they had to "become 'nurses' once again, and in many instances they . . . [were] held suspect by their peers as being no longer really a nurse."[105] These suspicions came not only from the fact that nurse scientists had been out of nursing for several years, but also because "they . . . [had] perhaps changed their views to looking at more basic highly circumscribed problems rather than looking at a whole individual or a whole family."[106] For many, the transition from conducting laboratory research during their doctoral degrees, where they had "become totally socialized" to the notion that "'good' research is that which can be rigidly controlled under experimental conditions," to conducting clinical research in the hospital or community setting, proved difficult. For these nurse scientists, "doing clinical research becomes difficult to achieve without feeling that you have compromised the scientific rigor of your work."[107] Reflected in these comments are two fundamental issues: 1) the assumptions held by non-nurse scientists that nursing practice was not a legitimate site of knowledge production, and 2) broadly held assumptions about the inherent value of clinical research in which laboratory-based, controlled experimental research is regarded as more reliable and objective than clinical observations. As discussed in chapter 2, it was this latter assumption that led academic physicians to develop the new science of clinical epidemiology, which applied the "scientific method"—typified by the well-controlled experiment—within the clinical setting.[108]

The Division of Nursing began phasing out the NSGTP in the early 1970s and terminated the final NSGTP grant in 1976 amid federal research budget cuts. During the 1970s, federal support of academic research and research training fell across all fields of science and engineering. Fellowship support, for example, which supported graduate education, dropped from a peak of $447 million in 1967 to $185 million ten years later.[109] In general, the health sciences were less severely impacted than the physical sciences and engineering. Between 1971 and 1981, as Hugh Davis Graham and Nancy Diamond note, "annual NIH obligations for academic research grew from $603 million to $2 billion, an increase in constant dollars of 55 percent," while "R&D support from all other federal agencies grew by only 12 percent" during the same period.[110] Despite ongoing support for the health sciences, nursing was hard hit by the federal budget cuts. As historian Joan Lynaugh has documented, under the leadership of Secretary Caspar Weinberger, the Department of Health, Education, and Welfare, which oversaw the Public Health Service's budget, "turned openly hostile toward nursing" and worked to severely limit Nurse Training Act funding.[111] By 1982, when for the eighth year in a row continuing federal support for nursing research was being debated in Congress, at stake was $5 million in nursing research grants and $1 million in research fellowships; these amounts were considerably less than the level of research funding available to other biomedical scientists.[112] The following year, for example, the NIH spent $32 million alone on predoctoral fellowships awarded to dual-degree MD/PhD students, and $2.8 billion on research grants.[113]

The Division of Nursing's decision to end the NSGTP was also shaped by a growing realization among nurse leaders that the program had served its purpose. By 1969, 109 nurses had completed doctoral degrees through the NSGTP.[114] The expectation, as Hildegard Peplau explained, was that the "nurse scientists who have earned PhDs can bring their knowledge back to nursing and use it to chisel out a PhD in nursing."[115] As the previous chapter detailed, by the 1970s, nurse theorists and researchers had made progress in defining "nursing science" as a distinct body of knowledge. And, as noted above, a growing number of nursing schools were establishing themselves within the postwar research economy. Thus, in the late 1960s, several nursing schools launched plans to establish nursing PhD programs. For nursing leaders, this was the next step to securing the equal standing of nursing schools within the postwar research university. After all, in the postwar research university, doctoral education was an integral component of the academic research enterprise.[116]

Establishing the PhD in Nursing

Although most nursing leaders viewed the research-based doctorate, the PhD, as the ultimate degree necessary to secure nursing's academic rank, several nursing leaders advocated the establishment of the clinical or professional doctorate, the doctor of nursing science (DNS/DNSc). In name, the DNS and nursing PhD were intended as different types of degree programs, with different objectives and end products. The primary emphasis of the PhD was research and scholarship, while the emphasis of the DNS was the preparation of "expert practitioner-scholars"[117] who would pursue "advanced clinical practice with the integration of research to improve nursing care."[118] In this rendering, DNS-prepared nurses would be well-positioned to serve as nursing's clinical researchers and (in today's parlance) translational scientists. Throughout these decades, nurse leaders debated the merits and drawbacks of each type of doctoral degree, asking what doctorate would better prepare would-be researchers for their future roles, what degree would secure nurses greater academic legitimacy and, ultimately, what type of degree program was feasible within their particular institutional context. As they did so, they looked to the other academizing practice professions—particularly engineering and clinical psychology—for guidance.[119]

As historians of engineering have documented, the American engineering profession had been engaged in a process of academization since the 1920s, which intensified in the postwar years as engineering science became the dominant emphasis in postwar engineering education.[120] Although the PhD became the preferred academic credential in engineering, initially some engineering schools had offered "professional" doctorates in engineering. These included the doctor of engineering, which reportedly stressed the practical or technical aspects of engineering, as well as the doctor of science in engineering, which was intended to integrate both practical aspects and theoretical and research aspects of engineering.[121] Given their experiences with the different types of doctoral programs, nursing faculty in this period often sought the advice of their engineering colleagues on how best to proceed in nursing. For example, as the nursing faculty at Case Western Reserve University began planning a doctoral program in the late 1960s, they met with Case Western Reserve University's dean of engineering. In addition to explaining the rationale that had led the engineering school to establish a PhD in engineering rather than one of the professional doctorates, the engineering dean also described the "relative proportion" of the PhD program "devoted to basic science courses such as physics and mathematics and that devoted to the practice of engineering and its attendant concepts."[122]

The postwar decades were also a critical period in the academic development of clinical psychology.[123] During the 1950s and 1960s, clinical psychology PhD students were educated in a "scientist-practitioner" model in which they received training both in clinical practice as well as "academic research design, methodology, and analysis."[124] By the mid-1960s, however, as increasing numbers of clinical psychologists entered private practice, the rationale for the integrated "scientist-practitioner" model was declining. In its place, clinical psychologists called for the establishment of a separate doctoral program that emphasized advanced clinical training, the professional doctorate, the PsyD.[125] The first PsyD program was established at the University of Illinois in 1968, and by the mid-1970s, the PsyD had emerged as a legitimate graduate program for training practitioners of clinical psychology.[126] By beginning with a PhD and transitioning to the professional doctorate, clinical psychology thus offered nursing a different model of doctoral education than engineering. As participants at a 1976 Midwest Invitational Conference on Doctoral Education noted, "We are at the same point that clinical psychology was a number of years ago with some of the same concerns. Now they are expanding all over."[127] For Luther Christman, dean of Rush University College of Nursing, the recent history of clinical psychology provided important lessons for nursing: "It was not so long ago that the clinical psychologist and all of psychology for that matter, admitted that they had most of their numbers prepared at the master's level, and that this was insufficient. They just pushed ahead and declared the doctorate as the professional degree." Although "there was some turmoil among the people holding master's degrees in psychology at that time and warnings that this was too much pressure on the profession—that they were going to price themselves out of the market," Christman continued, saying that clinical psychology "became a very productive enterprise, because graduates went out and did all the kinds of productive things."[128]

Through the early 1980s, nursing's leaders ostensibly advocated a pluralist approach to doctoral education, supporting the development of both PhD and DNS programs, yet they did so for strategic rather than intellectual reasons. Indeed, although intended as different types of degree programs, in practice, the distinction between the PhD and the DNS was "blurry," with a lot of curricular overlap between the two types of programs.[129] The University of Pittsburgh, for example, established a PhD in nursing program in 1954. Yet, the program's emphasis was that of a clinical doctorate: the program was premised on the belief that the nursing care of patients was "the origin and destination" of nursing research; students enrolled in the program spent "extensive periods of time in the clinical area of maternal or pediatric nursing," and their research focused "upon specialized problems in these clinical areas."[130] In this way, the "clinical component [was] the central programmatic focus; research emerge[d] from immersion in this clinical field." In contrast, the DNS programs at Boston University (established in 1963), UCSF (established in 1964), and Catholic University (established in 1968) all emphasized research, with the clinical component less clearly delineated.[131]

The blurred distinction between nursing PhD and DNS programs was typical of doctoral education more broadly. Writing about the differences between the EdD (doctor of education) and the PhD in education, a professor of education noted that while EdD programs were "ostensibly for those seeking a professional career, and the PhD for those seeking a research career in education," educators had, since the inception of the dual-track system, "engaged in endless rhetorical debates to justify the existence of the two degree programs. Their arduous efforts, it would appear, have been futile; for the passage of time has done little to resolve the issue of distinction between the two degrees."[132] Moreover, the president of the Council of Graduate Schools explained that while doctorates other than the PhD—for example, the doctor of music, the doctor of architecture, or the doctor of engineering—were "considered to be education and training for the 'practitioner,'" the "distinction becomes somewhat obscure in terms of the accepted comprehensiveness of the PhD." To his mind, there was "no reason" the PhD couldn't be offered as a "program suitable for turning out research workers, teachers, and professionals."[133]

Within nursing, however, the blurred distinction between PhD and DNS programs was due to the fact that nursing schools decided whether to establish a nursing PhD or a DNS program based primarily on institutional factors rather than on intellectual preferences or priorities. For example, for several years, the faculty at Wayne State University College of Nursing debated the merits of establishing a DNS program or a PhD program. As Virginia Cleland, who chaired the doctoral program committee, explained to Dean Margretta Styles in November 1973, while the "PhD has the advantage of being publicly recognized as a research degree," there were some potential benefits to moving forward with the professional doctorate. In particular, as a DNS program would be controlled by the College of Nursing, the faculty could make it "whatever we want it to be." A PhD, in contrast, would have to confirm to the standards and expectations of the graduate school. "I keep vacillating in my own thinking," Cleland observed, but in the end "would really prefer to see us go the route of the PhD." Cleland, however, was concerned that Wayne State University's Provost, Hank Bohm, would block this effort. Cleland wondered whether the provost's "desire of not wanting us to be outdone by University of Michigan and Michigan State University" would "make him more amenable to the idea of a PhD in Nursing."[134]

Some nursing schools, such as those at Boston University, UCSF, and the University of Pennsylvania, established DNS programs after university administrators opposed their plans for establishing nursing PhD programs.[135] At the University of Pennsylvania, nursing faculty viewed the DNS program as a stepping-stone to a nursing PhD program. The faculty hoped that after demonstrating the viability and research productivity of the DNS program, university administrators would look more favorably upon establishing a nursing PhD program.[136] The PhD degree was generally controlled by the graduate school and as such had to be "designed within the framework" and meet the standards "governing PhD study in other academic disciplines."[137] Because the DNS was described as a professional doctorate, clinically oriented as opposed to research-oriented, it did not fall under the purview of graduate schools. Instead, authority to confer the degree remained either solely within schools of nursing or jointly between the graduate school and nursing school. As a professional degree, the DNS could be "tailored to a particular professional rather than toward the more generally applicable format for the research doctorate."[138] As such, proposals to establish DNS programs faced significantly fewer obstacles than did proposals to establish nursing PhD programs.[139]

Even nursing schools that successfully established PhD programs faced significant institutional barriers because of gendered assumptions about nursing. At the University of Pittsburg, for example, the School of Nursing was academically located under the university's Council of Higher Education, while fiscally located under the Office of the Vice Chancellor for Health Professionals. To get approval for a PhD program, the nursing school needed to secure the approval of both entities. But as Florence Erickson, director of the University of Pittsburgh's NSGTP, explained, "I have no difficulty with my colleagues in other disciplines, but medicine does not see why nurses need PhDs."[140] In other schools, nursing faculty often had to overcome skepticism among their colleagues in the basic sciences who questioned whether clinical or applied courses were even the appropriate purview of doctoral programs.[141] At the University of Minnesota, for example, the nursing faculty faced opposition from their colleagues on the Health Sciences Policy and Review Council (which evaluated proposals for new PhD programs in the health sciences), who repeatedly questioned whether a body of nursing knowledge existed and whether nursing was an appropriate area of research. As a nursing faculty member recalled, the program didn't face much opposition from the schools of medicine, dentistry, or public health, but "from the basic sciences, because of their strong emphasis on research and how advanced they were. I think that they found it very difficult to find . . . an emerging profession and the need for a doctorate."[142] The committee was divided on the question of whether "nursing as defined in this proposal [is] a scholarly discipline which has evolved to the point where the offering of a PhD program is academically justified." For the committee, nursing was a "major health care profession which is presently dependent for a significant part of its instruction, practice, and research studies on the physical, behavioral, and social sciences."[143] Given this type of skepticism, Helen Grace, associate dean at the University of Illinois Chicago, explained, "Doctoral programs in nursing have had to provide proof that the focus is upon research, rather than upon professional practice to such an extreme that in most instances little or no attention has been devoted to delineating nursing content in doctoral programs."[144]

The efforts of nursing leaders to establish PhD programs were also undermined by the changing financial fortunes of research universities in the early 1970s. As described earlier, federal research support had begun to level off in the late 1960s. This, together with declining enrollments, led to substantial decreases in graduate student support during the 1970s. For example, in 1967, fellowship support had reached a high of $447 million, but by 1977 that figure had dropped to $185 million. At the same time, there was growing recognition among educators and policymakers that there were far more students earning PhDs than were needed to fill the available jobs. As a result, many universities began cutting back on graduate programs, which in turn led to a decline in the number of PhD degrees being awarded.[145] As a nursing educator noted in 1974, this "'no growth' or 'steady state period' of the past 5 years" made it "extremely difficult for academic administrators to maintain or reinforce their present educational commitments, much less initiate new programs."[146] At the University of Washington School of Nursing, for example, the faculty's efforts to establish a PhD program in nursing were delayed, in part by the university's moratorium on new doctoral programs and the limited availability of state funds.[147]

Given these institutional politics, as Madeleine Leininger urged, it was important for nursing leaders "to look carefully for university settings where there is encouragement and support and capitalize on them by helping them develop their resources."[148] Nursing schools' relationships with faculty in the already-established academic disciplines proved critical. Several of the nursing schools that successfully established PhD programs during the 1970s did so at least in part because they were able to build upon the collaborative and supportive relationships they had established with faculty in the biological, behavioral, and social science departments either through the NSGTP or through the FRDG. Faculty in these disciplines who had worked closely with nursing faculty (and students) testified to the research capabilities of nursing faculty and students and supported their academic arguments for the PhD.[149]

The establishment of the nursing PhD program at the University of Illinois Chicago in 1975, for example, built on the success of its earlier NSGTP and the connections the College of Nursing had forged with the departments of physiology, anatomy, and microbiology.[150] The College of Nursing's relationship with the Department of Physiology was especially strong. Several nurses had completed PhDs in physiology, working in particular with the stress physiologist, Sabath Marotta.[151] When the College established its PhD program, it demarcated research in stress physiology as a particular area of focus.[152] Among the faculty teaching in the PhD program were several faculty with doctorates and departmental appointments in the biomedical, social, or behavioral sciences.[153] While the PhD program at University of Illinois Chicago required students to take core courses in nursing theory, research design, research methods, and statistics, along with advanced nursing seminars in their designated clinical specialty, students were also required to take a significant portion of their coursework in the cognate disciplines. For example, a doctoral student with an MS in medical-surgical nursing and interested in researching the sleep patterns of patients who had suffered a myocardial infarction would take core graduate seminars in the cognate subjects of physiology of the heart, physiological psychology, behavioral pharmacology, and the physiological bases of emotion. In contrast, a doctoral student with an MS in psychiatric-mental health nursing and interested in researching problems related to drug use in adolescence would take graduate seminars in the cognate fields of criminal justice, psychology, and behavioral pharmacology. A doctoral student with an MS in maternal-child health nursing and interested in the genetic defects of children would take graduate seminars in genetics and population biology.[154] This approach of combining coursework in nursing theory and research with coursework in the relevant biomedical, behavioral, or social sciences was common among doctoral nursing programs in the 1970s.[155] However, as the previous chapter noted, the majority of nursing doctoral dissertations failed to include theory in general, and nursing theory in particular.[156] So too, as Helen Grace warned, "the richness of [the] interdisciplinary mix" within nursing doctoral programs, which sought to bridge a wide range of biological, behavioral, and social sciences, left most programs "struggling with problems of providing breadth and depth within one program format."[157]

By 1976, thirteen U.S. nursing schools had established doctoral programs in nursing; nine were PhD programs,[158] four were DNS programs,[159] and two were EdD programs.[160] Despite these early successes, as Rozella Schlotfeldt lamented, there was abundant evidence that doctorally prepared nursing faculty were still not "generally viewed by other members of the university community, by some health practitioner colleagues, and by many nurses with whom they work as [scientists]."[161] Indeed, nursing schools continued to struggle to justify the need for a PhD in nursing program. When the University of Florida College of Nursing set about establishing a PhD program in the early 1980s, the dean, Lois Malasanos, recalled, "What I heard here was, 'Why can you not do it in physiology?' for instance. It was wonderful because I was a physiologist and could speak immediately, saying, 'If I were a physiologist, these are the methods I would have to investigate this problem.' They cannot provide the answers. Really, the problems that nurses face are served by a variety of methods . . . We find out what a student's research is, and then the minor is to teach some new methods that will help to look at that problem."[162]

Meanwhile, nurses in practice remained unconvinced about the utility of doctoral education. For many nurses, nursing faculty were too "far removed from real life practice and problems" to provide adequate clinical education to students or improve patient care. Yet, as one nurse warned, "Although nurse educators function in a different sphere from practitioners, by their policies, they are affecting bedside care as surely as if they were there in person."[163] The frustration of another nurse was clear when she wrote to the *American Journal of Nursing*, "We in nursing should get up from our knees and stop worshipping science. The treatment for patellar bed sores" was not to be found in nursing science, but rather from "a double dose of renewed faith in ourselves."[164] Nurses in practice charged faculty with not preparing students for the realities of clinical practice but instead for idealized hypothetical situations. This of course resonates with the observations of the sociologist Andrew Abbott who, as chapter 2 notes, explains that the "perfected abstract knowledge system" of a profession, as developed by academics, "only exists in the world of professional textbooks," and is rarely applicable to working professionals.[165] As one nurse lamented, "It appears from a perusal of nursing curriculum that the faculty and students are getting father away from the patients."[166] Whether or not the faculty were doctorally prepared was not going to address what these nurses saw as a major problem facing nursing: the disconnect between education and nursing service. Rather, a potential solution was to have nursing faculty actually engage in clinical practice to ensure that the content of baccalaureate and graduate curricula reflected the realities and needs of clinical practice and provided students with adequate clinical education (discussed in detail in chapter 5).

The criticisms that nurses waged against educators was not a phenomenon unique to nursing but rather one experienced by other academizing practice disciplines.[167] In engineering, for example, the science-based reforms that engineering educators introduced in the mid-twentieth century led to complaints from engineers in practice about the balance of theory and practice within the new curricula. In the 1960s, "practicing engineers working on real problems were soon complaining about the gulf between their interests and those of the [engineering] faculty." Practicing engineers wrote letters to the editors of engineering journals complaining that their journals "contained little material of practical use," leading some engineers to drop their professional memberships.[168] Indeed, academic and industrial engineers eventually "developed different conceptions of engineering, and almost stopped talking to teach other . . . As a result of changes in research and practice, two subcultures had appeared in engineering."[169] Even some engineering reformers were troubled by the changes. As one such reformer lamented, by the 1970s there was an "overemphasis on science for its own sake" among engineering faculty. "The danger for engineers," he continued, "is that they can become too enamored of research for its own sake. A good engineer . . . must strike a balance between knowing and doing."[170] As engineering historian Bruce Seely, observed in the 1990s, a "now-common indictment of current engineering education voiced by many reformers is the fact that engineering students can leave college without skills essential to their functioning as professional engineers. Usually topping the list of missing capabilities is design, or the ability to solve problems."[171]

In nursing too, educational reformers were, by the late 1970s, raising concerns about some of the consequences of their push for doctoral education. In particular, they questioned nurses' motives for pursuing doctoral education, realizing that for some nurses the decision to get a doctorate was to ensure job security rather than to embark on a career as a nurse scientist. As nursing faculty without doctoral degrees found "their positions in serious jeopardy," Florence Downs warned, they "frequently [came] to view the acquisition of a doctorate as a credential, a kind of union card, that [would] permit them to retain a job." "One hazardous aspect of this situation," Downs continued, is that in "their anger and frustration, they are willing to accept any program that will permit them to enroll, regardless of its relevance to nursing or its quality. Most of these individuals will return to nursing, but the question here is, 'What will they return with that can be expected to exert a positive influence on the course of the profession?' " For Downs, it was imperative that nursing faculty "understand that the doctorate is preparation for scholarship but its demonstration is accomplished through continuous contributions to the state of the art. This is particularly true of faculty whose primary responsibility is at the graduate level and the sine qua non for those who work with doctoral students." [172] But as a survey of almost two thousand doctorally prepared nurses conducted by a team of nurse researchers at the end of the 1970s revealed, "Only 6% to 8% of doctorally prepared nurses were hired primarily for the conduct of research in either [their] first or current position."[173] This reflected the fact that, except for nursing schools that were part of research-intensive universities, particularly those within AHCs, most nursing schools at this time were not research-intensive and thus had little interest in or capacity to support faculty research.

Even as reformers like Downs questioned the motives of individual nurses who opted to pursue doctoral education, the same question could be asked of educational reformers' collective push for establishing nursing doctoral programs. What purpose were nursing PhD programs meant to serve? Were they a means of preparing new generations of nurse scientists who would conduct clinical nursing research that would ultimately improve patient care? Or were they merely an end for establishing the academic standing of the nursing profession?[174] Invariably, PhD programs were both things, even if the priority accorded to one over the other shifted over time and place. This reflected the persistent tension within nursing's academic project, that it was both an empirical project centered on producing knowledge to improve patient care *and* a political project to justify nursing's positioning within universities and academic health centers.

Conclusion

Nursing's academization efforts and the criticisms they provoked among nurses in practice and the older generation of nursing faculty must be understood within the context of the postwar research university. As historian of the postwar university Rebecca Lowen, has argued, "With salaries and even positions within the university dependent upon outside support, with promotion dependent on research, which required external support, with no institutional rewards for energies devoted to undergraduate instruction, academic scientists and scholars not surprisingly became avid seekers of grants and contracts." In doing so, Lowen continued, they "simply responded rationally to the university's system of rewards and penalties."[175] The situation was no different for the academic nurses who sought to make their way and secure the academic status of their discipline—nursing science—within the postwar research university. Nursing faculty sought to adapt to the postwar research economy by shifting their focus to securing external funding, engaging in research, and establishing themselves as the producers and disseminators of expert knowledge. Thus, just as in engineering and the physical, biological, and social sciences, nursing was transformed by the institutional context and patronage relationships of the postwar political economy.

But at what cost? For many nurses, the preoccupation of nursing leaders with the pursuit of credentials in the name of securing greater professional autonomy, recognition, and status for the nurse, had led nursing educators to lose sight of what mattered most—the patient. That sentiment was clearly expressed by Jessie May Scott, one of the most important nurse leaders of the second half of the twentieth century. Scott served as director of the U.S. Public Health Service Division of Nursing from 1963 through 1979, where she oversaw the implementation and operation of all federal nursing programs, including the FRDG and NSGT programs that proved critical to nursing's academic project. Scott was an advocate of nursing research and of improving the quality of nursing education and practice. But at a speech she gave in 1979, Scott voiced concerns about the current direction of nursing education:

The other day, I read some statements describing the characteristics of various types of nursing education programs. It was distressing to observe that scarcely any of the characteristics listed addressed the care of the patient or the "laying on of hands." The statements were global, rather than specific, and to the non-nurse reader, would have led to the conclusion that synthesizing, evaluating, and utilizing theory were what nursing is all about. I bring this to your attention because the people who read these articles/columns are the people who also support you in your institutions, in your State, and in your Federal government. I believe that we ought to have other ways in which to present ourselves and to describe ourselves to the public at large. The particular statements I read do not tell what nurses do in caring for people.[176]

Scott was not alone in sounding the alarm. In the 1940s and 1950s, Virginia Henderson had been something of a lone voice calling for nurses to engage in *clinical* nursing research rather than continue their almost exclusive focus on studies of nurses and nursing roles.[177] By the late 1970s, Henderson could acknowledge that the "emphasis *is* changing" as more nurses undertook clinical research. However, in her judgment, "nurses have scarcely begun to appreciate what Annie W. Goodrich [the founding dean of Yale School of Nursing] called the 'Social and Ethical Significance of Nursing'—the extent to which they might better the lot of mankind; the extent to which they might change health care in this, or any other, country." While Henderson could "rejoice and applaud" nursing's progress, particularly with its "present emphasis on 'sound research,'" and the fact that nurses were now able to compete for a part of the Department of Health, Education, and Welfare's $3 billion research and development budget, she also hoped "that future health-related research has humane goals. I hope that the hypotheses it tests are worth testing, that nurse researchers are more interested in improving practice than in academic respectability."[178]

Some nurses, particularly activist nurses, expressed concern that by focusing so heavily on nursing's academic project, nursing educators were undermining the nursing profession's potential for advocating radical change in the health care system. As members of the Committee on Nursing in a Society in Crisis wrote in 1972, "It is simply astounding to observe the degree to which so many nurses are preoccupied with questions of professionalism." This preoccupation, they argued, was "inordinately time-consuming and nonproductive." The committee instead called on nurses to reorient their priorities and focus their attention on the "interrelationship of sociopolitical issues and nursing." In particular, they hoped nurses would "provide leadership in the present acknowledged health care crisis" by taking "an active role" in tackling the "social forces" that "play an intricate part in the health of the population."[179] For nurse and civil rights activist Jane Kennedy, it was time for nursing faculty "to stop playing the academic game and to begin to transfuse urgency and relevance, whose pinnacle is service to the needs of the poor, into nursing education." For Kennedy, that meant getting faculty and students out of the university and its teaching hospitals and into community health centers where they could see firsthand the impact of social, economic, and environmental factors on health and work and intervene in them, whether by "lobbying with the poor at the state legislature for adequate food, clothing, and rent allotments" or working collectively "to eradicate the causes of poverty."[180]

Other nurses charged that nursing's "emphasis on 'credentialism'" was also undermining the nursing workforce by denigrating nurses who had been trained in hospital-based diploma programs and creating obstacles to educational and social mobility for the scores of nurses (including the majority of nurses of color) educated in diploma and associate degree programs.[181] By the 1970s, registered nurses throughout the country were pressuring their state legislators to facilitate career mobility for graduates of diploma and associate degree programs.[182] These legislators, in turn, put pressure on the state-funded nursing schools to resolve the problems of career mobility. They did so in the midst of state and regional concerns among health care leaders and policymakers about impending shortages of health care workers, including nurses. In response, as the next chapter shows, nursing leaders worked to balance nursing's academic imperatives against workforce needs, placing nursing's academic project and the politics of nursing education more broadly within the context of state health policymaking.

"Nursepower":
States and the Politics of Nursing
and Health Care in the 1970s

For state-funded nursing schools looking to establish doctoral programs in the 1970s, the state context mattered a great deal. As a nurse educator from the University of Arizona noted in 1974, "we have to realistically appraise which States would encourage the development of doctoral programs in nursing and proceed from there."[1] As chapter 1 details, the emergence of nursing's academic project occurred alongside growing state, regional, and national concerns among health care leaders and policymakers about shortages of health professionals, including nurses. Beginning in the 1960s, health care leaders and policymakers worked to increase both the quantity and the quality of the nursing workforce.[2] The demographic impacts of the baby boom generation, the health care needs of the aging population, the growth of employment-based health insurance, and the implementation of Medicare and Medicaid in 1966, all contributed to the expanding demand for health care services—and, thus, nurses—in the late 1960s and 1970s.[3]

The increasing complexity of patient care also created the need for better educated professional nurses (see chapter 1). By the mid-1960s, hospitals were increasingly organized into specialty units that grouped patients according to their critical care needs. These included intensive care units, cardiac care units, premature nurseries, dialysis units, and units dealing with postoperative care after open-heart surgery or neurosurgery.[4] The complex and dynamic needs of the patients in these units created demand for better educated nurses with the knowledge and skills "to make rapid, complex clinical decisions."[5] At the same time, the increasing incidence of chronic illnesses, which high-technology, hospital-based medicine was ill-equipped to cure, also contributed to greater demand for better educated nurses. For patients struggling with chronic diseases like heart disease, diabetes, and cancer, treatment often depended on the adoption of lifestyle changes. But not all patients were willing or able to make those changes. Nurses who were able to understand how and why patients made their health care decisions and were skilled in more effectively communicating with patients could facilitate the treatment of acute episodes of patients' illness and help patients more effectively manage their chronic illnesses.[6]

In this context, nursing leaders argued that BSN-prepared nurses were best equipped to care for and manage the increasingly complex needs of both hospitalized and ambulatory patients. In addition to being schooled in the biomedical sciences, BSN-educated nurses were educated in the behavioral and social sciences and newly developed nursing theories. This interdisciplinary education, as chapters 1 and 2 detail, equipped BSN-educated nurses with the knowledge, interpersonal, and analytical skills needed to understand and more effectively respond to patients' clinical and emotional needs. In addition, more and more complex patient care took place outside of the hospital, in outpatient specialty and primary care clinics, which, together with shortages of primary care physicians, especially in rural and underserved urban communities, created opportunities for nurses with advanced clinical education at the master's level to assume new expert clinical roles. Clinical nurse specialists were tasked with helping to manage increasingly complex patient care in hospital and outpatient settings, while nurse practitioners helped fill gaps in shortages of primary care physicians.[7]

The emergence of the quality assessment movement in health care was another factor contributing to the push for more highly educated nurses. In the 1960s and 1970s, as discussed in chapter 2, a series of studies by health services researchers documented troubling variations in the types and quality of care patients received across geographic regions, hospitals, and physician practices.[8] The result was the emergence of outcomes research, which "promised a more scientific approach to evaluating procedure-based treatments than currently existed."[9] Academic physicians joined health services researchers in calling for the collection and statistical analysis of data on physician practices, health services, and patient outcomes. Within BSN programs, nursing students were taught how to use quantitative and qualitative research methods and to analyze and interpret the results of that research. As such, BSN-prepared nurses were both well-placed by their proximity to patients and well-equipped to assist in the collection and analysis of data regarding the quality and effectiveness of clinical interventions. Moreover, nurses were themselves critical actors in the push to improve the quality of health care. As Jerome Lysaught, chair of the National Commission for the Study of Nursing and Nursing Education, asserted in 1970, "it is essential for the future of health care in this country to begin a systematic evaluation of the impact of nursing care in terms of objective criteria such as measurable improvement in patient condition, evidence of early discharge or return to employment, reduced incidence of readmission to care facilities, and lowered rates of communicable disease." Although it acknowledged that nursing was not "wholly responsible for these or any other factors in the qualitative measurement of health care," the Lysaught Commission believed "that nursing represents an important independent variable in our total health system."[10] And as chapter 2 documents, during these decades, PhD-educated nurse scientists were engaged in their own research efforts to evaluate the effectiveness of nursing interventions, improve the quality of nursing care, and improve patient outcomes.

During the 1960s and 1970s, health policymakers realized that the efforts by nurse educators to increase both the quantity and quality of nursing education were integral to the expansion of health care services and the quality improvement movement in health care. During these decades, in states throughout the country, health planners and legislators worried that the shortage of BSN, master's, and doctorally prepared nurses was undermining their state's health workforce and health care needs and looked for ways to support the expansion of nursing education. Shortages of qualified nurse faculty in particular were undermining their efforts to establish new, and expand existing, undergraduate and graduate nursing programs. In 1963, for example, when the Surgeon General's Consultant Group on Nursing warned that nursing schools needed to graduate 53,000 new nurses each year in order to meet the country's need for 850,000 professional nurses by 1970, the shortage of appropriately qualified nursing faculty was seen as a critical factor in the nursing shortage. As the Consultant Group on Nursing asserted, "More and Better-Prepared Faculty" were needed in order to meet future nursing needs.[11] The minimum educational requirement was the master's degree, but, as chapter 3 explains, by the late 1960s, nursing leaders were increasingly calling on nurse faculty to be doctorally prepared. In this context, nurse educators framed their arguments for the nursing PhD not only in terms of a new type of disciplinary knowledge (chapter 3) but also in the context of urgent nursing workforce concerns. By producing more doctorally prepared nurses, nursing educators argued, nursing schools could improve the quality of and expand the scale of master's, baccalaureate, and associate degree–level education. These more highly educated nurses, in turn, would play a vital role in the movement to improve the quality of health care. The mobilization of state health workforce arguments by nursing schools looking to establish PhD programs was critical as university administrators continued to question the value, legitimacy, and academic rigor of nursing PhD programs.

But even as nursing's academic project was imbricated within state health policymaking and the quality improvement movement, it was soon clear to nurses, educators, and policymakers that the academic project was itself undermining the nursing workforce in important ways. As nursing leaders sought to raise the educational preparation of nurses to the baccalaureate and graduate level, the graduates of diploma and associate degree programs were under pressure to upgrade their educational credentials. These nurses, however, frequently confronted significant financial, institutional, and social barriers to achieving so-called educational mobility. During the 1970s, graduates of diploma and AD programs, along with representatives from state nursing organizations, pressured state legislators to push state-funded nursing schools to establish programs (such as accelerated RN-to-BSN programs) that would facilitate nurses' movement from the lower levels of the educational hierarchy through the higher levels. They did so as policymakers at both the federal and state level instituted policies aimed at expanding access to higher education, particularly for women and minorities. As a result, state legislatures expected state-supported nursing schools to resolve the issues of educational mobility. In so doing, they shored up nursing's educational system as one characterized by differential pathways into nursing.

This chapter recasts debates that took place within nursing over entry into practice, educational mobility, and doctoral education as part of a series of much broader conversations taking place within higher education and health care in the 1960s and 1970s, particularly regarding the shifting terrain of higher education and student access and the politics of health care. In doing so, it highlights the ways in which these conflicts—and the broader state health and higher education politics they were situated in—shaped nursing's academic project.

The Policies and Politics of Higher Education in the 1960s and 1970s

In the 1970s, higher education policy was characterized by a new emphasis on "student access and egalitarianism."[12] Policymakers supported expanding access to higher education particularly for women and racial and ethnic minorities.[13] To be sure, policymakers had been committed to widening educational access since World War II (see chapter 1). At the federal level, the 1944 G.I. Bill provided educational opportunities to veterans and their family members, and the 1958 National Defense Education Act promoted educational opportunities in disciplines (particularly in science and engineering) that bore directly on national defense. The 1965 Higher Education Act, which was part of the Johnson administration's Great Society legislative agenda, authorized a program of federal scholarships to undergraduate students of "exceptional financial need" and provided federal grants to "developing institutions."[14]

Among state policymakers, educational access was also a priority during these decades. Throughout the 1960s, state higher education planners focused on expanding high school graduates' access to institutions of higher education. They did so by reducing geographic barriers to higher education by ensuring that community colleges and other two-year institutions were located "within commuting distance of most of the population of a state," while state universities were located in the major urban areas of a state. They also sought to remove academic barriers to access by offering "open admission" to states' publicly funded institutions of higher education. Finally, state planners also worked to "eliminate the economic barriers to a higher education" by providing part-time employment to students as a form of financial assistance, and by establishing state programs of student financial assistance that reinforced the student financial support provided through federal legislation.[15]

In the 1960s, the civil rights and women's liberation movements, together with campus protests for free speech and against the Vietnam War, had a transformative effect on higher education. Black and feminist student activists not only reinforced the importance of expanding educational access to an increasingly diverse student body, but they also helped create "a new understanding of higher education."[16] As historian Christopher Loss argues, this new understanding "prized the rights-bearing educated citizen" and recognized the importance of institutionalizing diversity within the curriculum.[17] The new understanding of higher education was also the result of changes in the legal and political status of students. For example, a series of legal decisions in the 1960s had overturned the long-standing definition of higher education as a privilege rather than a right. This legal change was due in part, Loss explains, to the widespread acceptance that "higher education was of inestimable financial benefit to individuals and society. That each degree earned appreciably increased earnings and occupational status."[18] The rights of students were further reinforced by ratification of the Twenty-Sixth Amendment in 1971, which lowered the voting age from 21 to 18, ensuring that almost all college students were eligible to vote.[19]

A series of national reports published in the early 1970s highlighted the continuing problems of lack of diversity and access, in spite of the passage of civil rights legislation and the Higher Education Act of 1965. In 1971, for example, the U.S. Office of Education published its *Report on Higher Education*, which called for more diversity and more opportunity of access, and

encouraged colleges and universities to develop new approaches to support the education of nontraditional students, such as those who were older
than typical college students.[20] Also that year, the Carnegie Commission on
Higher Education's report called on professions to "create alternate routes of
entry other than full-time college attendance, and reduce the number of narrow, one-level professions not affording opportunity for advancement, and
availability of a degree or other form of credit for students every one or two
years of their careers."[21]

With passage of the Education Amendments of 1972, policymakers extended the educational rights of women, students of color, and the poor,
which were initially promised by the Higher Education Act of 1965.[22] Title IX
of the amendments prohibited sex discrimination by any college or university
receiving federal aid. The amendments also prioritized the provision of federal support to students rather than to institutions and led to a major shift in
student aid from the graduate level to the undergraduate level.[23]

For state policymakers in the 1970s, educational access assumed even
greater import than it had in the previous decade. Like their federal counterparts, state policymakers were troubled by the assertions of civil rights and
women's liberation groups that women and people of color were routinely
discriminated against in state institutions of higher education. As John D.
Millett describes, state higher education planners "discovered" that while
"large numbers of black students . . . were enrolled in the open-door public institutions, particularly community colleges," the "state universities that
practiced selective admission" often engaged in racial discrimination. At the
same time, though, state policymakers struggled to reconcile the need to ensure equitable educational access with mounting concerns that states' open
access policies had "lowered the standards of expected student performance."
In addition, policymakers "were suddenly confronted with requests for appropriation support for remedial or development services to students," in the
wake of findings that "high school standards of performance left many students inadequately prepared for higher education." Beginning in the 1970s,
state policymakers looked to state boards of higher education and state-
supported colleges and universities to resolve these problems of educational
access and quality.[24]

Concerns about increasing access to, and reducing racial disparities within,
nursing education arose during these decades. The efforts of nurse educators
to recruit more women (and men) into nursing at both the undergraduate
and graduate level were both helped and hindered by the women's movement
of the 1960s and 1970s. Together with the civil rights movement, the women's
movement helped create new educational and employment opportunities for

women that, by the 1970s, had led to significantly greater numbers of women entering higher education. In theory, this provided nurse educators with an expanded pool of students to recruit from in their efforts to stem the nursing shortage. However, in practice, nursing schools encountered increased competition for students as women looked to pursue degrees in disciplines and training in professions that had previously opposed women's participation.[25] At the same time, many within the women's movement criticized the nursing profession for promulgating negative female stereotypes.[26] As Virginia Cleland reported in 1972, "when attending meetings on women's rights, I have heard nursing used time and time again as *the* illustration of discrimination. The assumption always is that if a nurse is intelligent, educated, and capable she is a nurse instead of physician only because of sex discrimination." As such, Cleland continued, "nursing is going to have an increasingly difficult time trying to recruit intelligent young women."[27] Indeed, nursing's recruitment efforts were explicitly undermined by feminists who called on women to reject careers in nursing in favor of careers in medicine, reflecting what Ellen Baer in 1991 called "the terrible paradox of feminism"[28]—that is, glorifying "women who emulate masculine behavior while virtually ignoring women who choose traditionally female roles and careers."[29]

Nursing schools, many of which had established affirmative action programs by the early 1970s, also struggled to not only recruit but also retain students of color in baccalaureate and graduate degree programs.[30] The majority of nurses of color graduated instead from associate degree programs, reflecting broader trends in higher education in which students of color were overrepresented in community colleges and heavily underrepresented in four-year colleges and universities. In 1972, for example, of the 2,735 African American students who graduated from U.S. nursing schools, 61 percent graduated from AD programs, 21 percent graduated from diploma programs, and only 17 percent graduated from BSN programs. Of the total number of students graduating from BSN programs that year, 5 percent were African American.[31] Of those graduating with master's degrees, 8.4 percent were from underrepresented groups, including 4.9 percent who were African American. At the doctoral level, M. Elizabeth Carnegie reported that of the 402 students enrolled in doctoral programs in nursing, only fourteen were African American, and only fourteen were American Indian or Asian. Of the twenty-seven nurses who received doctorates that year, only two were African Americans (including one man and one woman). That year, "no Spanish-Americans were admitted to, enrolled in, or graduated from doctoral programs."[32] Even as people of color were underrepresented as registered nurses, they were overrepresented in the lowest-rung occupations within nursing and health care, particularly as licensed practical nurses, nursing aides, and orderlies.[33] In 1969, for example, when African Americans constituted 11.4 percent of the U.S. population, only 5 percent of nursing students were African American, while 15 to 20 percent of those training to be practical nurses were African American.[34] As Black nursing leaders at the time—and historians since—have explained, the marginalization of Black nurses and nurses of color was the product not only of overt discrimination and segregation in nursing education prior to the civil rights legislation of the 1960s, but also of the "more subtle and sophisticated forms of institutionalized racism" that persisted thereafter.[35]

That the majority of nurses of color graduated from practical nursing, diploma, and AD programs subsequently limited their opportunities for career advancement, leadership, and faculty positions, all of which required, at minimum, a BSN. As Janice Ruffin (who served on the ANA's task force on affirmative action) noted, "the proportion of Blacks *decreases* sharply as the quantity and quality of education required for role performance *increases.*" Nursing's "emphasis on 'credentialism,'" Ruffin continued, was compounding the effects of institutional racism by "serv[ing] to cloud our view of competent practice in a population of nurses who, for reasons beyond their collective control, have been denied entrance to institutions of higher education." For Ruffin, "the continued channeling of a disproportionate number of Blacks into LPN, AA degree, and diploma programs is destructive to their creative potential. The results are that a disproportionate number of Black nurses are assigned low status in nursing, are rarely adequately assessed for their actual competence as practitioners, are often 'turned off' to pursuing higher education and are not equipped with the conceptual tools and wherewithal to maximize their contributions as Black people within the nursing profession."[36]

Black nursing leaders worked to convince nursing schools and nursing organizations "to develop strategies for reversing this trend."[37] But this was at a time, some twenty years after the formal integration of Black nurses into the ANA, when, as historian Darlene Clark Hine writes, "only imperceptible improvements had been registered in the actual status of black [*sic*] women within the profession."[38] As Rush University nursing faculty member Lucille Davis saw it, "In order to recruit and educate greater numbers of students from minority groups, there must be viable and successful role models for them. Attention must be directed toward not only increasing the numbers of minority practitioners on hospital staff and faculty, but also on increasing the types of positions held by those persons. The number of minority persons in leadership positions must be increased along with the necessary resources and support required for success within these roles."[39] In 1971, a group of Black nursing leaders led by Lauranne Samms established the National Black Nurses Association. Among its objectives were to advocate for improving the health care of Black Americans, to "set standards and guidelines for the quality of black nurses on all levels by providing consultation to nursing faculties and by monitoring for proper utilization and placement of black nurses," and to increase the recruitment of Black nurses.[40] On the issue of recruitment, Davis recommended educating high school counselors to recognize that Black students were not only capable of but well-suited to careers as registered nurses (thereby challenging the tendency of counselors to "often steer" Black students "into practical nursing programs because they [saw] blacks in subservient roles"), providing scholarships and loans to students of color so they could afford to attend four-year BSN programs, and improving the image of nursing within communities of color. As a nurse-turned-high-school-principal noted, the "menial image" of nursing had led "many black parents [to] resist nursing emphatically . . . They're happy to have their children become social workers, lawyers, or doctors—but not nurses!"[41]

In this context, the efforts of nurse educators, researchers, and theorists to establish nursing as an academic discipline—as evidenced by the creation of nursing PhD programs—was one way to overturn these and other negative stereotypes of nursing that circulated within communities of color as well as among feminist groups. But, as Ruffin warned, the very nature of nursing's academic project, by requiring nurses to secure higher and higher levels of educational preparation, stood to further marginalize nurses of color, a point to which we'll return later in this chapter.[42]

The Planning Movement in Higher Education and Health Care

The emphasis on expanding educational access during the 1970s took place amid declining state revenues, falling student enrollments, and reductions in federal research support. As described in chapter 3, the postwar growth of research universities and the related expansion of graduate education—underwritten by federal research funding—had led to increasing numbers of state universities awarding doctoral degrees. The postwar universities' emphasis on the capitalization of knowledge transformed research universities into drivers of regional economic development.[43] As such, in the 1950s and 1960s, state policymakers supported (often enthusiastically) the expansion of graduate education and research by state universities.[44] But as state revenues and federal research support began to decline in the late 1960s, state policymakers grew increasingly critical of the duplication that existed among their state's universities and colleges. In this context, states engaged in coordinated planning to "rationalize the program scope of various public institutions of higher education" by defining the "differential missions or prescribed purposes for the various state-supported institutions."[45] To facilitate planning, state governments established state boards of higher education to coordinate the multiple institutions of higher education within their state and to better match financial support of the state's higher education institutions to the state's perceived educational needs and resources.

State boards of education typically took their cue from what state planners had determined were the state's educational and workforce needs. In the arena of health care, this meant that state higher education policy intersected with state health planning and policy. Since the late 1940s, state legislators had looked increasingly to academic health institutions receiving state funds to expand educational opportunities and better coordinate the production and distribution of their state's health workforce (discussed in chapter 1). By the late 1950s, as Daniel M. Fox has documented, state health policy and state higher education policy had converged, with state governments throughout the country linking funding for health professions education to regional planning for health care services.[46] This coincided with the emergence of health planning as a major policy imperative. During the 1960s and 1970s, as Evan Melhado argues, health planners "aimed to make widely available health facilities and services, especially hospitals, and to foster their orderly and efficient development, that is, to meet need without duplication."[47]

The health planning movement was a response to the increasing costs of hospitals and other health care facilities, and, with postwar suburbanization, the growing number of hospitals located in suburban areas that increasingly competed with urban hospitals for patient revenue and health care workers. A series of federal legislation codified the planning movement. In 1966, Congress passed the Comprehensive Health Planning Act, which provided formula grants to states to engage in statewide comprehensive health planning under a single state agency, guided by a representative advisory council. The 1966 act also provided project grants to local public or nonprofit agencies to engage in comprehensive area-wide planning.[48]

Congress expected comprehensive health planning agencies to coordinate the existing federal health programs that required state or sub-state panning, particularly Hill-Burton, the Regional Medical Programs, and community mental health programs. The Hill-Burton program had been enacted by Congress in 1946 to provide funds for rural hospital construction. By the late 1950s, the program also provided federal funding for urban hospital construction and renovation.[49] With passage of the Heart Disease, Cancer, and Stroke Amendments of 1965, Congress authorized the implementation of

Regional Medical Programs (RMP). The programs were established "to encourage and assist in the establishment of regional cooperative arrangements
among medical schools, research institutions, and hospitals for research and
training, including continuing education, and for related demonstrations of
patient care."[50] It did so, as Fox explains, by offering incentives to health professionals and provider organizations "to improve the integration of primary,
secondary, and tertiary care for chronic disease under the leadership of medical schools and their principal teaching hospitals."[51] By the end of 1967, sixty-
one RMPs had been designated, and by 1970, fifty-four were operational.[52] In
1974, Congress consolidated Hill-Burton, Comprehensive Health Planning,
and the Regional Medical Program into the National Health Planning and
Resources Development Act, which created a new generation of state and local planning bodies.[53] Despite federal support for, and the subsequent enactment of, state and regional health planning in the 1960s and 1970s, as health
policy scholars have made clear, ultimately this series of health planning legislation lacked teeth, and the goals intended by the health planning movement invariably went unmet.[54]

The demise of health planning also coincided with the government's shift
to other cost containment strategies, particularly reform of the Medicare payment system and the turn toward managed competition in health care provision.[55] Both strategies reflected the growing influence of the Chicago school
of economics in the American political economy, with its commitment to
free markets and deregulation. In 1983, the Health Care Finance Administration, which had oversight of Medicare and Medicaid, introduced a new
system of Medicare reimbursement based on prospective payment. Instead
of paying physicians and hospitals for the services they had performed and at
the fees they charged, this system paid a set fee per case, determined by the
patient's diagnosis. Diagnoses were placed in one of 467 diagnostic related
groups (DRGs). If a hospital's costs were higher than the DRG payment, the
hospital suffered a loss, but if the hospital's costs were lower, they retained
the difference. In this way, the DRG system incentivized hospitals to provide
more cost-effective care by discharging patients more quickly and discourag-
ing physicians from overtreatment. Recognizing the dramatic cost savings,
private insurers soon adopted prospective payment based on DRGs.

Payment reform was one part of the government and private insurers' efforts to reign in health care costs. In the early 1970s, physician Paul Ellwood
proposed the establishment of health maintenance organizations (HMOs).
The HMO model, which was endorsed by Congress's passage of the HMO
Act in 1973, integrated health care financing and delivery and was intended
to increase efficiency and encourage preventive and comprehensive care. By

the early 1980s, the Reagan administration was promoting HMOs as a profitable investment opportunity, inviting a significant expansion in HMO plans, many of them for-profit. HMOs and other managed care organizations utilized a series of techniques to control spending. These included utilization reviews of the treatments ordered by physicians and the requirement that physicians acquire preauthorization for certain diagnostic procedures and treatment modalities. Primary care providers served as "gatekeepers," determining an HMO member's access to treatments and referrals to specialists. And, perhaps most importantly, HMOs introduced a new mechanism for paying physicians known as capitation, which paid physicians a set fee per patient.[56] By the early 1980s, large corporate employers had joined the federal government and third-party payers in the push for economic reform of the health care system. Alarmed by the escalating costs of employee health plans, corporations looking to assert more control over the costs of those health plans also advocated managed competition.[57] Collectively, the turn to managed competition and the corporatization of health care in the 1980s rendered the health planning of the previous decades obsolete.

Nevertheless, in the 1960s and 1970s, the enactment of state-level health planning and its convergence with state higher education policies shaped nursing's academic project. In this context, states viewed the size of the nursing workforce—what some termed "nursepower"[58]—as integral to meeting state health care needs, and by the late 1960s, initiatives to measure, evaluate, and fulfill current and future nursing workforce needs had emerged as a core component of state health planning mandates.[59] Indeed, during the 1960s and 1970s, state health planners across the country launched health workforce studies in order to document the current supply and project the future demand of health care professionals, including nurses. They then used this data to plan for and implement new educational policies and programs in an effort to match supply with demand. As part of this, state planners considered the ways in which nurses were being educated, the roles in which nurses currently were being utilized, and new roles in which nurses could be utilized in the future. The imperative for statewide planning in nursing education was reinforced by the National Commission for the Study of Nursing and Nursing Education. The Lysaught Commission, as it came to be called (named after its director, Jerome Lysaught of the University of Rochester), was established in 1967 to study problems in nursing education and nursing practice.[60] When the national commission published its report, *An Abstract for Action*, in 1970, it urged states to develop master plans for nursing and nursing education.[61]

The convergence of state higher education policy with state health policy presented state nursing schools with both a burden and an opportunity. As the dean of Boston University's School of Nursing explained, because state boards of education "[had] great control over the public institutions," it was important that nursing schools "be very sensitive to the role of elective legislators . . . as well as to the role of the Board of Higher Education."[62] In many cases, this meant that to garner support for its programming initiatives, it was in state nursing schools' interests to be responsive to the requests of the legislature.[63]

In the 1970s, state policymakers' interest in nursing education centered on three main issues. First, policymakers were interested in facilitating educational mobility for graduates of LPN, diploma, and AD programs seeking to move up the career ladder. This reflected policymakers' commitment to expanding access to and diversity within higher education, as well as their interest in increasing the number of nurses educated at the BSN level or higher in response to nursing leaders' assertions that higher levels of education for nurses would translate into the provision of higher quality of care. Second, state policymakers sought to introduce nurse practitioner programs (typically at the master's level) so as to increase the supply and utilization of nurse practitioners as a way of tackling the shortage of primary care physicians. Finally, state policymakers looked to increase the number of qualified faculty in order to support the establishment of new (and expansion of existing) AD, BSN, and graduate degree programs in nursing. The remainder of this chapter takes a close look at the state-level planning that took place regarding the education and supply of nurses. It reveals both the importance of state nursing school's responsiveness to the requests of the legislature, and the ways in which state nursing schools mobilized state health workforce concerns to secure support for their doctoral programs from university administrators. In turn, it makes clear the influence of nurses—working individually and collectively through their state nursing organizations—to affect state health and educational policies. Ultimately, it highlights the intersections of health planning with nursing's academic project.

Expanding Access and Educational Mobility for Nurses

As discussed earlier in this chapter, the expansion of educational access was a high priority among policymakers in the 1970s. This policy imperative had an important impact on nursing education in the 1970s, as legislators, in response to the demands of nurses in their districts and lobbying by state nursing organizations, pushed public colleges and universities to enhance opportunities for nurses to upgrade their education and expand access to undergraduate and graduate nursing education. As national and regional nursing leaders sought to raise the educational standards of nursing, the graduates of diploma and associate degree programs were under "constant pressure" during these decades "to upgrade their educational credentials in order to hold or advance in their jobs."[64] Possession of a BSN was necessary if a nurse wanted to climb the career ladder and move into administration or specialized practice, both of which increasingly required graduate-level education.[65] Graduates of practical nursing, diploma, and associate degree in nursing programs, however, frequently found their attempts to achieve "upward mobility to the better paying, more skilled positions . . . blocked by rigid educational requirements and the need for full-time study."[66] At the same time, "medical corpsmen returning from active duty were similarly indignant to find that the only kinds of jobs in nursing that recognized their experience were at the bottom of the status and economic ladder and that RN programs generally disregarded their previous health care education and experience."[67] In addition, as Helen Grace and Rozanne Spitzer (dean and assistant dean of nursing at the University of Illinois Chicago) explained, "educational mobility for nurses carries with it some special considerations. Practicing nurses most frequently are married, have children, and for a variety of reasons are placebound. Nurses wishing to complete baccalaureate or graduate degrees cannot uproot themselves for long periods of time to complete advanced educational programs. While many have made Herculean efforts to commute long distances to achieve educational mobility, the current increase in cost of commuting and a diminishing energy supply has made this solution untenable."[68]

The difficulty of educational mobility and the lack of articulation between the different levels of education made career progression in nursing inefficient and costly. Part of the difficulty centered on the lack of compatibility between diploma and collegiate nursing programs. As Bonnie Bullough and Vern Bullough explained, because "educational progress in the collegiate system is measured in units of academic credit and hospital schools are not authorized to issue such credit by themselves, the two systems are not compatible." The problem of articulating hospital and collegiate programs was thus "not completely one of quality because the quality of hospital nursing education [had] gone up in recent years to a reasonable level," but was "instead a problem of measuring course credits in the common denominator of academic units."[69] Another major obstacle identified by the authors was the NLN's recent ruling that for accreditation, the nursing major had to be concentrated in the upper division of the baccalaureate program. Because associate degree and diploma programs were classified as lower division, it "rule[d] out any easy articulation of the associate degree and hospital programs with baccalaureate ones."[70] But, as the Lysaught Commission observed, the lack of articulation between diploma, AD, and BSN programs was one of the major problems faced by nursing, and the Commission saw it as "essential that a planned and articulated curriculum be developed between the collegiate components" of nursing's educational system.[71]

Throughout the late 1960s and 1970s, the *American Journal of Nursing* printed scores of letters from diploma and AD graduates documenting their "stymied . . . attempts to further their educations."[72] In 1977, for example, a diploma graduate nurse wrote in the "sheer frustration . . . of the diploma school nurse who must start from scratch!" She asked, "Why shouldn't the diploma school nurse be entitled to those 90 credits which she *earned* over three years of hard work? As a result of not receiving the academic credit to which they are entitled," she continued, "many highly qualified, competent RNs are not interested in obtaining a BSN."[73] As another diploma graduate nurse wrote, "My attempts to upgrade my education have met with obstacles from the only university within commuting distance. It is time for people to stop inferring that diploma nurses don't want to better themselves." She went on to explain: "After six attempts to obtain a degree in nursing, I returned to college as an English major! It would have taken almost two years longer to obtain the nursing degree. With 2 years liberal arts in college and 10 years of nursing experience, it would take me almost 3 years to obtain a degree in nursing! This is why diploma nurses are not obtaining degrees in nursing— because of inflexibility of rules and complete disregard of previous training and experience by universities!"[74] Recalling similar difficulties, another RN called on "college programs to include better ways of testing nurses so that their valuable education in the real world could be transferred to college credit." After all, she continued, "Many diploma graduates want to continue their formal education but cannot afford to quit a job or pay tuition. Many are discouraged by the feeling that one must 'start all over' and that the knowledge and experience gained in the practice of professional nursing will not always be considered valid by educators."[75]

Another difficulty encountered by RNs seeking to upgrade their education was the limited number of RN-to-BSN programs that took their prior educational preparation into account and provided an accelerated curriculum. In 1976, for example, an AD graduate wrote that she was "finding it increasingly difficult to continue [her] nursing education because of a lack of baccalaureate programs available to registered nurses." Although most BSN programs, she found, accepted AD graduates without nursing training and with degrees in other fields, they were not open to AD nursing graduates. "Where does this leave registered nurses who want to go back to college to obtain a degree?" she asked.[76] A nurse educator raised similar concerns, calling for "much needed support for nontraditional programs committed to upward career mobility without loss of dignity for the registered nurse seeking a baccalaureate degree in nursing." She explained the difficulties encountered by nursing schools seeking to establish RN-to-BSN programs, noting that "attempts to provide realistic, quality programs leading to BSN degrees run into difficulties when the schools seek accreditation. There are some 60 programs for the RN sponsored by educational institutions, and, at present, only 9 are accredited." As she explained, "The conflict appears to be mostly philosophical rather than one of glaring flaws in the formulation or implementation of curriculums. We find ourselves attempting to be responsive to expressed needs of RNs and running afoul of traditional baccalaureate concepts." For this nurse educator, "The wheels of change turn slowly, and the burden of greasing them lies with those of us who are pioneering newer educational patterns of nursing. I believe that once we win the battle of philosophy, the profession will be free to concentrate its energy in providing reasonable academic pathways for nurses who wish to obtain baccalaureate degrees in nursing."[77]

Even when RNs were admitted into BSN programs, they were often disheartened by the expense of upgrading their education. A diploma graduate, "fortunate enough to find a college in the area that offered challenge exams to registered nurses and evening courses with only one full-time semester required," expressed dismay at the tuition, which "was a minimum of $4,200; maximum cost, $6,000! Since I had a toddler at home with future ones expected and a brand new 25-year mortgage along with umpteen debts, financial assistance was a necessity." But after completing the financial assistance paperwork, she learned that financial assistance was "reserved for those on welfare." At this time," she continued, I cannot afford to become 'professional.' "[78] As one AD graduate lamented, her college record and three years of clinical experience hadn't qualified her for scholarships. Furthermore, she said, "Any hopes for a federal or state grant have been turned down because my husband earns $17,000 a year for a family of four. This income will be impossible to live on once I stop working to attend school full-time, and it won't pay for tuition and books." She and her husband had decided to sell their house and move their family into an apartment. Even so, she continued, "We will have to go into debt to give me this opportunity to do what I feel I could do best—teach nursing." She accused nursing organizations of "preaching for change" but not being "willing to put their money where their mouths are."[79]

Of those nurses who had successfully navigated the process and achieved educational mobility, many questioned the value of their collegiate education. As one such diploma nurse who had gone on to get her AD wrote, "The diploma school taught me how to be a nurse, to care for my patients mentally and physically. The associate degree program taught me little more than how to study. The graduates could quote their textbooks, but needed a lot of experience working in the hospital situation." She had been frustrated that as an AD student, she had had to repeat most of her "nursing arts" courses "since [she] could not challenge them . . . The thought of having to repeat nursing arts classes *again* is a strong factor against my going on for a baccalaureate degree. Many graduates of diploma schools might continue their education more quickly if they had transferrable credits."[80] A diploma graduate currently enrolled in a BSN program similarly questioned the value of her collegiate education, finding the "education at the baccalaureate level [was] sadly lacking in relevancy."[81] For other nurses though, the value of the additional education was clear. As a diploma graduate who had recently completed her BSN wrote, "The courses in the nursing curriculum are geared toward developing a practitioner who thinks critically, applies the nursing process, utilizes the decision-making process, and demonstrates accountability to the consumer of health care." She considered herself "fortunate to be among the new breed" of nurse.[82]

Since the mid-1960s, nursing leaders had been pushing to establish the BSN as the minimum educational requirement for entry into professional practice, initially codified in the ANA's 1965 position statement on education (see chapter 1).[83] In the late 1970s, this push was further reflected in the New York State Nurses Association's proposal that by 1985, the BSN should be the basis for licensure of registered nurses and the AD the basis for licensure as a practical nurse.[84] Despite the ongoing efforts by nursing leaders to restrict entry into practice, diploma and AD-educated nurses continued to assert the importance of maintaining multiple educational pathways into professional nursing. An AD graduate wrote that AD programs provided critical opportunities for social mobility, noting, "Many women and men who enter associate degree programs are older and more mature than the eighteen-year-olds who have just graduated high school. Some have already worked in a health-related field for several years. Most already have family or financial responsibilities that prevent them from entering a four-year program." She thus argued against the New York State Nurses Association's proposal that would bar AD graduates from being licensed as professional nurses. "When we're understaffed and overworked," she asked, "why eliminate persons who are eager to join our ranks?"[85] Another nurse who had begun her educational experience in an AD program followed by two years in practice, two years in a RN-to-BSN program, five additional years in practice, and finally, a master's degree, wrote, "At each level, I benefitted more from the educational process because of my experience in the practice of nursing." As a result, she extolled the virtue of "a system of multiple entry and exit points" that enabled "alternating education with actual work experience." This nurse wondered "why nursing [was] trying to do away with its own system of multiple exit and entry routes" and when the profession would "accept that sometimes we do things better than other professionals." She continued, "We must give up the fantasy that one's goals never change and that with proper counseling all will be channeled into the appropriate program from the beginning. Instead, we must clearly delineate performance expectations for each level and continue with our efforts to identify ways of evaluating these levels. Then we can allow formal credit for both previous knowledge and experience and allow caregivers to advance in flexible ways."[86]

The difficulties of career mobility significantly impacted nurses of color who entered nursing predominantly through diploma and associate degree programs.[87] In Illinois, for example, the Illinois Board of Higher Education reported that the majority of minority students entered nursing and other health care professions through associate degree programs. As the dean of nursing at the University of Illinois Chicago, Helen Grace, explained, "the way in which minorities enter the field, serves to handicap them at each stage of the educational level." Reflecting the systemic racism within higher education and nursing, she said, "Most minority students enter the system through the community college system," which was less well financed and supported than the four-year college and university system. For example, Grace wrote, many of the AD programs "that have large numbers of minority students [were] nonaccredited and of poor quality." She went on to say, "Although a nurse may complete these programs with little difficulty and a high grade point average, the graduate frequently experiences difficulties in passing state board examinations." If the graduate then entered a baccalaureate completion program, the student might have "difficulty in passing entry exemption examinations over basic nursing content, and in mastering the content of the program . . . Poor performance at the baccalaureate level [made] it difficult for these graduates to obtain access to graduate education." The result was "a very small proportion of minority nurses with graduate preparation and occupying leadership position[s] both in clinical practice settings and in educational programs."[88]

As recognition of both the importance and difficulty of educational mobility in nursing, several nursing schools, the NLN, and other nursing and educational organizations launched a series of initiatives over the course of the 1970s to make such mobility more readily available.[89] In some cases, nursing schools granted credit for certain levels of previous educational preparation. Monmouth College in New Jersey, for example, granted graduates of Ann

May Hospital School of Nursing one hundred credits to apply toward their BSN.[90] At Russell Sage College in New York, registered nurse students could obtain up to fifty-four credits through proficiency examinations.[91] Several state legislatures, including those in Ohio, North Carolina, and California, proposed legislation that would grant diploma and associate degree graduates blanket credit (often one to two years of credit) to put toward baccalaureate degrees in state universities.[92]

Other measures included the introduction of innovative curricula that facilitated educational mobility. Arizona State University College of Nursing, for example, established a "continuous process curriculum" that provided students with the opportunity to progress through the curriculum according to their individual ability. All students were admitted to the nursing major in their junior year having either completed at least sixty credit hours at Arizona State University or transferring those credits in from other colleges or universities. The students could "challenge any course in accordance with university policy" and they could "obtain upper division credit for knowledge and skill they [could] demonstrate."[93] The nursing curriculum was divided into four levels, designed to be completed, usually, in four semesters. Each level had designated objectives, which all students needed to achieve before moving on to the next level. Registered nurses, though, were often able to obtain credit by challenge for many of the objectives within each level. As of 1973, twenty-one registered nurses had enrolled in the continuous process curriculum, with most finishing in less than four semesters.[94]

Several initiatives responded to the Lysaught Commission's call for "planned and articulated curriculum" across different levels of the collegiate system. In Iowa, for example, the dean of the University of Iowa College of Nursing, Laura Dustan, developed "a statewide network of private, community, and state colleges" that offered "a carefully articulated science and liberal arts base" for the University of Iowa's BSN program. In particular, Iowa's articulation project developed "'feeder' or lower-division transfer curriculums" in five private colleges, five community colleges, and two Iowa state universities, which articulated "directly with the upper division major in nursing offered" by the University of Iowa College of Nursing. The project recruited "students from all social classes," and provided "a wider geographic scatter of educational opportunities so that more scholastically able high school graduates" would select the BSN "as their entry point into nursing."[95] Although the project was designed for high school graduates who would "enter a local articulation project college, and then transfer to the [University of Iowa] after completing the two years of prerequisite courses," the program had also attracted "local nurses who wanted to upgrade their education and earn the

BSN degree." The program appealed to diploma and associate degree graduates because "all but one calendar year of work for the bachelor's degree could be completed in one of the cooperating colleges scattered across Iowa."[96] Although there was evidence that the articulation project had helped to increase recruitment of lower income white students into the BSN program, the recruitment of students of color was significantly limited. Indeed, within the project's first five years, only one student from an underrepresented group entered the BSN program through the articulation project. This reflected a "weakness of the program," which stemmed in part from the fact that the "two Iowa cities with the largest racial minorities, Des Moines and Waterloo, are not represented by colleges in the program."[97]

In Southern California, a consortium of five community colleges, three universities, and one medical school collaborated to establish a "five-level articulated program," with funding from the W. K. Kellogg Foundation. This "unique multiple-entry, multiple-exit career ladder" provided nursing education at five levels: nurse's aide, licensed vocational nurse (known in other states as the licensed practical nurse), associate degree in nursing, BSN, and a master's degree with advanced preparation as a nurse practitioner or clinical nurse specialist. The five community colleges of the consortium developed programs for the nurse's aide and the licensed vocational nurse, while California State University, Fullerton established a BSN program that was only open to registered nurses, especially AD graduates of the consortium's community colleges, and California State University, Long Beach, reorganized its curriculum to facilitate the entry of registered nurses, in addition to generic BSN students. California State University, Long Beach, also established a master's degree program in cooperation with the UCLA Medical School, which prepared nurse practitioners and clinical nurse specialists in pediatric, adult, and family medicine.[98]

In 1972, the NLN launched the Open Curriculum Project with funding from the Exxon Education Foundation.[99] The project followed a selected number of programs with open curriculum components, defined by the project's staff as "an educational approach designed to accommodate the learning needs and career goals of students by providing flexible opportunities for entry into and exit from the educational program, and by capitalizing on their previous relevant education and experience."[100] The NLN project also provided information about current programs, and planned the development of guidelines for nursing faculty interested in starting open curriculum programs. In 1973, the NLN held a conference in which nursing faculty involved in thirty-two open curriculum projects representing twenty-one schools reported on their experiences.[101]

It this context, the issue of educational mobility for the state's nurses emerged as high priority among state health planners in the 1970s. In Minnesota in 1970, for example, the comprehensive health planning agency's advisory subcommittee on nursing recommended that the faculty of BSN programs at the University of Minnesota and other state and private colleges in Minnesota, either individually or collectively, "develop validating examinations to allow for advanced placement of registered nurses seeking Baccalaureate degrees." Similarly, the subcommittee urged the faculty of the state's AD nursing programs to "provide examinations to permit entry of LPNs at an appropriate level in the Associate degree programs." The subcommittee also supported the State College Board's recent "Credits in Trust" proposal, which would enable diploma graduates to receive credits toward a baccalaureate degree.[102] Minnesota's Higher Education Coordinating Commission (HECC), which was responsible for coordinating and approving new educational programming in the state's two- and four-year colleges and universities, also regarded the facilitation of career mobility for nurses as a key priority of the state. In 1973, HECC's advisory committee on nursing education called on faculty at undergraduate nursing programs to direct effort toward curriculum articulation so as to meet "the needs of students . . . seeking to increase their professional competence through additional" education. The advisory committee also urged nursing faculty to "increase opportunities for career mobility in Minnesota" by providing qualified candidates with "credit for previously educational and work-related experiences."[103]

The issue of educational mobility among registered nurses resonated strongly with state legislators. In Minnesota, as in other states throughout the country, the state's legislators were under pressure from RNs to facilitate educational mobility for graduates of diploma and AD programs.[104] These legislators, in turn, put pressure on the University of Minnesota, as the state's land-grant institution, to resolve the problems of educational mobility. In April 1971, for example, state representative Verne Long wrote to the University of Minnesota's vice president for legislative affairs, Stanley Wenberg, asking the university to help resolve a current problem in nursing education. Long held considerable political and financial leverage at the university as chair of the Minnesota house's higher education committee and vice-chair of the appropriations committee. His attention to the problem of nursing education was in part a response to the "many letters, calls, and visits" he had received since the beginning of the legislative session from nurses who were troubled by the difficulties they had faced in their efforts to attain advanced training. In making his request to Wenberg, Long reminded him, "Several times in the past weeks you have pointed out specific needs and asked us, as legislators, to address and appropriate dollars to specific programs. I would now like to ask you to direct your *immediate attention* to the problem of challenge exams. . . . If, in fact, the solution to these problems can be found . . . then I want to say in the most forceful manner I know how—let's have the answers forthcoming soon."[105]

Like many state legislators throughout the country, Long was unconvinced about the necessity of higher education in nursing, given that diploma, associate degree, and BSN graduates all had to pass the same state licensing exam. "How great can the difference in education be?" Long asked. He was frustrated by the "pat answers" of nurse educators and the "snail-pace and fuss about developing challenge exams." He continued, "I think it's a put off and it's the darned old power game between degree and diploma nurses which stymies the procedure." Long urged Wenberg to "Please tell Dr. French [the vice president for health sciences] of this situation about the credits in trust and the challenge system. Perhaps the Chancellor's office also. I'm so darned mad."[106]

For the University of Minnesota, Long's interest in and frustration with the delays in improving educational mobility in nursing were significant. As Wenberg wrote to his colleagues in the university's central administration, it was important they take seriously Long's request for definitive action. He asked, "Is there some way we can get an answer to [Representative Long] that responds to his concern that the University ought to give a little leadership in trying to multiply approaches to better utilization and training of health manpower particularly in paramedical fields [such as nursing]?"[107] In January 1972, several of the state's nursing leaders, including Isabel Harris, dean of the School of Nursing, testified before the Minnesota House of Representative's Medical Education Subcommittee, which was chaired by Verne Long. Long was still concerned about the problems associated with career mobility in nursing and asked Harris about "the progress you have made in the areas of those that are trying to upgrade their education." Harris explained that the School of Nursing had developed challenge exams for the first-year nursing courses and for half of the physiology course of the junior year, and was continuing to work on developing challenge exams for the other courses in the junior year of the BSN curriculum.[108] Six months later, the School of Nursing submitted a legislative special request to secure legislative funding to develop "a special, two year curriculum for associate and diploma graduates leading to a baccalaureate degree in nursing."[109]

The issue of career mobility was, then, highly political. As Mariah Snyder, a faculty member in the University of Minnesota School of Nursing, recalled, "Because of the two-year programs being in rural communities or outstate, legislators were not going to do away with the schools in their cities."[110] The Minnesota Nurses Association (MNA) was also opposed to restricting access to professional practice by closing diploma or associate degree programs. As Snyder explained, "The [MNA's] largest membership was two- and three-year grads, so they weren't going to get behind this effort" to close two- and three-year programs.[111] As a result, the state's registered nurses and the legislators that represented them expected the state's four-year colleges, particularly the state's flagship University of Minnesota, to take the lead in facilitating the educational mobility of the state's nurses.

Nurse Practitioner Education and the Crisis of Primary Health Care

During the 1970s, state health planners also viewed the development of programs to prepare nurse practitioners as a high priority. As discussed in chapter 1, several collaborative initiatives between nurses and physicians in the 1960s and 1970s led to the development of new expert clinical roles for nurses with advanced education, including the nurse practitioner and the clinical nurse specialist.[112] For example, public health nurse Loretta Ford, in collaboration with her physician colleague, Henry Silver, introduced the first nurse practitioner program at the University of Colorado in 1965. The program was a postbaccalaureate curriculum for pediatric nurses providing "total health care" to children in private physicians' offices and in low-income urban and rural areas of Colorado that lacked adequate health care services.[113] The program prepared students to "provide comprehensive well-child care to well children and identify, appraise, and temporarily manage certain acute and chronic conditions of the sick child" in physicians' offices, clinics, and other facilities without adequate health services for children.[114] Nurse practitioner programs were soon established at other nursing schools across the country, and by the late 1970s, the education of nurse practitioners (along with clinical nurse specialists) increasingly took place at the master's level.[115]

The nurse practitioner movement emerged as the passage of Medicare and Medicaid in 1965 exacerbated existing concerns about the urban and suburban concentration of specialists and shortages of primary care physicians, especially in rural and underserved urban communities.[116] Medicare, in particular, heightened the economic disparities between general practitioners and specialists and strengthened the institutional basis of specialization. Medicare's reimbursement model built upon existing fee-for-service reimbursement systems that reimbursed specialists, particularly those who were procedure based, at significantly higher rates than general practitioners and, increasingly, physicians in the other primary care specialties of internal medicine, pediatrics, and family medicine. Medicare—along with the passage of Medicaid the same year—expanded the number of people able to afford private health care, putting further strain on the shrinking primary care physician workforce.[117] By the early 1970s, a series of national and state-level reports reaffirmed the critical role to be played by nurse practitioners and other so-called physician extenders (such as physician assistants) in helping to resolve the problems of inadequate health care access related to the physician shortage.[118]

In Minnesota in 1966, for example, the Health Manpower Study Commission had documented the shortage of primary care physicians in the state. As a predominantly rural state, Minnesota had a particularly high demand for primary care physicians willing to work outside metropolitan Minneapolis and Saint Paul.[119] By 1970, state planners looking to "expand the primary care capacity in the State" made "training and educational programs directed toward such care," including those preparing nurse practitioners, "a high priority."[120] As the advisory council of the state's comprehensive health planning agency argued, nurse practitioners "could help to expand our capacity to deliver primary health care in this state."[121] The Northlands Regional Medical Program began funding demonstrations of the nurse practitioner role in Minnesota.[122]

In the 1970s, the University of Minnesota was the only school in the state and upper Midwest region that offered nurse practitioner programs. The nurse practitioner programs were under the purview of public health nursing, which at the University of Minnesota was located in the School of Public Health.[123] By 1972, the university offered three nurse practitioner programs underwritten by grants from the U.S. Public Health Service's Division of Nursing and the Northlands Regional Medical Program. The first program was a master's in public health nursing program in which students could specialize as a family nurse specialist, pediatric nurse associate, or adult nurse associate. Graduates of the program were prepared to practice in primary care settings. The second program was a nine-month postbaccalaureate program producing pediatric nurse practitioners who were trained "to exercise sound nursing and medical judgment" and to "function without close supervision" in ambulatory care settings.[124] The third program was a five-month continuing education program preparing adult and geriatric nurse practitioners able to "function as associates to physicians delivering adult and geriatric care in those geographic areas where these services are limited."[125] The adult and geriatric nurse practitioner program was implemented as an off-campus rural nurse practitioner certificate program in an effort to increase health care services to the state's "medical underserved populations," particularly rural communities that had a shortage of physicians.[126]

At that time, the majority of registered nurses in rural Minnesota were "women with families who were committed to the agricultural community of which they were a part." In 1972, seventy percent of these rural nurses were "diploma graduates with limited access to continuing professional education." In the majority of cases, these nurses were working in communities in which there was a shortage of physicians. As such, many rural nurses "were forced to develop expanded role skills 'on the job'" in order to meet the health care needs of the community. Through the adult and geriatric nurse practitioner program, the public health nursing faculty would provide rural nurses with the training necessary to competently perform in an expanded and independent clinical role. The program provided "classroom and clinical learning experiences in history taking, physical examination, data analysis, and management of patients with minor acute illnesses and stabilized chronic diseases." Through the program, students were "prepared for health maintenance, primary prevention, and patient/family teaching and counseling."[127] To facilitate participation by registered nurses already working and living in rural communities, rather than have the program located on the Twin Cities campus, the public health nursing faculty taught the classroom material at selected sites throughout Minnesota, while students gained clinical experience in their home communities under the preceptorships of physicians.[128] By 1973, twenty-three students had completed the university's adult and geriatric nurse practitioner program in Thief River Falls, St. Cloud, and the Twin Cities; twenty-two students were currently enrolled in classes in Grand Rapids and in the Twin Cities area; and a new class of students was planned for the Wadena area beginning in 1974.[129]

In 1973, the state's senate subcommittee on medical care, chaired by John Milton, launched a study of the state's primary health care system. The investigation sought "to determine what primary health care is available, whether residents have access to that care, whether they use it and whether they can pay for it."[130] As part of its study, the subcommittee considered the potential role of nurse practitioners in facilitating expanded access to health care services. To this end, Alma Sparrow, director of public health nursing at the University of Minnesota, and William Fifer, director of the University of Minnesota Area Health Education Center,[131] urged legislators to support the nurse practitioner concept and provide state funding to increase the education of nurse practitioners and reorganize the primary care delivery system in the state to facilitate expanded use of nurse practitioners in the delivery of rural health care.[132] In doing so, they emphasized both the cost-effectiveness of nurse practitioner education and the critical role already being played by the university's nurse practitioner programs. As Fifer noted, when "compared to the very high cost of training physicians from scratch," the cost of training nurse practitioners was "inexpensive because it builds on the already considerable knowledge the nurse acquired in her nurses' training," and because the programs "use[d] existing educational physical facilitates and faculty." In light of the "considerable evidence" already marshaled from the experiences of the graduates of the University of Minnesota nurse practitioner programs, "nurse practitioners were well accepted by patients and . . . able to deliver high quality patient care under defined conditions."[133] Given the early success of the adult and geriatric nurse practitioner program, Sparrow and Fifer urged state senators to increase funding of the University of Minnesota's nurse practitioner programs. This funding would be used to expand the size of the university's existing nurse practitioner programs offered and increase the number of master's-prepared nurse practitioner faculty available to implement and teach additional nurse practitioner programs established throughout the state.[134]

Senator Milton was persuaded. In 1974, he recommended that training be expanded in the state for "the nurse practitioner, the pediatric nurse associate, the midwife, and the school nurse specialist" as the most effective way to tackle the shortage and maldistribution of physicians in the state. He admonished the University of Minnesota, however, for its "'go-slow' approach to allied health expansion," which, he said, appeared to be premised on four assumptions: "1) Physicians are not ready for it. 2) Nurses aren't ready for it either. 3) The public isn't ready for these allied health persons. 4) There aren't enough faculty to do the training."[135] Milton's comments refer to the ambivalence—and in some cases outright opposition—among many physicians and some nurses throughout the country to the nurse practitioner role. As Milton argued, just because "physicians are not ready for it" was not legitimate cause for delay. Rather, he asserted, "The health care needs of Minnesotans should not be directly dependent on medical traditions and prerogatives." Furthermore, the subcommittee had heard from nurses throughout the state that they *were* ready for expanded roles and that "surveys of public attitudes toward allied health professionals indicate[d] widespread acceptance of an expanded role." For the subcommittee on medical care, there was clearly a demand for nurses to fulfill expanded roles in the state of Minnesota. To help facilitate the expansion of nurse practitioner education in the state, Milton highlighted the importance of tackling the shortage of faculty necessary to expand graduate education opportunities for nurses. As such, Milton called on the University of Minnesota to "a. Request the money for faculty salaries and student stipends; b. Fight as hard for this appropriation as for medical school buildings; c. Hire the faculty if you succeed in b, above, and d. Turn the faculty loose in outstate Minnesota."[136]

In the end, the state legislature endorsed the University of Minnesota's nurse practitioner programs, authorizing a special appropriation to ensure their sustained support. By the end of the decade, the gains of this legislative support were evident. In 1979, ninety graduates from rural areas had completed the university's adult and geriatric nurse practitioner program, 88 percent of whom remained employed in rural communities. Of those remaining in rural communities, 73 percent reported that they were working in a nurse practitioner role, while the remainder were serving in administrative and educational roles in their rural communities.[137] In Minnesota, as they did in other states throughout the country, state health planners and policymakers recognized that by increasing the supply and utilization of nurse practitioners they were able to increase access to primary health care services among rural and underserved urban communities.[138]

The Need for Qualified Faculty and the
Argument for Doctoral Education

The shortage of appropriately qualified nursing faculty was seen as a critical factor in the nursing shortage. Indeed, as the Surgeon General's Consultant Group on Nursing had asserted in 1963, "More and Better-Prepared Faculty" were needed in order to meet future nursing needs.[139] Three years later, in 1966, the U.S. Public Health Service Division of Nursing noted that less than one-third of all nurses occupying positions as faculty, administrators, supervisors, and clinical specialists held the minimum preparation for their specialty. In particular, the Division of Nursing called attention to the persistent shortages of qualified nursing faculty. Citing data from 1966, the Division of Nursing warned that "174 associate degree programs reported 114 unfilled faculty positions and 27 positions occupied by persons with no preparation to teach." That same year, 196 baccalaureate programs reported 302 unfilled faculty positions.[140]

The problem of faculty shortages was exacerbated by the fact that the majority of nurses were still being trained in hospital-based diploma programs and that "the educational preparation of the teachers for hospital schools, and cooperating agencies, [fell] far below the faculty qualification in junior and senior colleges." For as long as "the least qualified teachers of nursing [were] preparing the majority of [nurses]," it would be difficult to improve patient care. As such, the Division of Nursing regarded an "increase in both quantity and quality of teachers" as "essential for the delivery of adequate nursing services to the people of this Nation." In particular, it was of "utmost importance" that nurses holding faculty and administrative positions be prepared at "educational levels comparable to other professional positions of equal responsibility." The implication, then, was that nursing faculty, like their colleagues in medicine, dentistry, and, increasingly, pharmacy, should be doctorally prepared.[141] This was not only a political argument—that of establishing parity with other health professionals; it was also empirically driven. Nursing leaders maintained that doctorally educated nurses—that is, the creators and custodians of nursing's abstract knowledge system—were best equipped to educate new generations of professional nurses in the nursing theories and research that constituted that knowledge system.[142] After all, nursing leaders hoped, improvements in nursing practice would derive from advances in nursing science. Thus, they saw doctorally educated faculty as essential to raising the educational standards of professional nurses and improving the quality of patient care.

To be sure, concerns about shortages of doctorally prepared faculty was expressed across academic disciplines beginning in the 1950s and continuing through the 1960s. One reason for the shortage was demographics: education leaders worried, in particular, about the pending growth in enrollments once the baby boom cohort graduated from high school and pursued higher education in the 1960s. Another reason was the relatively low number of faculty with doctorates, which by the 1950s was seen as the desirable qualification for teaching at the collegiate level. As Roger Geiger notes, "A survey in 1953 estimated that just 40.5 percent of the college teachers possessed doctorates, [and] roughly 30 percent of new entrants to the profession had their final degree." These factors, Geiger continues, "gave rise to the conviction, which persisted into the late 1960s, that a crisis was at hand: a vastly larger number of doctorates were thought to be needed to avoid a decline in the quality of college instruction." As a result, throughout the 1960s, the shortage of doctorally prepared faculty "provided a powerful incentive" to universities to establish or expand doctorate programs.[143] "As long as taxpayers were willing to foot the bill," Geiger writes, "there were few negatives associated with entering the doctoral lists."[144]

In many states, health planners perceived the shortage of qualified nursing faculty as undermining the state's health workforce and health care needs. Beginning in the mid-1960s, as states engaged in comprehensive health planning, nursing leaders' calls to establish doctoral programs in nursing became an effective political tool to mobilize against retrenchment and institutional opposition within state-supported universities. In 1966, for example, the College of Nursing at the University of Illinois Chicago initiated plans for a doctoral program in nursing "to meet the dire needs of the State for nurses prepared for University teaching and for research for improvement of nursing care."[145] The previous year, the Illinois League for Nursing and the Illinois Nurses Association had established the Illinois Study Commission on Nursing, a two-year project "to assess Illinois' nursing resources and needs, present and projected to 1980, and develop a program of action to meet the state's needs for nursing services." The Commission on Nursing was chaired by Mary Kelly Mullane, dean of the University of Illinois Chicago College of Nursing, and was composed of fifty-five members "widely representative of the professional and public groups concerned with the provision of adequate nursing care in Illinois."[146]

The commission's study, which was completed in 1968, documented the serious nursing shortages that already existed. As of 1966, for example, "20 percent of all budgeted positions for nurses in . . . hospitals, clinics, community health services and other agencies employing nurses were vacant." With this vacancy rate, Mullane warned, Illinois "is not prepared for the increased services resulting from Medicare and other expanding community health service programs." The shortages of appropriately trained nurse leaders in Illinois were even more profound. The commission found that as of 1966, 88 percent of all working nurses in Illinois had "completed no training beyond the basic hospital school" and only 12 percent of Illinois nurses were college graduates. Among nurses holding senior administrative positions—directors of nursing and chiefs of in-service education—only 66 percent had completed educational preparation beyond their RN training. The nursing faculty in the state's nursing schools were also found to be "ill-equipped." At that time, only 27 percent of the state's nursing faculty had "completed the Master's Degree, the basic qualification for high school teaching; 49% . . . completed only the bachelor's degree; 22% [had] nothing more than their RN training."[147]

For the commission, the first priority was to upgrade the educational preparation of the state's nursing faculty, directors of in-service education, and administrators and directors of nursing services in the state's health care institutions.[148] Indeed, the commission's findings stated, "The greatest single deterrent to the quality of education that will produce needed nursing leaders is the lack of available qualified faculty in baccalaureate and graduate programs." As such, the commission called for a significant expansion of educational resources in the state. To this end, the commission created a "blueprint" for nursing education in Illinois (the Illinois Plan for Nursing Education), intended as a statewide planning guide for schools of nursing and other educational institutions. The blueprint called for the number of BSN programs offered by nursing schools in the state to double by 1980; the number of schools offering master's programs to increase from four in 1968 to six by 1980; and "at least one Illinois university offering a doctorate designed for nurses to provide faculty for master's programs and for research." At the time, no Illinois university offered such a doctorate.[149] On the basis of the commission's report, the Illinois State Board of Higher Education recommended that the University of Illinois Chicago College of Nursing establish a doctoral degree in nursing that by 1980 would graduate fifty doctorally prepared students per year.[150]

The University of Illinois Chicago College of Nursing subsequently framed its proposal for a PhD program in the context of the state's nursing workforce needs (for additional discussion of University of Illinois Chicago's doctoral program, see chapter 3). The proposal, which the college submitted to the University of Illinois Medical Center Graduate College in 1974, argued that the "urgency" of Illinois's nursing workforce situation necessitated the establishment of the nursing PhD program. The proposal cited, in particular, the "plight" of the state's "senior and junior college nursing programs" as they struggled "to find qualified faculty" to expand undergraduate and masters-level education. "Prospective employers" in hospitals, clinics, and other service agencies were also reporting that they planned to hire double the number of doctorally prepared nurses by 1980. As of 1974, Illinois needed thirty additional doctorally prepared nurses, but it was expected that seventy-six would be needed by 1980. Regionally the demand was even greater. In 1974, the north central states of Illinois, Indiana, Iowa, Michigan, Minnesota, Missouri, Ohio, and Wisconsin needed an additional 212 doctorally prepared faculty; by 1980 that number was expected to increase to 588. At that time, Case Western Reserve University had the only doctoral program in the region, and as of 1974, only two students were enrolled in it.[151]

The state workforce argument proved particularly compelling at a time when state-supported universities across the country faced declining state and federal support for graduate education. As noted earlier, in the early 1970s, federal support of academic research and graduate education decreased and states struggled, in the midst of rising inflation and the economic crisis, to balance their budgets. In this context, many universities were forced to cut back on the establishment of new PhD programs.[152] Indeed, when the College of Nursing submitted its proposal, Illinois was operating under fiscal constraints, and as a result, the state's Board of Higher Education placed a moratorium on all new doctoral programs.[153] Nevertheless, as the college's dean, Mary Lohr, explained, the proposal for the nursing PhD program received overwhelming support from its reviewers, each of whom "expressed the belief that the impact of graduates of the program upon health care delivery in Illinois and the Midwest would be so significant that the moratorium on new doctoral programs was lifted so plans to offer the program could proceed."[154]

The University of Illinois Chicago College of Nursing's PhD in nursing program was approved in May 1975 and enrolled its first students that fall.[155]

Nursing schools also utilized state health workforce concerns to convince reluctant university administrators to endorse their application for a doctoral program in nursing. In the early 1970s at Wayne State University, for example, the provost, Hank Bohm, suggested the College of Nursing proceed "cautiously" with its plans for a PhD program, expressing concern about the research productivity of the college and uncertainty about how a doctoral program would be financed.[156] To overcome Bohm's reluctance, however, the dean of graduate studies and the chairman of the graduate council's committee on new PhD programs advised the college to make clear in their proposal that the college would be preparing "nurses for faculty positions in the State." Such a strategy would be particularly effective, they argued, given that the University of Michigan, the state's land-grant school, did not currently have a doctoral program in nursing and reports from the University of Michigan School of Nursing indicated that the school had "decided doctoral program may be unfeasible at this time in their school."[157] This state workforce argument, together with the supportive connections the College of Nursing had forged with faculty in the behavioral, social, and biomedical sciences (see chapter 3), led to the university approving the PhD in nursing in the spring of 1975.[158] That same year, the University of Michigan School of Nursing also launched its PhD in nursing.

When the University of Minnesota School of Nursing began planning for a doctoral program in the early 1970s, the nursing faculty confronted "considerable opposition within the general University faculty," who questioned whether nursing had the theoretical underpinnings and a distinct body of knowledge to justify the PhD, and whether the nursing faculty had the research capabilities to conduct scholarly research.[159] However, ongoing concerns about the state's nursing workforce, exacerbated by the shortages of qualified nursing faculty, generated substantive support for the nursing PhD among the state's nursing leaders, health planners, and policymakers.

In 1980, the American Nurses Association Council on State Boards was planning to implement a new policy that required all faculty teaching in basic nursing programs to hold at least a master's degree. In Minnesota in 1977, only 23 percent of the faculty in baccalaureate programs held a BSN as the highest earned credential and less than 5 percent of the state's BSN faculty had a doctoral degree. In the state's AD programs, 51 percent of faculty held either a BSN or AD as their highest earned credential.[160] The Advisory Committee on Nursing Education of the Minnesota Higher Education Coordinating Commission warned that five hundred additional nurses prepared at the master's level were currently needed, both for faculty and for advanced practice and clinical leadership positions in hospitals and health care agencies, but the state's only two master's programs at the University of Minnesota were "unable to accommodate all qualified applications."[161] The committee put it at a "conservative estimate" that 150 doctorally prepared nurses were needed in the state. As of 1978, there were "fewer than twenty-five nurses" in Minnesota who were "known to have doctoral degrees."[162]

Given these figures, nursing schools throughout the state were struggling to recruit appropriately qualified faculty. In 1977, Edna L. Thayer, acting chairperson of the Division of Nursing at Mankato State University, wrote to the dean of the University of Minnesota School of Nursing, Irene Ramey, reflecting on "the extreme difficulty in recruiting a chairperson with a doctoral degree" to the nursing program at Mankato State. The school was also interested in employing nursing faculty with doctoral degrees who could provide "expertise in clinical nursing, curriculum design, research, and evaluation," which was "needed among the faculty to continue to improve the quality of the nursing educational program." Thayer noted that in addition to herself she knew "of many other nurses in Minnesota who would like to pursue a doctoral degree but [were] restricted geographically from reaching this goal." Instead, she and her colleagues were forced to "continue in positions which should be filled with people having more academic preparation because there [were] no applicants who qualif[ied] academically."[163] The Department of Nursing at Gustavus Adolphus College was also struggling to recruit qualified faculty. As the department's chairperson, Hazel M. Johnson, wrote to Dean Ramey in 1977 regarding the eight years Johnson had served as chair of nursing, explaining, "Only once have I been able to choose from three qualified applicants for a full-time position. For the other vacancies (probably 12) there has been one person available and in two of these situations we did not have anyone with a master's degree apply."[164] Thayer and Johnson, along with scores of other nurse educators throughout the state, strongly supported the University of Minnesota School of Nursing's efforts to establish a PhD program, which would prepare the faculty needed not only to sustain but also to expand the state's existing nursing education programs.

The University of Minnesota School of Nursing mobilized this support and the argument that its PhD program was essential to meeting the state's need for both a larger and higher quality nursing workforce in its final proposal for the PhD program.[165] Despite ongoing ambivalence among some of the proposal's reviewers, the School of Nursing's proposal was narrowly approved by the Health Sciences Policy and Review Council and eventually, through a series of other university committees, by the Board of Regents in the spring of 1982. The School of Nursing admitted its first three doctoral students in the fall of 1983.[166] In Minnesota, as they did in Illinois and Michigan and a host of other states, nursing educators were joined by health policymakers in calling for the establishment of nursing PhD programs so as to increase the state's supply of doctorally prepared nursing faculty. By producing more doctorally prepared nurses, they persuasively argued, the state's nursing schools could improve the quality and expand the scale of masters, baccalaureate, and associate degree–level education.

Conclusions

State nursing workforce and health care needs were thus critically embedded within nursing's academic project. Over the course of the 1970s, in states throughout the U.S., health planners and policymakers worked with state-funded nursing schools to facilitate educational mobility for graduates of LPN, diploma, and AD programs; to develop and expand nurse practitioner programs; and to increase the number of qualified nursing faculty in the state. These examples reveal the ways in which state policymakers looked to state-funded AHCs and the health professional schools within them to produce enough of the "right type" of health care professionals willing to work in underserved regions of the state. These examples also make clear the tensions that characterize state-funded nursing schools and the AHCs of which they are part: tension with the states that fund them, the state and federal health policies that direct them, and the professional and educational imperatives of their constituent faculty.

As nursing schools and nursing organizations worked to resolve some of the difficulties of educational mobility for diploma and AD-trained nurses, debates over those measures—and about the merits of maintaining multiple educational pathways into nursing—continued. Nevertheless, nursing leaders were unwilling to give up the multiple pathways for entry into practice because of the stakes involved for those institutions currently preparing nurses at the diploma, AD, and BSN level, and for the nurses who earned these degrees—*and* because the multiple pathways into practice enable social mobility for "nurses who may have chosen the wrong path for entry into nursing, or who now have the resources to pursue advanced education."[167] Indeed, by the early 2000s, the importance of those multiple pathways to increasing the diversity of the nursing workforce and to improving access to higher levels of education particularly among underrepresented populations, were readily apparent. As historian Patricia D'Antonio has documented, the "numbers of nurses earning a bachelor's degree or higher over a lifetime rose from 9 percent in 1960 to 47 percent in 2004," which far exceeds the proportion of American women in general who earned baccalaureate degrees over their lifetime through 2004. "The advantages accrued to American nurses of color," D'Antonio continues, "are even more pronounced." Although data on the numbers of women of color earning baccalaureate degrees prior to the civil rights movement is problematic, D'Antonio writes, "data from both 2000 and 2004 suggest that the current proportion of nurses of color with bachelor's degrees earned over a lifetime is greater than that for white nurses, still the predominant group of American nurses." For example, "in 2004, only 46 percent of white nurses had earned a bachelor's degree at some point in their lives. By contrast, 52 percent of African American nurses and 72 percent of Asian or Pacific Islander nurses could point to such an accomplishment. Hispanic nurses match their white colleagues at 46 percent."[168] More recent government data confirms that nurses of color "are slightly more likely than their white counterparts to obtain a baccalaureate or higher degree during their careers."[169]

In the early 2000s, the entry into practice debate took on a new spin. The introduction of a new practice doctorate, the doctorate of nursing practice (DNP), shifted the focus to entry into specialty practice. The DNP, many nursing leaders argued, should replace clinical master's degrees and designate entry into advanced nursing practice.[170] The conclusion to this book describes the efforts by nursing educators to establish a professional doctorate comparable to the professional doctorates in medicine, dentistry, and pharmacy, introduced initially as a postbaccalaureate entry-level generalist degree in the late 1970s, and subsequently, in the late 1990s, as the advanced practice degree. The next chapter, however, highlights another consequence of nursing's postwar academic project: an essential severing of the relationship between nursing education and nursing's practice base. Because the faculty in baccalaureate and graduate nursing programs rarely held clinical appointments in the teaching hospital's nursing service, the nursing content of baccalaureate and graduate curricula were often divorced from the realities and needs of clinical practice. And as we saw in earlier chapters, nurses in practice often complained that nurse scientists were not asking research questions relevant to practice, and that nurse theorists were failing to develop and test their theories in practice settings.

Beginning in the late 1950s, a small group of nurse educators began calling for the establishment of academic leadership in nursing. Predicated on the medical model of professional education, nursing faculty would participate in the tripartite academic mission of research, education, *and* practice, and nursing schools would have responsibility for and authority over the quality of nursing education, care, and research that took place in teaching hospitals and clinics. Academic leadership in nursing would, they argued, lead to improvements in nursing education, ensure the clinical relevance of nursing research and theory development, and secure nursing's equal status among the other health professions within academic health centers. The development of a professional doctorate was integral to this effort. In addition to putting the professional nurse on equal footing with the other doctorally prepared providers in the room (physicians, dentists, and pharmacists), advocates of the professional doctorate argued, the degree also provided nurses with the knowledge, skills, and expertise to serve as clinical leaders in a new era of patient-centered care and as clinical scholars able to both translate nursing science into improved patient care and identify areas in need of nursing research.

Academics in the Clinic

One of the consequences of nursing's academic project was an essential sev-ering of the relationship between nursing education and nursing's practice base. In hospital diploma programs, education and practice occurred in the same space and were overseen by the hospital's nursing service. In baccalau-reate programs, by contrast, education took place on university or college campuses and was directed by nursing faculty, while nursing practice took place in the university's teaching hospitals, overseen by the hospital's nursing service. Nursing faculty rarely held clinical appointments in the teaching hos-pital's nursing service. Indeed, for some nurse educators, a strict separation between education and practice was seen as essential to establishing nursing as an academic discipline. The education-service gap (as it came to be called), however, had profound implications for nursing's academic project: the nurs-ing content of baccalaureate and graduate curricula were often divorced from the realities and needs of clinical practice; nurses in practice complained that nurse scientists were not asking research questions relevant to practice, and nurse theorists were failing to develop and test their theories in practice set-tings. At the same time, the absence of nursing faculty from teaching hospi-tals meant they had little contact with physicians, which disadvantaged them as they sought to claim their rightful place as equals within the interprofes-sional health care team and within academic health center governance.[1]

For several nursing leaders, the location of a nursing school within an academic health center (AHC) afforded nursing faculty with both opportuni-ties and responsibilities. Within AHCs, health profession faculty had, in gen-eral, responsibility for education, research, and patient care. However, as the dean of Case Western Reserve University's (then Western Reserve Univer-sity) Frances Payne Bolton School of Nursing, Rozella Schlotfeldt, lamented in 1965, to date the role played by most nursing faculties within AHCs was "that of guest in the center's treatment and care facilities." Because nursing faculty did not have appointments within the AHC's teaching hospitals and clinics, they did not have "authority for establishing standards of nursing care in the university health centers." As a result, "neither patients nor students" were "well-served." It also meant that without guaranteed access to patients they had not had access to clinical research populations, and as a result, "inquiry into nursing practice problems ha[d] been impeded and advancement of knowledge in the field" was "woefully inadequate." It was time, Schlotfeldt argued, for nursing faculties to "become integral parts of the university health centers and to fulfill the three distinct functions that uniquely characterize[d] those centers, those of education, patient care, and research."[2]

Schlotfeldt was part of a small group of nursing leaders who saw the integration of nursing education and nursing service as critical to nursing's academic project. Beginning in the 1960s, this small but growing group of nurse educators began calling for the establishment of academic leadership in nursing, or what in the twenty-first century is referred to as academic nursing practice.[3] Predicated on the medical model of professional education, nursing faculty would participate in the tripartite academic mission of research, education, *and* practice, and nursing schools would have responsibility for and authority over the quality of nursing education, care, and research that took place in university's teaching hospitals and clinics. Academic nursing practice would, they argued, lead to improvements in nursing education and ensure the clinical relevance of nursing research and theory development. It would also ensure that nursing had an equal and parallel role to the other health professions within academic health centers. When the National Commission for the Study of Nursing and Nursing Education published its report in 1970, it echoed these calls for academic leadership in nursing and a "rapprochement" between nursing service and nursing education.[4] Academic leadership in nursing—in health care delivery, higher education, and policymaking— was also an early concern of the recently formed American Association of Deans of College and University Schools of Nursing, renamed the American Association of Colleges of Nursing in 1972 (see chapter 1).[5]

The nursing schools that experimented with unification in the 1960s and 1970s sought to bring academic nursing closer to the structural model of academic medicine. As Loretta Ford reflected in 1985, "Perhaps schools of nursing have tried so hard to be accepted in academe that they have followed the arts and science model," leading to the gap between nursing education and service.[6] For Ford, unification reflected academic nursing's first efforts to move nursing toward the "professional school model," typified by medicine.[7] But as the early unification efforts at the University of Florida, Case Western Reserve University, the University of Rochester, and Rush University made clear, academic medicine had its limits as a model for academic nursing. Most significantly, nursing faculty, unlike their colleagues in medicine, could not be reimbursed for nursing care services.

Because physicians billed for the services they performed and were reimbursed by third-party payers, they had the ability to generate substantial clinical income for medical schools and AHCs. As discussed in chapter 3, the passage of Medicare and Medicaid in 1965 greatly increased the availability of clinical income for physicians, which led medical schools to hire greater numbers of clinical faculty and helped underwrite the expansion of clinical research and undergraduate and graduate education in medical schools. The introduction of prospective payment and managed care in the 1980s, which reduced physicians' reimbursement rates, put greater onus on the clinical faculty of medical schools to increase their volume of clinical work.[8] Nurses, however, were salaried employees and were not directly reimbursed for their services. Instead, the costs of nursing care were wrapped into the total cost for hospital services, making it difficult to tease out the contributions of nurses to the bottom line of hospitals. For nursing faculty to be compensated for their clinical practice required that nursing deans and faculty negotiate individually with the hospital and other service agencies. But as neither public nor private insurers directly reimbursed nurse practitioners, clinical nurse specialists, or other advanced practice nurses (to say nothing of registered nurses) for their services until the late 1990s, these negotiations invariably generated mixed results.[9] Thus, at least until the late 1990s, academic nurses who engaged in clinical practice had no mechanism for generating clinical income. The revenue for most nursing schools instead came from state support, tuition, and grants. Within AHCs, however, schools whose faculty were able to bring in substantial research funding or generate clinical revenue—or both, as was the case of medical schools—had greater budgetary flexibility and institutional power with which to expand and innovate.

The model of academic medicine also proved limited in facilitating interprofessional collaboration among nurses and physicians in education, practice, and research settings. The academic nurses who worked to rebuild the connection between education and practice, and establish academic nursing as parallel and complementary to academic medicine, also confronted resistance from physicians and hospital administrators all too comfortable with the gendered and hierarchical status quo within academic health centers.

Enter the Clinical Nurse Specialists

The ability of nursing schools in the 1960s and 1970s to establish integrated models of education, research, and practice depended on the implementation of an educational hierarchy within nursing, and on two key roles: the clinical nurse specialist and the practitioner-teacher. During the 1960s, several nursing educators conceptualized the role of the clinical nurse specialist (also referred to as the clinical specialist or nurse clinician). This was a nurse who had undertaken advanced clinical education in a specialty area and was prepared for leadership positions within service agencies and educational institutions. At the University of Florida, founding dean of nursing Dorothy Smith introduced the clinical specialist, an expert clinician responsible—within each patient care unit of the hospital—for planning the patients' nursing care and distributing the components of each nursing care plan to the members of her team, matching levels of skill with complexity of task. The clinical specialist carried these responsibilities twenty-four hours a day, seven days a week.[10] At New York Medical College, the dean of nursing Francis Reiter developed the nurse clinician role, drawing upon the experiences of Smith at the University of Florida. Reiter's nurse clinician was responsible "for *coordinating* all the various services relating directly to the patient's welfare," as well as "for *continuity* of care" for the duration of the patient's hospitalization, discharge, and follow-up. She was also responsible for collaborating with the physician and other members of the patient's health care team so as "to achieve the therapeutic, restorative, and rehabilitative goals set for the patient."[11] In practice, the nurse clinician was to have the "authorized responsibility for nursing practice within a given area," comparable to the responsibility of the physician for medical management of the patient. "Like the physician," the nurse clinician "might be on 24-hour call—for consultation and decision-making whenever nursing practice problems occur."[12] Reiter's concept of the nurse clinician thus built upon Dorothy Smith's concept of the clinical specialist.

At Cornell University-New York Hospital School of Nursing, Laura Simms developed the clinical nurse specialist role as an expert clinician to ensure the continuity and comprehensiveness of nursing care given to patients. As with Smith's clinical specialist and Reiter's nurse clinician, Simms's clinical nurse specialist was responsible for developing and implementing the nursing care plan for each patient and coordinating each patient's care with all members of the patient's health care team. Through the coordination and leadership of the clinical nurse specialist, the patient would "experience hospitalization and follow-up care as a continuous whole rather than a series of isolated activities."[13] Simms first introduced the clinical nurse specialist role on the cardiac surgery unit, but soon added additional clinical nurse specialist positions in other units in the hospital.[14]

In all three cases, this expert clinician was to assume leadership for patient care within hospitals and other service institutions. In addition, Smith and Reiter argued that this expert clinician also had a vital role to play within nursing education. In their view, the clinical nurse specialist was to have responsibility for clinical education within the service institution and as such should hold a faculty position in the nursing school. For both Reiter and Smith, nursing school faculty should combine the two responsibilities of practice and of teaching. As Reiter asserted, "I do not believe you can do one without the other."[15]

Although the terms *nurse clinician*, *clinical specialist*, and *clinical nurse specialist* were used interchangeably during the decade, by the end of the 1960s nursing leaders had settled on the title of clinical nurse specialist. So, too, nursing educators had determined that the advanced education of clinical nurse specialists would take place in clinical master's degree programs. As discussed in chapter 1, Hildegard Peplau had first called for the specialized clinical training of psychiatric nurses at the master's degree level in the 1950s, and by the end of the 1950s a handful of nursing schools had established clinical master's programs in psychiatric nursing. The clinical master's degree program was to replace the functional master's degree that prepared nurses for roles as administrators, educators, or clinical supervisors. Beginning in the 1960s and intensifying during the 1970s, nursing schools introduced clinical master's programs in a growing range of specialty areas, including maternal-child health, medical-surgical nursing, oncology, nephrology, and critical care nursing.[16]

By creating a leadership role for the clinical nurse specialist within academic nursing, unification of nursing education and service facilitated the development of and reinforced the need for clinical master's programs. In turn, clinical nurse specialists emerged as critical figures in the clinical education of the nursing students who trained within their service institutions, and in the translation of new nursing knowledge into transformed practice. As the University of Illinois Chicago's Helen Grace elaborated, "it is not enough to be developing a core of nurse researchers who are directed toward developing a body of nursing knowledge. This must be coupled with a group of equally prepared expert clinicians who take this body of knowledge into the clinical practice arena, apply it in the care of patients, and test out the effects of new approaches in the patient care situation. In this systematic way, nursing can begin to demonstrate that application of nursing knowledge does make a profound difference upon the quality of the life experience."[17] In other words, clinical nurse specialists had an integral role to play in demonstrating the improvements in health outcomes achievable through the research of nurse scientists. They were also critical to the efforts of nurse leaders to unify nursing education and nursing service.

The Service-Education Gap

The relocation of nursing education from hospitals to university and college campuses after World War II had essentially severed the relationship between nursing education and its practice base. In nursing schools during this period, nursing faculty rarely held clinical positions in the teaching hospital's nursing service. For Dorothy Smith, who was dean of nursing at the University of Florida during the late 1950s and 1960s, the situation "was so bad" that "anyone who worked with students in a clinical area was called [a] clinical instructor and they usually did not have very much education. They were second-class citizens." Meanwhile, the education-oriented nursing faculty "were standing in classrooms telling people what they ought to do, and screaming about how bad things were in the hospital because the nursing staff did not know anything."[18]

Some nurse educators regarded a strict separation between education and practice as essential to establishing nursing as an academic discipline. As Mary Kelly Mullane, dean of nursing at the University of Illinois Chicago, acknowledged, in the postwar decades, nursing education and nursing service "had to be separated . . . in order that each might develop its unique purpose without distraction or hindrance from the other."[19] As described in earlier chapters, nursing faculty in this period were expected to focus on teaching, curriculum development, and educational administration; effective teaching was the primary marker for university promotion. Some educators argued that by taking time away from these educational roles, faculty engagement in clinical practice would only undermine nursing's academic goals. The outcome, the University of Iowa's Myrtle Aydelotte noted, was that many faculty members "have virtually withdrawn from practice settings and are no longer seen has persons knowledgeable about nursing care."[20]

By the 1960s, nursing leaders—in education and in practice—warned of the dangers of separating education from practice. Because faculty and students were separated physically, psychologically, and experientially from clinicians, the nursing content of baccalaureate and graduate curricula was often divorced from the realities and needs of clinical practice, and as such, students were receiving inadequate clinical education.[21] As Schlotfeldt saw it, the fact that nursing faculty "have largely withdrawn from personal involvement in nursing care and thus have divested themselves of responsibility for the quality of the clinical learning environment . . . has had adverse effects on both faculty and students and has been the single greatest deterrent for the development of nursing science."[22]

Nurse supervisors similarly lamented the quality of nursing education, complaining that BSN graduates arrived for their first clinical appointments inadequately prepared for the realities of practice. For example (and as described in chapter 1), at the University of Minnesota in the 1960s, members of the University Hospital's nursing service criticized the nursing faculty for not providing nursing students with adequate clinical education, particularly in the biomedical sciences. As Duke University's Thelma Ingles summarized the tensions in 1962, "Unfortunately, the 'degree' nurse is not wholeheartedly accepted" by physicians, hospitals administrators, or diploma-trained nurses. "Doctors are concerned about her because she does not 'mind' as well as the good old nurse; hospital administrators and nursing service staffs are concerned about her because she does not contribute as many hours of work as former students." Furthermore, Ingles continued, "Many service nurses who themselves graduated from hospital schools, criticize her 'new-fangled' concepts of nursing care."[23]

The problem came down to a difference in expectations. In classrooms, nursing faculty were teaching students "one set of facts and values—that as a nurse she is to be concerned with the *total* care of her patients, with the psychological, social and physiological ramifications of illness as they affect each patient. Equipped with a modicum of basic information from the psychological, sociological and physiological sciences, she is told that she is to care for the whole patient." But once nursing students entered the hospital, they confronted a different set of expectations. Nursing service personnel were "concerned with the tasks which must be accomplished in order to keep the [ward and hospital systems] running smoothly. Beds must be made, pills passed, treatments given." As Ingles saw it, nursing staff "seem more concerned with the composite needs of the ward than with the needs of individual patients."[24]

In order to succeed in the hospital environment, nursing students were expected to comply with the nursing service values and expectations and disregard those of the faculty. At the same time, nursing students confronted the differing expectations of nursing faculty and hospital physicians. While the faculty were teaching students "to see beyond the disease process per se, to look at patients in their total social context," many physicians remained concerned, primarily, "with the management of the specific physiological problems of their patients, with the treatment of disease."[25] "This conceptual difference in patient care," along with the differential values and expectations between nursing faculty and nursing service personnel, was, Ingles concluded, creating "not only a schism between nurses and doctors and nurses and hospital administrators, but an even more devastating schism between nurses and nurses." Thus, nursing students in university programs in the early 1960s were, Ingles concluded, "caught in the inexorable 'squeeze' of a changing system."[26] Given all this, as the dean of the University of Illinois Chicago Mary Kelly Mullane argued at the end of the 1960s, the "time has come for reunification of nursing practice (not nursing service) and nursing education in the teaching hospitals and agencies that constitute the practice and research laboratories for nursing students and professors."[27]

The University of Florida College of Nursing was the first university-based nursing school to pursue unification. As a case study, it makes clear that the integration of education and service depended on replacing the traditional administrative hierarchy in nursing service with an educational hierarchy, and on the role of practitioner-teachers and the newly emergent role of the clinical nurse specialist. It also highlights the tensions that characterized the effort to unify nursing education and service, particularly those between the nursing faculty and the teaching hospital's staff nurses, and those between the nursing and physician leadership within the teaching hospital. It also reveals the challenges that confronted academic nurses as they pursued leadership within academic health centers.

Unifying Nursing Service and Nursing Education at the University of Florida

In 1956, the founding dean of the University of Florida College of Nursing, Dorothy Smith, had seen the integration of education and service as critical to the successful education of future nurses and the advance of the profession. For Smith, "the crux" of the "traditional friction between nursing education and nursing services [lay] . . . in the lack of belief that each group [was] equally important . . . and in the failure to recognize expertness and experience in nursing practice with the same economic and social rewards accorded to nurse educators."[28] Smith saw in unification the opportunity to overcome that friction by making it clear that service and education were equally important and integrally related.[29]

When Smith arrived at the University of Florida, the AHC was being established. Organizationally and administratively, the deans and the hospital administrator were granted equal authority and institutional responsibility within the health center.[30] With the support of the other health science deans, the provost, and the university president, Smith was able to implement her vision for nursing education, which was premised on the unification of the university school of nursing with the university hospital nursing service. Smith took as her model that of academic medicine in which the dean of the medical school was also chief of the teaching hospital's medical staff, the medical school's department chairs were also chiefs of the specialty medical services in the teaching hospital, and the medical faculty held clinical appointments and engaged in faculty practice within the teaching hospital.[31]

To this end, the unification of nursing was enacted through a series of dual appointments between the college and the hospital. Smith, as dean of the College of Nursing, was also chief of the hospital's nursing service with responsibility for nursing education, nursing research, and professional nursing practice. An assistant dean for nursing practice, a position held from 1959 through 1967 by Lucille Mercadante, served as chief of the nursing staff at the teaching hospital. Each unit within the hospital was led by a Nurse II who held a dual appointment in the hospital and a faculty appointment in the College of Nursing.[32] The Nurse IIs reported to the head of the clinical specialty section within the College of Nursing.[33] There were five clinical specialty sections—medical-surgical, pediatric nursing, psychiatric nursing, maternal and infant nursing, and public health nursing—all of which were headed by faculty members who were clinical experts in their designated specialty. While some nursing schools were beginning to move away from a department structure premised on the medical specialties, Smith "deliberately chose the medical set up because that is where the patients were and that is where the doctors were."[34] For Smith, it was important to establish a parallel structure to the College of Medicine in order to facilitate collaborative practice between medicine and nursing. For example, "'If we had a section of adult nursing,' she explained, 'Where would you go to find your patients and your doctors[?] It would have been a mess.'"[35] At the same time, it was a departmental model that the university recognized and accepted.[36]

Central to Smith's unified model of nursing was the elimination of the traditional administrative hierarchy in nursing, in which nurses moving up the hierarchy—from assistant head nurse to head nurse to nurse supervisor—invariably moved further away from direct patient care toward personnel management and other administrative responsibilities.[37] In its place, Smith instituted an educational hierarchy in which the best educated nurses would be closest to the patient.[38] As part of this, Smith established the role of clinical specialist. As discussed earlier, this nurse was an expert clinician responsible for planning the patients' nursing care and distributing the components of each nursing care plan to the members of her team. The Nurse IIs were to be clinical specialists and, within each patient care unit, were responsible for planning the patients' nursing care and distributing the components of each nursing care plan to the members of their team, matching levels of skill with complexity of task.[39] In this way, the Nurse II's responsibilities paralleled those of the attending physician, who was likewise responsible for consultation and decision-making related to the patient for the duration of the patient's admission to the hospital.

To ensure that nurses' time and talents were being used for nursing care activities rather than for non-nursing activities, Smith developed and implemented a unit manager system. In this system, the hospital assigned a non-nurse unit manager who was administratively responsible for the management of the entire nursing floor, which included maintaining supporting services to nursing and ensuring the unit had adequate supplies and material resources.[40] The hospital also appointed ward clerks to perform all clerical work related to the functioning of the unit, such as transcribing physician orders and routine requisitions, and answering the phone.[41] By freeing up the "best prepared" nurses to focus on bedside nursing, the unit manager system was integral to Smith's unified model of nursing and the educational hierarchy on which it was predicated.[42]

The faculty's "dual responsibility" as teacher-practitioners was also critical to the unified model and its educational hierarchy.[43] To this end, all of the faculty taught at least one clinical course and also taught "some kind of nursing on the units" in the teaching hospital. In addition, the faculty would "select certain patients whom they will carry themselves in order that they learn more about nursing or in order that they help some of the nursing service people with problems."[44] In some cases, particularly when the assistant dean for nursing practice was unable to find appropriately qualified staff nurses, faculty were appointed as Nurse IIs.[45] Nursing staff, in turn, helped the faculty teach the nursing students.[46]

In several of the clinical specialty sections, including the maternal-infant, pediatric, and psychiatry / mental health sections, the faculty in charge of the section worked "beautifully together" with the Nurse II.[47] In other sections, such as medical-surgical nursing, however, the collaborative effort, as Mercadante recalled, "did not quite click off as well." Difficulties stemmed from "power struggles" between the faculty, who were master's- and, in some cases, doctorally prepared, and the Nurse IIs, very few of whom had master's degrees. As Mercadante explained, the "power struggle" centered, in large part, on who was "better qualified" or "better educated to make these decisions." But the power struggle was also a result of a dismantling of the traditional administrative hierarchy in nursing in which the head nurse (a position now reframed as the Nurse II role) had held full authority and control over nursing activities on her unit. In the traditional model, a faculty member would have to negotiate with the head nurse to secure access to patients, either to provide bedside care or for the clinical education of students. In the new educational hierarchy, the Nurse IIs worked *with* the faculty to ensure the quality of nursing care on the unit.[48]

There were also tensions between the faculty and the Nurse Is, who were the staff nurses of the traditional nursing service hierarchy. Although Smith pushed for an all-BSN staff, many of the Nurse Is, especially in the early years of the University of Florida model, were diploma-trained nurses. This often led to friction between the faculty and the Nurse Is. As Mercadante explained, "You would get graduates from the diploma schools who would have had ten, twelve, fifteen years of experience, practicing, taking care of patients, if you will. And along comes a faculty person with a Master's degree, maybe one year of experience. There was this feeling," among the Nurse Is, "of you are going to tell me what to do? This is my patient, I have the experience."[49] Edna Mae Jones, a faculty member in medical-surgical nursing, recalled that the diploma-trained nurses who worked in the teaching hospital also questioned the quality of education being given to the BSN students. Because the students were not in the hospital all the time, the diploma-trained nurses assumed the students would "never know how to do anything" because they were not receiving the same number of clinical hours the diploma-trained nurses had received as students. "It was difficult for the student to work around" nurses who held that attitude, Jones explained.[50] Smith frequently lamented what she called the "diploma school mentality" and worked with Mercadante to hire an all-BSN staff at the teaching hospital.[51] They encountered persistent difficulties with recruitment, however, because of the "terrible" salaries at the teaching hospital.[52]

Smith's system not only relied upon but also established the basis for nurses educated in clinically based master's degree programs.[53] Smith needed clinically expert faculty to lead the college's clinical specialty sections and clinical nurse specialists to serve as Nurse IIs in charge of the specialty clinical units. Initially, the University of Florida College of Nursing had established a traditional functional master's degree that prepared students for roles in administration or education, but in 1964, Smith and her faculty established clinical master's programs in psychiatric-mental health nursing, pediatric nursing, and medical-surgical nursing.[54] By valuing and providing a clear leadership role within the teaching hospital and university for the expert clinical nurse specialist, Smith's unification model validated the expansion of clinically oriented graduate education.

In Smith's unified model, nursing and medicine shared control for patient care, with each contributing their respective clinical expertise to ensure comprehensive patient care.[55] The effectiveness of collaborative patient care, however, depended on the individuals involved. While physicians in obstetrics and pediatrics were responsive and collaborated well, others were resistant.[56] Pauline Barton, who chaired the section of pediatric nursing, recalled, "Our pediatricians really supported us in what we were doing . . . We did not fight the battles that some of the other nursing faculty had to fight."[57] Some of the most challenging "battles" took place on the surgical units. For example, in the early 1960s, cardiac surgeon Myron Wheat Jr. heavily criticized the ways in which the College of Nursing was educating nursing students and staunchly opposed nursing leadership within the teaching hospital.[58] As Betty Hilliard recalled, "There were a lot of doctors—a lot of people, but particularly, the doctors—were vocal. They used to say that we were training psychological nurses" who "wouldn't be able to do anything." But what this vocal group of physicians wanted, Hilliard believed, was to have "their handmaidens back; that was all they needed. So they just didn't go along" with the changes that Smith was implementing.[59]

Despite the resistance Smith encountered among her colleagues at the University of Florida, nursing leaders from across the country and outside the U.S. visited the university to learn about its unified model and the unit manager system.[60] This included Loretta Ford and Luther Christman, who each went on to establish unified models at the University of Rochester and Rush University in Chicago, respectively.[61] Smith and her colleagues also wrote to and visited colleagues throughout the country, describing the system at the University of Florida.[62] As faculty member and anthropologist-in-residence Carol Taylor pointed out to Smith in 1968, "It seems ironic that the innovations for which you and the Teaching Hospital have become famous continue to be subjected to periodic attack."[63] But as Smith later reflected, it was the very "success of [their] mission" that "became a threat to the medical and hospital establishment."[64]

For as long as Smith's chief supporters and fellow advocates of the unified model remained in place in the health center, Smith was able to overcome the dissenters. As Betty Hilliard recalled, through the mid-1960s, "the key people" in the health center, including Dorothy Smith, Russell Poor (the first provost), George Harrell (the first dean of the College of Medicine), and Samuel Martin (who was chair of the Department of Medicine prior to being appointed the health center's second provost in 1962), "all were in agreement that what was happening, should happen. And so they were all supporting it and making it happen."[65] However, by 1969, Poor, Harrell, and Martin had left the University of Florida and had been replaced by leaders within the College of Medicine and the health center "who came from, say, more traditional backgrounds" and did not share Smith's commitment to an integrated model of academic nursing.[66]

By 1969, this included the chief of staff at the Shands Teaching Hospital, cardiac surgeon Myron Wheat. As noted earlier, Wheat had long been critical of the unified model and the nurses it was educating. Wheat argued that as chief of staff he, rather than the College of Nursing, should be responsible for nursing services in the hospital.[67] Things came to head when Wheat, in a written statement he asked to be read at a public meeting, criticized a grant proposal written by members of the nursing faculty to support the development of a clinical nurse specialist program at the health center. Wheat used the opportunity to attack the quality of the nursing service.[68] Smith wrote to the provost, Edmund Ackell, after the meeting, objecting to Wheat's actions and alerting Ackell, "This is the kind of behavior to which nursing is being subjected day in and day out."[69] Smith continued, "I suppose this kind of tactic is meant to 'wear us down,' and there is some indication that the objective is being met."[70] As Julie Fairman has written of the situation, this episode was one of many that "kept Smith and her faculty preoccupied with the politics rather than the practice of patient care."[71]

By that time, Smith was also facing growing opposition among many of the nurses who worked in the teaching hospital, led by a new assistant dean for nursing practice who, immediately after being hired, worked to replace the educational hierarchy with the traditional administrative hierarchy, reintroducing the roles of head nurse and nurse supervisor, and to eliminate the unified model in which Nurse IIs had served on the faculty.[72] Smith was also finding it ever more difficult to secure resources for nursing. In 1969, Smith wrote to Ackell requesting an increase in nursing salaries in order to tackle the high nursing turnover the hospital was facing. Smith was frustrated that she was "expected to produce miracles yet [saw] very little evidence that the priorities of the hospital, including nursing, [were] being considered in a realistic way." Smith warned Ackell, "[If the] needs of the Medical School and of the physicians continue to take priority . . . the end result will be that not even Medicine can continue to function well. We all suffer—including the patient."[73] Six months later, in 1970, Smith wrote again to Ackell protesting "the steady decline in support services for nursing." Smith called on Ackell to provide "equitable funding" to the hospital's "care functions." "It will be a catastrophe," Smith argued, "if this Health Center does not try to demonstrate both aspects of healing (care and cure) through some kind of equitable funding." Raising broader concerns about the ever-growing emphasis being placed within health care on high-tech, interventionist medicine, Smith continued, "More and more machines, more and more beds, more and more emergency admissions—without care aspect—make this place a poor environment for students to learn the fundamentals of supposedly service professions."[74]

By that summer, as tensions between Smith, the College of Medicine, and the hospital administration continued and financial support for nursing languished, Ackell separated the College of Nursing from the hospital's nursing service, thereby disbanding Smith's unified model of nursing. In response, Smith wrote that the college did "not wish to take advantage of the '6 month trial period' which allows the College of Nursing to be administratively involved in nursing service." For Smith, this arrangement was "unrealistic." She wrote, "It has been made very clear that the Hospital Director and the Chief of Staff are opposed to the College of Nursing involvement, and we no longer wish to be engaged in this kind of power struggle."[75] In January 1971, Smith resigned her position as dean, effective October of that year.[76] Although she remained on the faculty for several years, the era of unified nursing at the University of Florida was over.

Although the integrated model at the University of Florida was short lived, the Frances Payne Bolton School of Nursing at Case Western Reserve University during the 1960s, and the nursing schools at Rush University and the University of Rochester during the early 1970s, established integrated models of nursing education, research, and practice with their university teaching hospitals.[77] They all did so at the same time that their universities were establishing academic health centers.[78] This enabled the nursing schools' leaders to capitalize on—as Smith had done at the University of Florida—their university's commitment to shared governance among the health professions schools and teaching hospitals on their campuses.[79] In all three cases, the deans of nursing drew upon Smith's experiences at Florida, modeling their own experiments in academic nursing practice upon those at Florida. Indeed, all three experiments centered on implementing an educational hierarchy within the teaching hospitals' nursing service and on the integral roles of the clinical nurse specialists and practitioner-teachers.

Models of Academic Nursing Practice

In 1961, the Frances Payne Bolton School of Nursing at Case Western Reserve University entered into a collaborative arrangement with the University Hospitals of Cleveland. Unlike the fully unified model implemented by Dorothy Smith at the University of Florida, the model implemented by Case Western Reserve University's dean of nursing, Rozella Schlotfeldt, was one of institutional collaboration. While at the University of Florida the College of Nursing and the hospital were under one administration and one budget,

Case Western Reserve University and the University Hospitals of Cleveland were two private, independent organizations, each with their own administration, governing board, and budget. In this institutional context, it was not feasible to fully unify nursing education and nursing service. Instead, Schlotfeldt hoped that by establishing a structure in which the nursing faculty and nursing service administrators and personnel worked together, they could still effectively bridge the gap between the two groups.[80]

The plan, which Schlotfeldt described as "academic leadership for nursing," granted the School of Nursing responsibility for and authority over the quality of nursing education, nursing care, and nursing research that took place in the University Hospitals.[81] In this way, the nursing faculty would join the faculties of the other health professions schools at Case Western Reserve University (which included medicine and dentistry) in assuming authority and "responsibility for the quality of patient care, education, and research in all of the agencies used for education of health science students."[82] This responsibility would be exercised through a series of joint appointments. Nurses (holding a minimum of a master's degree in nursing) in leadership positions in the University Hospitals were appointed to the School of Nursing's clinical faculty and were "accountable for the quality of care provided in the clinical setting," ensuring that it was of a high enough quality for students to be taught and observe. As clinical faculty, they could participate in teaching, serve as preceptors for students, provide consultation to students and staff, and participate in curriculum development and committee work in the School of Nursing.[83] In turn, all tenured and tenure-track faculty members whose teaching, practice, and research activities required use of the clinical resources of the University Hospitals were given a hospital appointment.[84] These faculty were responsible for "influencing the quality of nursing care" to ensure it was of "the caliber desired for students to observe and emulate."[85] Reflecting the value placed by the school on faculty practice—and seen by the dean as essential to ensuring academic leadership for nursing—faculty participation in clinical practice was recognized and rewarded as a legitimate part of the faculty role within the system of promotion and tenure.[86]

In the early 1960s, Schlotfeldt and her faculty pilot tested the project in psychiatric nursing at the University Hospitals. Following the success of the pilot project, Case Western Reserve University secured funding from the W. K. Kellogg Foundation to implement the concept of academic leadership for nursing throughout all clinical areas.[87] The subsequent five-year demonstration project was led by Jannetta MacPhail.[88] Although measurable outcomes were difficult to assess, for McPhail, a major outcome of the experiment was that there was "no longer a sense of 'we' and 'they' but rather 'us.'" Instead of only being concerned with education, the nursing faculty had "a sense of responsibility for the quality of nursing practice and maintaining their own competence."[89]

For the faculty who engaged in clinical practice, the expectations of the new role could be highly rewarding. For example, as two faculty-clinicians reflected, "Rather than being drawn apart by the demands of two systems, the stems are themselves pulled together by the activities of the clinician." In this way, they continued, the faculty-clinician "bridges the two systems by encouraging relevant educational experiences for nursing students while serving as a role model for practitioners."[90] MacPhail also reported "evidence of a more scholarly approach to nursing practice, questioning, and testing new ideas."[91] After five years, the School of Nursing and University Hospitals of Cleveland deemed the model sufficiently successful and decided to continue the joint endeavor.[92]

During the early 1970s, the nursing schools at the University of Rochester and Rush University also established integrated models of nursing education and nursing service. Both schools were established as equal and parallel units within newly organized academic health centers.[93] The University of Rochester School of Nursing was founded in 1972, with Loretta Ford as its first dean. As Julie Fairman has described, from its conceptualization in the late 1960s, the school was premised on a unified model of academic nursing.[94] The school had complete responsibility for nursing education, practice, and research, and as dean, Ford also held the position of director of nursing in the University of Rochester's teaching hospital, Strong Memorial Hospital. Within the new academic health center, the School of Nursing was established "on a par with" the School of Medicine and Dentistry.[95] Within the University of Rochester Medical Center, nursing's organizational structure paralleled that of medicine and hospital administration. Ford had visited the University of Florida in the 1960s to learn about Smith's unification model and Smith's ideas clearly influenced Ford's thinking. Indeed, the organizational structure within the school was similar to that implemented by Smith at the University of Florida. Nursing leadership within the medical center consisted of "clinical nursing chiefs, associate chiefs, and nurses holding the title of clinician II, all of whom hold faculty appointments. They are joined," explained Margaret Sovie, University of Rochester's associate dean for nursing practice, "by nurses who hold the title clinician I, and their assistants, both of whom manage and direct each patient care unit."[96] Every nurse in the medical center carried "responsibilities for nursing education, practice, and research."[97]

The unification model instituted by Luther Christman at the College of Nursing at Rush University also drew upon Smith's experiences at the University of Florida. Like Ford, Christman had visited the University of Florida in the 1960s to learn about the system in place there.[98] When the College of Nursing opened in 1972, Christman held the position of dean as well as vice president of nursing affairs in Rush-Presbyterian-St. Luke's Medical Center. In turn, the nursing faculty were responsible for education, service, and research, occupying all nursing leadership positions (including doctorally prepared department chairpersons; program directors for research, service, and education; and masters-prepared clinical nurse specialist unit leaders) within the medical center, and with a large number engaged in direct patient care.[99]

While there were structural differences among the integrated models implemented at Case Western Reserve University, the University of Rochester, and Rush University, they all shared with Smith's unified model several core components. First, all three replaced the traditional administrative hierarchy within the teaching hospital's nursing service with an educational hierarchy that rewarded nurses "for staying closely involved in patient care and becoming increasingly competent in practice."[100] As part of this, each school implemented the unit manager system within the teaching hospital to ensure that nurses' time and talents were being used for nursing care activities rather than non-nursing activities.[101]

Second, all three schools implemented an organizational structure that paralleled that of academic medicine, the goal of which was to establish with medicine shared responsibility and authority for patient care and to foster interprofessional collaboration in patient care, education, and research. Third, the integrated models implemented at Case Western Reserve University, the University of Rochester, and Rush University—like the University of Florida's unified model—all hinged on the pivotal role of the clinical nursing chiefs (ideally, doctorally prepared faculty), which paralleled that of the clinical chiefs in medicine, and on the work of clinical nurse specialists who functioned, in parallel, to medicine's attending physicians.[102] As such, unification relied upon and reinforced the need for master's-prepared clinical nurse specialists and for doctorally prepared, clinically competent faculty. In parallel, then, with the organizational changes, all three schools introduced doctoral programs (1972 at Case Western Reserve University, 1977 at Rush University, and 1979 at the University of Rochester) and expanded their clinical master's programs to encompass the clinical specialties within their teaching hospitals.[103] Doctoral and clinical master's programs were not only essential for producing the type of faculty who would take on the academic leadership of nursing within the academic health center, but also for development of the knowledge and clinical research base of advanced nursing practice.[104]

Fourth, each model utilized the system of primary nursing, which, in contrast to the team nursing model of care then dominant, assigned a specific nurse to a specific patient for the duration of the patient's hospital stay. The system of primary nursing was formally developed and introduced by Marie Manthey and colleagues at the University of Minnesota Hospital and Clinics in 1968, but it shared similarities to the system of nursing implemented by Smith at the University of Florida.[105] The primary nurse would, with the help of an associate (often a licensed practical nurse), be responsible for planning, implementing, and evaluating care for the patient. In this way, Ford likened the primary nurse "to the attending physician: he responsible for medical care and she for nursing care."[106] Indeed, for Christman, the system of primary nursing was essential if nursing was to share power within academic health centers. "Each nurse," Christman argued, "has to be exposed to the same responsibility for each patient as do our physician colleagues." Primary nursing did this by holding nurses accountable for the patient care they provided. "It is impossible," Christman continued, "to devise a consistent care plan for each patient unless the same nurses and the same physicians are planning together daily and then implementing their respective portions cooperatively. One cannot expect to be given power (rights and privileges) without accountability (obligations)."[107]

Finally, each model relied upon, validated, and prioritized the practitioner-teacher role first conceptualized by Smith at the University of Florida. Indeed, as Christman explained in 1985, "It is the concept of the practitioner teacher that holds the system together."[108] For Christman, the practitioner-teacher role was the "organizational means of enabling nurses with faculty qualifications to portray, in varying amounts, the components of the full professional role."[109] To be sure, the roles and responsibilities of individuals occupying the practitioner-teacher role would vary. For example, the practitioner-teacher might hold a leadership position in the hospital nursing service, engage in direct patient care, consult on patient care problems with the nursing staff, serve as a preceptor for graduate students in a particular area of expertise, conduct clinical research on a patient unit, or conduct in-service education in their area of clinical competence. No matter the nature of their practice, the practitioner-teacher served as a role model in the delivery of high-quality, professional nursing care or in clinical nursing research for students and nursing staff alike.[110] As Schlotfeldt explained, appropriate role models were in "extremely short supply" for nursing students in undergraduate and graduate nursing programs in which faculty were not engaged in practice.[111]

The practitioner-teacher was also instrumental to ensuring that what students were learning in the classroom was reflective of and responsive to the realities of clinical nursing. For example, Christman argued, the practitioner-teacher role ensured that the "scientific theory a teacher expounds in the classroom is clearly translated into the empirical science he/she applies in the clinical setting." Observing this process, students "become attuned to the subtleties and the sophistication of clinical judgments as they see their teachers function as primary nurses committed to the welfare of patients."[112] At the University of Rochester, Ford had been concerned that the "clinical and theoretical competencies of the faculty as a group were imbalanced," with more emphasis being placed on the psychosocial as opposed to the physiological and physical aspects of nursing care. Removed from the practice setting, it was easy, Ford contended, "for faculty to criticize nursing service personnel as functionaries and at the same time to prepare new graduates without testing out their efficacy, efficiency, or economics, much less be certain of their 'fit' with the changing health care demands." For Ford, nurse educators needed to be engaged with nursing practice and the health care system in order to be aware of the "phenomenal changes" in health care, and develop baccalaureate and graduate curricula that took account of and prepared graduates for these changes.[113]

Practitioner-teachers who engaged in research were critical to promoting clinical nursing research and bridging the gap between nursing research and nursing practice. Nurse researchers often had great difficulty carrying out clinical research that required access to patients. Without an appointment in the hospital or clinic, nurse researchers did not have a population of patients on which to conduct their research. In this situation, they usually had to secure permission from physicians to conduct patient research. And because nursing faculty were not involved in patient care, when they entered the hospital to carry out research, the nursing staff often viewed them as intruders who disrupted the work of the unit. Patients often viewed nurse researchers suspiciously, seeing them as being uninterested in their care and only interested in collecting data from them.[114]

In the integrated models at Case Western Reserve University, the University of Rochester, and Rush University, however, the faculty not only held hospital appointments but also engaged in clinical practice. In such cases, it was hoped, faculty researchers were less likely to be viewed by the nursing staff as disruptive or by patients as suspicious. Moreover, Christman noted, the research problems identified and undertaken by faculty who were engaged in practice would be "of a different order" because those problems came "from the real world of practice [rather] than the speculation of the classroom," helping to ensure that nursing research remained relevant to nursing practice.[115] Because faculty researchers in the integrated models would be engaged in sustained interactions with the hospital's nursing leaders and personnel, advances in knowledge acquired through research could promptly be translated into new and improved nursing care practices in the hospital. In such an integrated model, Ford explained, "the people who know things, who are discovering things [the researchers] are working with people in practice who are putting it all together in some kind of model of advanced practice."[116] In this way, the faculty's research activities would help ensure that the nursing care practiced in the hospital was up-to-date, high-quality, and evidence based.[117]

Obstacles to Academic Leadership in Nursing

The integrated models of nursing at Case Western Reserve University, the University of Rochester, and Rush University raised a series of challenges, including some that Smith had encountered at the University of Florida. Given the dearth of both clinically competent and doctorally prepared nursing faculty, Case Western Reserve University and the University of Rochester struggled to recruit faculty for the positions of chair or chief of the clinical nursing specialty services. For example, at Rochester, the position of chief of surgical nursing remained unfilled for several years.[118] The faculty who were successfully recruited to these leadership roles were, as both MacPhail and Ford described them, "risk-takers" who were "dissatisfied" with the traditional system and were "eager to effect change in control of the clinical learning environment and quality of care."[119] But in the 1960s and 1970s, there were few such risk takers among appropriately qualified nursing faculty. Indeed, recruitment was made all the more difficult by the complex and demanding nature of the role, which often led to role strain among the clinical nursing chiefs.[120]

Recruitment difficulties also extended to finding clinical nurse specialists able to fill the other leadership positions in the hospital. At Case Western Reserve University and the University Hospitals of Cleveland, for example, not only were clinical nurse specialists in short supply, the majority of nurses who had held leadership positions in the hospital prior to the implementation of the experiment had received advanced education in functional rather than clinical roles and thus lacked the clinical expertise required to fulfill the new leadership positions. In turn, most of the nurses who had recently earned a master's degree in a clinical specialty area were "relative neophytes when it comes to directing clinical nursing service."[121]

The integrated model also provoked criticism from nurses and physicians. At Case Western Reserve University, for example, diploma-trained nurses accused the school of "downgrading the diploma graduate" by prioritizing the BSN graduate in the hospital nursing service's new educational hierarchy. Counter to these accusations, MacPhail maintained that she and her colleagues believed strongly that graduates of each type of basic nursing program "have a very worthwhile, albeit different, contribution to make." MacPhail deplored "the intense competitiveness and anti-intellectualism that has been and continues to be engendered by many nurses."[122]

The Case Western Reserve University and University Hospitals of Cleveland model also faced criticism from physicians. Although physicians supported the concept of nursing faculty practice, they were, as a whole, less receptive to the changes integrated within the hospital nursing service. Physicians were particularly critical of the new requirement that nurses in leadership positions have preparation as clinical specialists, rather than the old expectation that they would have functional preparation as administrators or teachers. As MacPhail noted, "some physicians seem to prefer the old type of nurse role which engendered subservient relationship and acceptance of his word as law, rather than fostering questioning and collaboration."[123]

Although integration was intended to promote interprofessional collaboration, the outcomes were often less clear. The unification model at the University of Rochester, for example, was organizationally structured so as to facilitate collaboration with physicians and other health personnel. The parallel structures at the clinical chief level, Ford argued, were particularly important for "planning, implementing, and evaluating" the specialty programs "in patient care, the education of nurses and physicians, and research." The effectiveness of those interprofessional collaborations, however, ultimately depended on "the personalities and styles of the medical and nursing chiefs, and the availability of resources." Ford explained, "Some Medical Chiefs (all are men) recognize nursing as an independent, autonomous professional group," which formed a basis for effective collaboration. Other medical chiefs, however, "view[ed] nurses as handmaidens to physicians," and this had led to "friction and conflict." In these situations, the physicians struggled to adapt to the parallel organization structure and instead, considered themselves "'in charge and responsible for everything' including nursing."[124]

After more than ten years of experience at Case Western Reserve University, MacPhail felt that it was "easier to achieve" collaboration with physicians in the service setting than between the schools of medicine and nursing. In the service setting, MacPhail credited the "appointment of qualified leadership nurses in the hospital setting" who had at minimum a master's degree and sometimes even a doctoral degree, as having "contributed greatly to promoting communication and collaboration between medicine and nursing." However, she cautioned, "It is true that the power that can be gained by nursing may indeed be a threat to medicine if the physicians in control of the service wish to make all the decision[s]."[125]

In the educational setting, interprofessional collaboration was more challenging. Because each school had its own curriculum design and "its own priorities," MacPhail explained that it had proved "difficult to work out joint learning opportunities for students of medicine and nursing." In the school's efforts to establish interprofessional courses, MacPhail said, "A major impediment to their success has been the demands of the curriculum in which students are enrolled and the priorities given to courses in their respective schools, rather than to joining in interdisciplinary efforts which have been electives." MacPhail noted that the most interest in interprofessional courses had been shown by nursing and social work students, while medical and dental student interest had been much more limited.[126]

Efforts to implement interprofessional education were also difficult "because of the discrepancies in the educational background of most nursing students and medical students." While nursing students were baccalaureate students, medical students already held a baccalaureate degree and thus were learning at the postgraduate level. In this context, requiring nursing students "to have a college degree for entry into nursing school is one means of promoting a more common educational base" and enhancing interprofessional education. In fact, this argument was one factor that led Case Western Reserve University School of Nursing to introduce an entry-level professional doctoral degree, the doctor of nursing (ND) in 1979 (discussed in the conclusion). Indeed, MacPhail felt strongly that interprofessional collaboration at the undergraduate level "would only be possible if the students in both schools [nursing and medical] ha[d] a similar educational base, namely liberal arts education required for entry into professional program. Even with this requirement," though, "a collaborative approach to education [was] certainly not guaranteed." While there was evidence that graduate nursing students and graduate medical students "appear[ed] to work well together," such collaboration was "not done to any great extent." Again, this was in large part due to the fact that the residency requirements did not as yet allow time for, or place value on, collaborative practice.[127]

The faculty at Case Western Reserve University also faced obstacles when they tried to participate in collaborative research with physicians. In particular, they frequently confronted physicians who neither understood nor valued nursing research. As had become "very clear to nurses serving on the Hospital Research Review Committee," MacPhail explained, physicians struggled "to understand behavioral science research since most [were] oriented to experimental design and biological type research." She suggested, "One way that might help to promote collaborative [research] endeavors is to have more understanding of each other's interest and respect for each other's difference in focus and type of clinical investigation."[128] Ultimately, for inter-professional education, practice, and research to succeed, MacPhail argued, "there must be a commitment to promoting interdisciplinary collaboration in both educational opportunities and in practice," and this could "only be done ... [with] a commitment from the deans and the heads of departments" in all health science schools. "Even then," MacPhail said, "it will be difficult to achieve, but it should be given priority."[129]

The integration of practice into the faculty role—embodied in the new practitioner-teacher role—ultimately introduced new fracture points within nursing schools. As MacPhail had argued in 1979, it was important "that practice not pre-empt the functions of teaching and research, particularly research which is in relatively early stages of development." Thus, while it was necessary to redefine faculty role expectations—and the requirements for promotion and tenure—to include practice, teaching, and research, it was imperative that an appropriate balance be struck between the three roles. After all, MacPhail said, "It is very difficult for faculty to do everything."[130] The establishment of clinical faculty appointments was one approach to resolving the related issues of role overload and balancing the role expectations of regular (tenured or tenure-track) faculty.

In this model, which Case Western Reserve University adopted, nurses holding leadership positions in the clinical agencies used for student practice would be giving clinical appointments in the nursing school. While the same criteria would be used for appointment, reappointment, and promotion, clinical faculty were not eligible for tenure. As a result, MacPhail explained, "the time requirements for moving from one rank to another do not apply to them." And while research and publications "are promoted, encouraged and rewarded," she said, the "requirements may not be as high as for promotion and tenure of regular faculty." Instead, the "major responsibility of clinical faculty [was] to ensure the quality of care provided patients in the clinical setting [was] of the caliber desired for students to observe and emulate."[131] However, as Dorothy Smith pointed out, there was a risk in establishing a "system where the 'clinical' faculty [were] treated differently from the 'research' faculty. That seems to go back to the time when clinical faculty were considered second-class as compared to 'classroom' teachers." For Smith, this was unacceptable. Instead, she felt, faculty who engaged in practice should be "rewarded" and "held in high esteem."[132]

Mindful of this risk, at Rush, Christman had made the decision not to award tenure in nursing as part of a deliberate strategy to avoid the creation of "a two-tier faculty system" between regular (tenured or tenure track) and clinical faculty. Inherent within the two-tier system, Christman argued, were "problems of role strain, role derogation, covert obstructionism, and similar undesirable by-products of structural inequality." Without the institutional parameters, pressures, and expectations of the tenure system, department chairs were better able to manage and allocate the workloads among their faculty members. In place of tenure, the college had a system of "rolling contracts according to academic rank." The faculty were clearly satisfied with this approach, Christman noted, having "voted unanimously" on "three separate occasions" not to establish tenure, "taking the position that it has undesirable effects."[133]

Despite the challenges to unification encountered by Case Western Reserve University, the University of Rochester, and Rush University, by the early 1980s, a growing number of nurse leaders regarded "clinically based and focused teaching and faculty practice" as a "restored nursing ideal."[134] In 1979, for example, the deans of twelve leading nursing schools and the director of the American Association of Colleges of Nursing (AACN) published a "Statement of Belief Regarding Faculty Practice," in which they asserted, "Nursing's fullest potential in the delivery of health care is contingent upon the unification of nursing service and nursing education. Unification is the mechanism to enhance the quality of care, stimulate research into nursing practice questions, infuse curricula with clinical realities, provide exemplary learning opportunities for nursing students, and facilitate entry for nurses prepared for both basic and advanced practice."[135] Over the next two years, the American Academy of Nursing, the American Nurses Association, and American Association of Colleges of Nursing made similar resolutions calling for the unification of nursing service and education.[136]

New Models, Ongoing Challenges

As more nursing schools worked to implement academic nursing practice in the 1980s, they did so in the midst of the managed care movement, which prioritized the provision and utilization of efficient and cost-effective health services, and which conceptualized of nurse practitioners "as a cheaper alternative to physician care."[137] In this changing political economy, nursing schools that were part of AHCs experimented with different structural relationships between nursing schools and nursing service agencies. At the University of Pennsylvania School of Nursing, for example, after struggling for several years to come up with a workable integrated organizational structure, Dean Claire Fagin and her colleagues established a partnership plan between the School of Nursing and the Hospital of the University of Pennsylvania Division of Nursing. The plan centered on a newly created role—the clinician-educator—which, they hoped, would overcome some of the limits of the previous integrated models, including that of the two-tier faculty problem.[138]

The clinician-educator position, similar to the practitioner-teacher model first introduced by Dorothy Smith at the University of Florida, was modeled upon the already well accepted clinician-educator positions in the University of Pennsylvania's medical school, dental school, and school of veterinary medicine.[139] Faculty members appointed as clinician-educators held a joint appointment between the School of Nursing and the Hospital of the University of Pennsylvania or another clinical agency, where they performed in a specified clinical role. They were also expected to engage in scholarly activities, including publications, and their teaching was typically practice oriented.[140] Different from the earlier practitioner-teacher roles, however, the clinician-educator was a fully-fledged member of the School of Nursing's standing faculty, which also consisted of tenured or tenure-track faculty who were expected to be "investigators/educators whose primary interests [lay] in clinical or basic research."[141]

As standing faculty, clinician-educators enjoyed all the same rights and privileges of the tenured or tenure-track faculty except they could not vote on tenure or the compensation of tenured faculty. If initially appointed at the assistant professor level, they had ten years to achieve the rank of associate professor. To be sure, either of the standing faculty positions could include teaching, research, and practice, "but the emphasis on each of these roles [was] expected to vary from one position to another."[142] As Joan Lynaugh, who had been a faculty member at the University of Rochester in the 1970s and in 1980 joined the faculty at the University of Pennsylvania, explained, "Each nursing faculty member needed to think through the personal implications of focusing on research and publishing." It meant that "being an expert teacher would not be enough to warrant promotion for tenure-track faculty. In importance, research and scholarship moved in from the margins and became central to the school." But it also meant that faculty on the tenure track would not have to be expert clinicians. Rather, "the most expert clinicians would be in the clinician-educator track."[143]

The clinician-educator role ostensibly eliminated concerns that the integration of nursing education and nursing service would create a two-tier faculty structure. But for many schools of nursing, conflicting objectives between nursing schools and nursing service agencies were another impediment to integration and academic nursing practice.[144] In an effort to resolve this, some nursing schools established their own academic, nurse-managed clinics. There was some precedent for doing so. In 1963, Lydia Hall had established the Loeb Center for Nursing and Rehabilitation at Montefiore Hospital and Medical Center in the Bronx. The eighty-bed clinic was entirely nurse-run and offered a range of services and programs to people needing rehabilitation following hospitalization.[145]

At the University of Florida in the late 1960s, the maternal-infant nursing faculty (with encouragement from the medical school's chair of obstetrics) had established a nurse-led prenatal clinic separate from the physician-led obstetrics clinic at Shands Teaching Hospital. The Carver Clinic was open one to two days a week in a predominantly Black neighborhood of downtown Gainesville. After an initial visit with an obstetrician, and as long as the obstetrician detected no problems, a pregnant woman would be transferred to the nurse-led prenatal clinic where she could continue to receive her care for the duration of her pregnancy. As faculty member Betty Hilliard recalled, "They were our patients and you know, they wanted to come back."[146] At the end of each clinic, the nurses would conference with the obstetrics resident at Shands Teaching Hospital about their patients and if the resident had any concerns, the patient would be transferred back to the obstetrics clinic.[147]

The Carver Clinic provided the maternal-infant nursing faculty and staff with, as Hilliard put it, "the opportunity to do the kind of care we thought nurses ought to be doing."[148] Hilliard explained that at the hospital obstetrics clinic, the nurses provided an "assembly line" type of prenatal nursing care: after taking the patient's blood pressure, weight, and urine samples, the nurse would send the patient "into a room to wait for the doctor." The nurses' contact with patients was limited and ended as soon as the patient finished meeting with the physician. At the Carver Clinic, Hilliard continued, "we wanted the students to do some different kinds of things in the clinic besides doing the weights and blood pressures . . . We wanted them to have some mothers that were theirs. That they could see, each visit and maybe go up when they were in labor and delivery—really follow them through."[149] The students also had the opportunity to practice health education by holding small prenatal classes and question and answer sessions with groups of patients.[150]

During the 1970s and early 1980s, other nursing schools followed suit, establishing academic nurse-managed clinics—entities owned by nursing schools, managed by nurses, and providing direct nursing care to clients.[151] Nursing schools did so in order to provide clinical teaching sites for their undergraduate and graduate nursing students, to serve as research sites for their faculty and doctoral students, and to provide needed health services to underserved communities. Many of these clinics were initially funded by grants from the U.S. Public Health Service Division of Nursing or from private foundations, and in some cases, they were supported by city, county, or state funds. For example, in 1977, Arizona State University College of Nursing established a nurse-managed family health clinic that offered "family planning, maternity care, immunization, and referral to other community resources for acute and serious medical, social, and psychological problems." It was initially funded by a U.S. Public Health Service Division of Nursing grant, with subsequent support provided by the city of Scottsdale (where the clinic was located), the Maricopa County Health Department, and "contributions, grants, fees, and the College of Nursing." The clinic served primarily low-income women and children living within four miles of the clinic.[152] In Mansfield, Connecticut, the University of Connecticut nursing school established a Wellness Center, with initial funding from the U.S. Public Health Service Division of Nursing and county health department, to provide preventive screening, health maintenance, counseling, and health education services to Mansfield residents over fifty-five years of age. The nursing school established the center, initially, as a site of research and in response to the "need for a health promotion program for older citizens." By 1984, however, the center was in search of ongoing funding.[153] The University of Kentucky College of Nursing organized its first revenue-generating practice in 1985, establishing a nurse-managed clinic for homeless adults. Initially conceived in 1981 as a volunteer student project, the clinic became operational in 1985 with funding from a local nonprofit organization that provided services to the homeless. Between 1986 and 1989, the clinic was funded by a federal U.S. Public Health Service Division of Nursing Special Projects Grant. Until the funding ran out, the clinic was run by the college's nursing faculty and provided clinical "learning experiences for BSN and MSN students, and research opportunities for doctoral students and faculty."[154]

The idea of academic nurse-managed clinics or centers spread rapidly in the 1980s.[155] By 1988, there were "more than 60 schools of nursing with NMCs [nurse-managed centers]."[156] In the era of cost containment, nurse-managed clinics had much to offer. The introduction of the prospective payment system and capitation incentivized hospitals to restrict admission criteria and discharge patients sooner, creating greater demand for patient care in community settings. This was the type of care that nurse-led clinics could provide, along with preventive and primary care services. And by prioritizing the provision of care to underserved populations, nurse-led clinics promised to reduce hospitalization costs caused by delays in treatment due to barriers to accessing care. But as these few examples show, the financial feasibility of academic nurse-managed clinics was precarious, contingent on philanthropic and grant funding. Often when the funding ran out, the clinics ended.[157] Other difficulties included issues of "licensure, certification, and other regulations that govern nursing practice within each state. These include the legal definition of nursing, advanced scopes of practice as described in nurse practice acts, prescriptive authority, and direct reimbursement of nursing services by third-party payers."[158] In the latter case, public and private third-party payers would either fail to cover or would reimburse nurse practitioners at a lower rate than physicians, undermining the financial viability of the nurse-managed clinics. In the context of the managed care movement, nurse-managed clinics offered the potential to provide high-quality and cost-effective primary care services. But it was incumbent on nurse researchers to demonstrate "provider competency, productivity and efficiency, accessibility of services, [and] comprehensiveness of services."[159] In other words, they needed to demonstrate the ability and cost-effectiveness of nurse-managed clinics to improve health outcomes.

Conclusion

Despite the growing number and role of academic nurse-managed clinics and centers, and despite the successful introduction of the clinician-educator position at the University of Pennsylvania and other experiments in integrating nursing service and nursing education, the full potential of academic nursing practice continued to go unrealized in American nursing. As Joan Lynaugh reflected on these early efforts to integrate nursing education and nursing practice, the models implemented at the University of Florida, Case Western Reserve University, Rush University, and the University of Rochester were not "some panacea for the dilemmas" of academic nursing. Lynaugh explained, "Trying to meet higher standards for faculty appointment in colleges and universities, greater demands for more sophisticate[d] school work, and increasing pressures for clinical competence while trying to build nursing research with under-funded budgets ensured that efforts to link academic nursing with the practice of nursing would continue to be difficult."[160]

One of the major structural limitations to nursing faculty practice was the lack of reimbursement for nursing care services. In this way, the model of academic medicine was of limited use because physician faculty were not only routinely reimbursed for clinical services, but their clinical practices also generated substantial revenue for medical schools. As Case Western Reserve University's Jannetta MacPhail had lamented in 1979, "The fact that nurses cannot be reimbursed poses a particular problem in trying to work out means of getting paid for faculty practice. In some settings where nursing clinics have been set up, care is given without payment." In others, MacPhail continued, "the payment is to physicians with whom the nurses work since this is the only means whereby reimbursement can be obtained."[161] Until the late 1990s, advanced practice nurses were not able to receive direct reimbursement through Medicare and received very little from Medicaid reimbursements.[162] Academic nursing's efforts to institute academic nursing practice were also undermined by the lack of prescriptive authority granted to advanced practice nurses in many states until the early twenty-first century, as well as by other regulatory issues.[163] Even with the resolution of some of these regulatory and reimbursement issues, the financial implications of and structural barriers to nursing faculty practice are still largely unresolved.[164]

Conclusion

By the end of the twentieth century, American nurses had made substantial gains in their academic project. They had developed a science of nursing that underpinned a patient-centered model of care. The nursing model considers patients holistically and in relationship to their environments, attends to patients' physical, psychological, sociocultural, and emotional needs, and prioritizes the agency of patients in shaping their health. So, too, nurse scientists had demonstrated their capacity to conduct patient-centered research that could shape health care practice, inform health policy, and improve health outcomes. The legitimacy of nursing—and the importance of ongoing nursing research to expand the knowledge base of nursing science—was reflected in the establishment of the National Center for Nursing Research at the NIH in 1986, followed by its designation as the National Institute of Nursing Research (NINR) in 1993. At the end of the twentieth century, the NINR was critical to raising the legitimacy of and amount of funding available for nursing research in the U.S.[1] And as the previous chapters detail, academic nurses had also navigated the institutional, interprofessional, and gender politics of higher education and secured their roles within research-intensive universities and academic health centers.

Thus, in the early twenty-first century, American nurses provide essential care to patients in hospitals (which includes providing most of the critical care in intensive care units), in long-term care facilities, and in their homes.[2] Nurses also engage in innovative research, the fundamental framework of which is to focus on the lived experiences of patients, families, communities, and clinicians during times of disease, illness, and health. This means that when new infectious diseases emerge, as happened in late 2019 with the emergence of COVID-19 caused by the new coronavirus, SARS-CoV-2, nurse scientists provide critical research on the impact of disease on caregivers, family members, and communities; and on the differential effects of disease among different populations, such as the elderly, the housing insecure, those already living with chronic illness, and those at increased risk of intimate partner violence. They research the impact of preventive measures like social distancing, or delayed routine primary care or symptom management appointments, on the experiences and health outcomes of people living during an epidemic or global pandemic. And they research the experiences of, and the health impacts on, nurses and other health care workers who practice in underresourced and understaffed hospitals and nursing homes. As they undertake this research, nurse scientists focus on improving care not only during the acute phase of illness, but also for those who, in the aftermath of epidemics, continue to experience the chronic effects of infection and the various disabilities that can result from them.[3]

Yet in spite of the gains that academic nurses have achieved, in the early twenty-first century, nursing's academic project remains incomplete. Despite repeated calls to establish the bachelor of science in nursing as the minimum educational requirement for entry into practice, nurse leaders have been unwilling to give up the multiple pathways for entry into practice because of the stakes involved for those institutions preparing nurses at the diploma and associate degree level and for the nurses who earned these degrees, and because the multiple pathways into practice enable social mobility for "nurses who may have chosen the wrong path for entry into nursing, or who now have the resources to pursue advanced education."[4] In 2010, the Institute of Medicine (IOM, now National Academy of Medicine) called for the proportion of nurses with baccalaureate degrees to increase from 50 percent to 80 percent by 2020.[5] It did so in response to more than a decade's worth of compelling evidence that hospitals with higher percentages of BSN-educated nurses had better patient outcomes.[6] Nevertheless, the IOM recognized that the associate degree remained a critical entry point into nursing, particularly for people from rural areas, disadvantaged backgrounds, or underrepresented populations.[7] Four years later, the institute reaffirmed the importance of maintaining and strengthening the different educational pathways into nursing.[8]

In the early twenty-first century, as it has in the past, racial inequities persist in nursing, especially within academic nursing, where, still, 82 percent of full-time nursing faculty are white.[9] Among registered nurses, 73.5 percent are white, while 84 percent of advanced practice nurses are white.[10] Indeed, ongoing systemic racism has meant that Black, Indigenous, and other people of color continue to face barriers accessing higher education in nursing. This is reflected in the continuing marginalization of women of color in low-paying, low-status, direct-care occupations, such as nursing assistants and home health aides.[11] During the global COVID-19 pandemic, nurses of color have been disproportionately impacted, reflecting the broader disproportionate impact of COVID-19 on communities of color. As of September 2020, National Nurses United found that 58 percent of the 213 registered nurses it had identified as dying due to COVID-19 and related complications were nurses of color, including 32 percent who were Filipino nurses and 18 percent who were Black nurses.[12] Thus, much more work is needed to address these racial inequities and increase diversity within nursing, particularly at the highest educational levels. Providing support and resources for educational mobility within nursing—from the role of home health aide all the way through to the advanced practice role—via articulated educational pathways and the implementation of career ladders is part of this work.[13]

The work of addressing racial inequities in nursing is urgent. Diversification of the health workforce is integral to improving access to and quality of care, particularly in underserved communities of color.[14] For example, recent studies on racial concordance between clinician and patient have shown that Black newborns do better when there is racial concordance with the delivering physicians.[15] Although researchers have yet to study whether the race of nurses matters to the outcomes of newborns, they have documented the important ways in which birth workers of color, including midwives, provide racially concordant perinatal care to patients of color.[16] This has implications for tackling historical and persistent racial disparities in both infant and maternal mortality.[17] According to the Centers for Disease Control and Prevention (CDC), pregnancy-related mortality is two to three times higher among Black, American Indian, and Alaska Native women than white women,[18] and Black infants have mortality rates twice that of white infants.[19]

The boundaries of nursing science are still contested. As academic nurses reassert the importance of nursing's "core disciplinary knowledge," they are also debating whether and how to incorporate knowledge and skills derived from emerging sciences such as omics, big data, and biomedical and health informatics into nursing science.[20] Moreover, while nursing theory is infrequently used to frame nursing research, theoretically oriented nursing research is dominated by theories from psychology and sociology. This is raising questions about the degree of nursing science content in PhD education.[21] As part of this, academic nurses are also debating the role of interdisciplinary scholars in the development of nursing science and as faculty members in schools of nursing.[22] As Sheria Robinson-Lane characterizes the issue, "When nurses or other interdisciplinary scholars working in schools of nursing ask scientific questions rooted in non-nursing frameworks, though the results of their work might improve health outcomes or service delivery, the science they are building is debatably not nursing but rather the discipline from which the framework was derived. However," as Robinson-Lane continues, "it is possible to move borrowed models and theories into nursing by intentionally seating them within a nursing frame of reference."[23] As this book makes clear, these ongoing debates over what types of research, which types of theories, and which types of researchers can contribute to the development of nursing science, revisit and rehash the debates of the 1960s and 1970s, when academic nurses first sought to define and erect boundaries around nursing science and demarcate who should be permitted to contribute to nursing's epistemological project.

As in the past, the degree of research funding available for nursing science is impacting the field. Relative to other types of health science and biomedical research, nursing research is poorly funded. Between 1988 and 2014, the NINR provided more funding for nursing research than any other federal agency (followed closely by the Division of Nursing in the Health Resources and Services Administration). However, for more than a decade, NIH support for nursing research has remained relatively flat, representing just 0.5 percent of the total NIH budget, and the NINR remains the lowest-funded institute within the NIH. Nurse scientists often struggle to compete for funding from other centers and institutes within the NIH and other federal funding agencies because, Mary Kerr suggests, they are "not communicating the significance of their research or describing their scientific approach in a way that resonates with grant reviewers." For Kerr, it is time to examine whether the scientific approaches and models taught in nursing schools "are reflective of contemporary funding expectations."[24] But as historians of science have shown, the research priorities of funding agencies can ultimately shape what becomes valued within a discipline.[25] The enduring preference among funding agencies, including the NINR, for data-driven empirical research continues to make it difficult for qualitative nurse researchers to secure funding for their work and also threatens to devalue philosophical, conceptual, and theoretical inquiry within nursing PhD programs and the continued advancement of nursing science.[26]

Academic nurses have yet to achieve full partnership in health care delivery, education, and research. As noted in the 2016 American Association of Colleges of Nursing report, *Advancing Healthcare Transformation: A New Era for Academic Nursing*, academic nurses have "minimal meaningful participation in health system governance," nursing faculty are not integrated into health system leadership roles and are only marginally integrated into clinical services, and nurse scientist research is siloed within nursing schools.

Included among the barriers to full integration are the "tuition-dependent structure of academic nursing" and the paucity of nursing faculty practice. Because nursing faculty, unlike physician faculty in medical schools, have been unable to develop robust faculty practices, the majority of PhD-prepared faculty have not engaged in clinical practice. As such, academic nurses, the report concluded, are "not positioned as a partner in health care transformation."[27]

How are we to understand and explain the mixed results of nursing's academic project? As this book has argued, nurses had two main rationales when they undertook their academic project to raise the educational level of professional nurses, construct a science of nursing, and establish PhD programs in nursing to prepare new generations of nurse scientists and sustain advancements in nursing science. The first rationale was empirical: to better understand patients in order to more effectively respond to their health care needs, and, ultimately, to improve patient care and health outcomes. The second rationale was political: to establish nursing as an academic discipline, underpin the legitimacy of the nursing profession, and secure the status of nurses within the postwar research university and academic health centers. Even as academic nurses have demonstrated the improvements in health outcomes made possible by nursing's academic project, the effectiveness with which academic nurses made their claims reflects the influence of various intersecting politics.[28] On the one hand, this history shows the impact of disciplinary, institutional, and interprofessional politics—and the shaping of those politics by gender and race—on the making of a new discipline. On the other hand, this history also reveals the importance of the intersections of health and higher education policy—and the politics of state policymaking—on the education of America's health care professionals.

As the previous chapters have detailed, nursing's academic project has been shaped by the politics of academia and the interprofessional politics of health care. Within the postwar research economy, medical schools—and the physician-scientists that taught in them—were particularly effective at capitalizing on the postwar research economy.[29] Nursing schools operated within the same political economy, but as relative newcomers to university campuses, nursing schools and their faculty confronted significant challenges to establishing their discipline and securing their status in the postwar university and research economy. Some of these challenges were gendered; others, however, were epistemological in character.

Several historians of science and technology have documented the transformative effect of the postwar research economy on the physical, biological, and social sciences.[30] Others have examined the academization of practice professions like clinical psychology, engineering, and computing in the postwar decades.[31] These were disciplines and practice professions that through-out these decades were composed primarily of male scientists, engineers, and practitioners. Yet as Margaret Rossiter has documented, women scientists faired especially poorly in the postwar research economy.[32] While Rossiter and other historians of gender and science have described the postwar de-mise of predominantly female disciplines like home economics, they have also analyzed the efforts of women scientists—particularly following the civil rights and women's liberation movements of the 1960s and 1970s—to establish themselves within traditionally male disciplines previously closed off to them.[33] As a still-predominantly female profession, nursing's trans-formation in the postwar university is a compelling counterpoint to these other histories. Although its transformation was indelibly shaped by gen-der, nursing was able to secure a footing, however tenuous, within the post-war research economy. The transformation of nursing—and the experiences of nurse scientists—within the postwar research university thus provides new insights into the experiences of women scientists and the intersections of gender, knowledge production, and discipline formation in the postwar decades.

But the status of academic nurses and of nursing science in the postwar research economy has also been shaped by the relationship to and changes within biomedicine. While rejecting the medical model and seeking to distin-guish nursing science from the biomedical sciences, academic nurses opted to construct nursing science as a theoretical and empirical discipline, one that drew heavily upon the theoretical frameworks and qualitative research meth-ods of the social and behavioral sciences. They did so at the same time that academic physicians were establishing the empirical and statistically derived discipline of clinical epidemiology and asserting the primacy of the random-ized controlled trial for generating the most objective and reliable knowledge. In this context, academic nurses' path to knowledge development—partic-ularly, their reliance on the development of new, nursing-specific, theories and qualitative and quantitative research methods thought to generate less objective, reliable evidence than the randomized controlled trial—contributed to the undervaluing of nursing science and the siloing of nurse scientists within the research economy and academic health centers.

This history thus makes clear the processes, stakes, and limits involved in the boundary work that constitutes the formation of new disciplines.[34] As the sociologist Andrew Abbott has explained, the development of an abstract system of knowledge is an integral part of constructing a new discipline. This process of abstraction demarcates the "borders of professional jurisdiction with utmost clarity," making "obvious what is and what is not part of the professionally claimed universe of tasks."[35] But as Abbott also noted, there is a limit to that abstraction. As the history of nursing science makes all too clear, too much abstraction can dilute core jurisdictional claims. Too often, the theories developed by academic nurses neither resonated with nor were legible to their health science colleagues in universities and AHCs, who neither understood nor saw the need for nursing theory. Furthermore, the degree of abstraction necessary for asserting jurisdiction depends on the values of the broader culture.[36] Academic nurses staked their jurisdictional claims on the development of distinct and unique nursing theories, at a time when the broader research and biomedical culture valued statistically backed empiricism over theoretically informed empiricism. As such, academic physicians, biomedical scientists, and national funding agencies not only struggled to understand the content of and need for nursing theory, they also did not place high evidentiary value on nursing research informed by theory, be it nursing theory or the theories of other disciplines.

To be sure, though, the history of nursing's boundary work also makes clear the racialized nature of nursing's epistemological project. The work of drawing boundaries in the construction and maintenance of disciplines is about making rules about what and whose knowledge counts, and thus who is allowed to contribute new knowledge to the discipline. Since the introduction of trained nursing in the late nineteenth century, only people granted entrance—first to hospital-based training programs, later, to undergraduate nursing education, and, eventually, to doctoral nursing programs—were permitted to contribute to the science of nursing. Because of the long history of segregation and racial discrimination in nursing, health care, and higher education (as well as gender discrimination in nursing), those able to contribute to nursing science have been primarily white women.[37] As a result, the construction of nursing science has been a racialized and gendered project in which the knowledge, perspectives, and experiences of those who have not acquired the educational credential of the BSN or PhD in nursing have either been ignored, dismissed, or seen as an epistemological threat to the discipline. This has contributed to a tendency toward insularity within academic nursing, whereby knowledge and knowledge workers from outside of nursing are perceived as threat to the integrity of nursing science. The recent debates over the role of interdisciplinary scholars in the advancement of nursing science, as noted earlier, is just the latest iteration of this boundary work.[38] And in the efforts of academic nurses to construct a science that was legible within the postwar research economy—to access to doing science-as-it-was-currently-done, so-called normal science—academic nurses have privileged Western scientific ways of knowing, reifying, unwittingly or otherwise, white privilege and the systemic racism that is embedded within and reinforced by Western science.[39]

The history of academic nursing also reveals the ways in which the intersections of state and federal policymaking impact academic health centers, particularly those at state-supported universities. As the previous chapters detail, nursing's academic project has existed in tension with nursing's workforce needs and as such, has been both shaped by and shaping of the politics of state health policymaking. While the existing literature acknowledges the importance of federal health care legislation like Medicare and Medicaid to recent American history, far less attention has been paid to the influence of state governance on America's health care system.[40] As this book has shown, since the 1950s, state legislators have looked increasingly to academic health institutions receiving state funds to expand educational opportunities and better coordinate the production and distribution of the state's health workforce. During the postwar decades, state health planners across the country launched health workforce studies in order to document the current supply and project the future demand of health care professionals, including nurses. They then used this data to plan for and implement new educational policies and programs in an effort to match supply with demand. State policymakers were also concerned, during these years, about racial inequities in higher education. Their concerns extended to the barriers accessing undergraduate and graduate nursing education experienced by students and nurses of color. State policymakers thus looked to state-supported nursing schools to not only provide enough professional nurses to meet states' health care needs but also resolve problems of educational access. *Dr. Nurse* has put the state back into the history of American health care, providing scholars and policymakers with a case study of the ways in which state governments—in concert with state-funded nursing schools and academic health centers—have worked to address disparities in the distribution of health care resources.

The history of academic nursing offers valuable lessons for understanding recent changes in (and the politics of) health professions' education.[41] At the turn of the twenty-first century, the IOM issued a series of reports describing serious problems with the American health care system and health professions education. In 1999, the IOM Committee on the Quality of Health Care in America released its first report, *To Err Is Human*, which addressed issues related to patient safety and laid out a national agenda for reducing errors in health care and improving patient safety.[42] Two years later, in 2001, the committee released its second report, *Crossing the Quality Chasm*, which called for a restructuring of the health care system focused on providing care that was evidence based, patient centered, and systems oriented.[43] As part of this restructuring, the IOM called for "a major overhaul" of clinical education, which it detailed in its third report, *Health Professions Education*, published in 2003.[44] In particular, the IOM urged that all health professionals be "educated to deliver patient-centered care as members of an interdisciplinary team, emphasizing evidence-based practice, quality improvement approaches, and informatics."[45] These reports, with their focus on reducing errors, increasing accountability, improving patient safety, and increasing quality within the American health care system, reflected the continuation of the quality assessment movement in health care and the importance of health professions education to that goal.[46]

This series of reports provided the context in which nurse leaders, at the turn of the twenty-first century, advocated a new vision for the education of advanced practice nurses: the establishment of practice-focused doctoral programs—the doctor of nursing practice (DNP)—to "prepare graduates for the highest level of nursing practice."[47] As Elizabeth R. Lenz, dean of Ohio State University College of Nursing explained in 2005, the IOM reports called attention to the "increasing need for insightful visionary nursing leadership in practice with the educational credentials necessary to be accorded a place at the table in high level health care management and policy decisions."[48] The DNP was intended to prepare advanced practice nurses to provide evidence-based, patient-centered care that was systems oriented and quality improvement focused; provide leadership in health care systems and in the health policy arena; and to provide expert clinical teaching.

The call for the DNP (and the ensuing debates over it) reflected and reinforced the claims and stakes that had long shaped nursing's academic project. As with earlier calls to raise the educational preparation of nurses, the arguments made by advocates of the DNP for increasing the educational preparation of advanced practice nurses were both empirical, with the goal of improving patient care and health outcomes, and political, with the goal of securing parity for professional nurses within the health care team. But as with the history of nursing's academic project, the calls for the DNP also resurfaced the marginalization and exclusion that had long defined nursing's history and threatened to exacerbate existing inequities within nursing, the health care system, and universities.

Academic nurses had actually been experimenting with a new type of doctoral degree, the practice doctorate, since the late 1970s. In 1979, the Case Western Reserve University Frances Payne Bolton School of Nursing introduced an entry-level professional doctoral degree, the doctor of nursing (ND). This was a three-year postbaccalaureate doctoral degree, modeled on, and intended to be equivalent to, the postbaccalaureate doctoral education received by physicians, dentists, and pharmacists. While MD and DDS programs were four years in length, PharmD programs, which were first introduced in the 1960s, ranged from two to three years in length. With equivalent doctoral preparation, the professional nurse would, like her colleagues in medicine, dentistry, and pharmacy, have the knowledge "to act independently" and the "competence" to execute her "own responsibilities" and work "interdependently" with the other members of the health care team "in planning, providing, and evaluating programs of care and in evaluating the total health care system."[49]

The Case Western nursing faculty cast the ND as "a solution to the health care crisis"[50] and the future of professional nursing: not only would it raise the expertise—and thus the professional standing—of professional nurses, putting them on equal footing with the other doctorally prepared providers in the room (physicians, dentists, and pharmacists), but it would also provide them with the confidence, knowledge, and skills to lead the interprofessional health care team in a new era of patient-centered care. In this way, the nursing faculty sought to position their ND graduates as the ideal professionals to lead patients and other members of the health care team through a period of crisis. This was a crisis characterized by rising health care costs without any apparent improvement in the quality of health care; persistent shortages of all health care professionals and ongoing disparities in access to, and the quality of, health care services; and growing criticism among patients in general and health feminists in particular about the paternalism and reductionism of medical care and the physicians who delivered it.

The ND program's "scholarly, professional approach" would prepare each graduate to be both a clinician *and* a clinical scholar, one able "to use and test concepts, models and theories; to use and explicate the rationale and data for clinical nursing decisions; to critically analyze nursing phenomena and evaluate clinical situations; and to systematically study a selected area in order to advance practice in that area."[51] As such, this "scholar-clinician" would be well-placed to translate new nursing science into innovative clinical practice and develop evidence-based nursing practice. By incorporating "newly developed nursing knowledge into nursing practice and . . . [suggesting] new areas of investigation for nursing research," the ND graduate could better integrate nursing research with nursing practice and help tackle the schism between nurse researchers and theorists and clinical nurses.[52]

The ND, however, was not the panacea that the Case Western nursing faculty had hoped for. In the Cleveland area alone, nursing educators, hospital administrators, and physicians remained skeptical about the value added (and the added expense) of the ND-prepared nurse.[53] Nationally, the ND failed to gain traction. In 1990, the University of Colorado College of Nursing was the only other school to establish an entry-level professional doctorate in nursing (Rush University and the University of South Carolina also established ND programs, but they were not entry-level professional doctorates but advanced specialty practice doctoral degrees).[54] A 1987 survey of the deans and directors of baccalaureate and graduate degree nursing programs concluded, "Given the difficulty of attaining consensus for requiring the BSN for entry into practice, it is not surprising that even those who support the ND concept do not view it as a realistic entry level degree in the near future."[55] For all intents and purposes, the ND was a failed educational innovation; by the mid-2000s it was no longer offered by any nursing school. Instead, the ND had been replaced by a new type of practice doctorate, the DNP—an advanced graduate degree that many nursing leaders argued should designate entry into advanced practice nursing.

In 1999, the AACN appointed a task force charged with revising the quality indicators for doctoral programs and addressing differences among PhD, doctor of nursing science (DNSc/DNS), and doctor of nursing (ND) degrees.[56] At that time, only six nursing schools offered some version of a practice-focused doctorate, including Case Western Reserve University, the University of Colorado, Rush University, and the University of South Carolina, all of which offered the ND degree; the University of Tennessee, Memphis, which offered a practice-focused DNS; and the University of Kentucky, which offered a DNP.[57] Sandra Edwardson, Dean of Nursing at the University of Minnesota, chaired the task force. "As we got into it," Edwardson recalled, "we thought, this whole area of clinical doctorates is so confused."[58] That confusion was experienced as much within nursing as it was by the public, particularly "regarding the competencies of graduates and the roles within the health care delivery system they were prepared to fill."[59] As a result, the task force recommended to the AACN Board of Directors that they appoint a second task force to study clinical, or practice-focused, doctorates. Edwardson was also appointed to this new task force.

One of the task force's first recommendations was to change the terminology "from clinical [doctorate] to practice [doctorate] because the practice was more than clinical."[60] Practice included public health and community health nursing, as well as "organizational and professional leadership, management, health policy, and nursing/health informatics"—those areas of practice that support patient care.[61] In 2004, the AACN Task Force on the Professional Clinical Doctorate recommended that a practice-focused doctoral program, the DNP, be established as "a distinct model of doctoral education" that would "prepare graduates for the highest level of nursing practice" and for leadership in nursing practice.[62] The task force also recommended that the DNP "be the graduate degree for advanced nursing practice preparation, including but not limited to the four current APN [advanced practice nursing] roles: clinical nurse specialist, nurse anesthetist, nurse midwife, and nurse practitioner."[63] They also recommended the DNP as the "ideal preparation and credentialing for clinical teaching."[64]

In October 2004, the AACN brought the proposal for the DNP to a vote of member deans at its fall deans' meeting. Although the deans present at the meeting voted to move forward with establishing the DNP as the required credential for advance practice nursing, the vote was contentious and mired in politics. Only the 266 deans who were present at the meeting were permitted to vote; absentee voting or voting-by-proxy were not permitted. At the time, there were more than five hundred deans of AACN member schools, meaning that almost half of the AACN members were not given the opportunity to vote on the proposal. Of those deans present at the meeting, 160 deans voted in support of establishing the DNP, while 106 deans voted against doing so.[65]

The nature of the vote and its outcome were influenced by both politics and economics. First, for deans of non-research-intensive nursing schools with neither the research capacity nor resources to establish a PhD program, the ability to establish a DNP program offered a way to earn legitimacy for their schools within their universities. Second, the DNP was a way for state-supported nursing schools to generate new revenue at a time of precipitously declining state appropriations.[66]

Nursing schools had long been dependent on tuition revenue, and were never more so than at the turn of the twenty-first century. Federal funding and state allocations to public universities had been declining since the late 1970s, even as the costs of education increased. At the University of Minnesota, for example, between 1978 and 2008, state funding remained relatively flat even as the state budget had grown significantly.[67] Through the 1990s, most states determined their funding allocations for higher education using funding formulas that were input-based, driven by student enrollment, as well as faculty salaries and student/faculty ratios. But in the 1990s, many states shifted away from such demand-driven funding models toward performance-related funding models that reflected both inputs (including enrollments) and outcomes (for example, graduation rates, licensure pass rates). The shift in state funding priorities had a substantial impact on the budget of state-supported nursing schools.[68] For example, at the University of Minnesota in 2000, the School of Nursing got 37 percent of its revenue from the state; by 2003, that figure had fallen to 26 percent.[69] At the University of Colorado School of Nursing in 2003, amid shrinking state appropriations, the state rescinded 36.7 percent of the funding to the school.[70]

As federal and state support declined, nursing schools, like other academic units on university campuses, became increasingly dependent on tuition revenue to support the costs of increasing educational quality and expanding the size of its educational programs. Nursing schools, however, could not raise tuition to offset rising costs in their baccalaureate programs, because baccalaureate tuition rates were set by the university and standardized across all baccalaureate degree programs. This meant that although it cost more to administer nursing programs, in any given university the tuition for a baccalaureate nursing degree was the same as the tuition for any other baccalaureate degree, such as English, biology, or philosophy. In this context, the introduction of a new type of doctoral program promised nursing schools a much-needed source of new enrollment and thus tuition revenue (as well as a higher funding allocation in state funding models). Perhaps most significantly, as a professional degree, nursing schools were able to determine their own tuition levels for their DNP programs, which meant they could charge closer to what it cost to administer the program. Thus, despite the costs involved in developing and implementing a new graduate program, DNP programs offered nursing schools a much-needed new source of tuition revenue.[71]

The ensuing debates over the introduction of the DNP reflected the tensions between the empirical and political rationales within nursing's academic project. DNP advocates argued the new degree was both necessary for providing patients with evidence-based, patient-centered, high-quality care (the empirical rationale), and for finally securing parity and equity for nurses—specifically, advanced practice nurses—with other doctorally prepared members of the health care team (the political rationale). By the early twenty-first century, this not only included physicians, dentists, and pharmacists, but also a growing list of health care professionals now educated to the doctoral level. In the early 2000s, as physical therapy, occupational therapy, optometry, and audiology began establishing practice doctorates, "proponents of the DNP suggest[ed] that nurses should be included in this trend."[72] For example, as Ellen Olshansky argued in 2004, although nurses "are equal players with a wide range of expertise . . . we cannot ignore the social context in which we live, a context in which titles often precede the person. In such a context, nurses must be recognized through titles that reflect their expertise to others."[73]

The introduction of the DNP, however, resurfaced familiar gendered interprofessional politics. The DNP faced considerable opposition from physicians, particularly national organizations representing physicians, whose concerns centered on titling and scope of practice. Physicians were concerned that nurses were overreaching their professional expertise. In 2011, Roland Goertz, MD, the board chairman of the American Academy of Family Physicians asserted that physicians were worried about losing control over the title of "doctor" and that the use of the term would confuse patients. In several state legislatures, physician groups opposed to nurses being called "doctor" pushed for legislation that would restrict who would be able to use the title "doctor."[74] In 2010, the AMA launched a "Truth in Advertising" campaign that was "designed to ensure health care providers clearly and honestly state their level of training, education, and licensing."[75] In addition to advocating truth in advertising legislation, the AMA also released a widely published advertisement in opposition to advanced practice nursing, particularly the DNP.[76]

The introduction of the DNP also reignited long-simmering debates within nursing about the types of education needed to deliver high-quality patient care. This raised questions among some nurse leaders as to whether the push to establish the DNP as the requisite credential for entry into advance practice nursing roles was just more of the same "emphasis on credentialism" and its attendant marginalization of those denied access to the educational ranks that Janice Ruffin had warned of in the 1970s.[77] Given nursing's "long history of marginalization," Afaf I. Meleis, dean of the University of Pennsylvania School of Nursing, and Kathleen Dracup, dean of the UCSF School of Nursing, asked whether nursing was "intentionally creating the potential for another set of marginalizing credentials." This time, they questioned the potential "devaluation of the MS-prepared advanced practice nurses who [were] slated to be obsolete and replaced by the new DNP graduates."[78] In response, though, DNP advocates held up the fact that clinical master's programs were usually twice as long (requiring twice as much course credit) as all other master's programs, and in fact were already almost equivalent to the amount of credit and preparation expected of other practice doctoral programs.[79] So rather than saying master's degree programs were not good enough to prepare nurses for advanced practice roles, DNP advocates instead argued that the extensive educational preparation that advanced practice nurses undertook in MSN programs was not being adequately valued and that the DNP was a way to appropriately credit nurses for work they were already doing.

For some nurse leaders, the DNP also threatened the hard-fought gains that academic nurses had made to establish the discipline of nursing science and the place of nurse scientists within universities and AHCs.[80] In 2005, Meleis and Dracup argued that "going ahead with the DNP [was] a major mistake" for the nursing profession and the "discipline of nursing knowledge." In their view, efforts to develop the DNP were "derailing our efforts to become equals in universities of higher learning, and . . . setting the stage for developing second-class citizens [in universities] who are marginalized." As Meleis and Dracup explained, academic nurses had "participated painfully" for more than thirty years "to justify, provide rationale for, and present evidence that growth in nursing science depends on providing a degree that equals other terminal degrees in the university," that is, the PhD. Thus, nursing faculty had fought long and hard to "become equal partners in universities," the outcome of which was not just "confidence and self-confidence of faculty but, more importantly, the ability of nursing faculty to become part of the decision-making bodies of universities and affect policies, budget, and the future of universities." The ability to offer an equal terminal degree, the PhD, "that [was] acknowledged and respected by all disciplines" was essential to nursing's ability to emerge "out of academic marginalization." DNP advocates argued that the DNP should be the requisite credential for clinical teaching, but DNP-prepared nursing faculty would have neither the same status nor standing within university governance as the PhD-prepared faculty, their roles limited to nontenured, nonvoting status. Meleis and Dracup thus asked, "With such a history of struggle and marginalization, why repeat it?"[81]

Another concern raised about the DNP was that it would further limit the number of nurses pursuing the PhD and careers as nurse scientists. For Meleis and Dracup, given the shortage of nurse scientists, the profession's priority should be "to prepare and train those who can combine and integrate advanced nursing expertise with a scientific knowledge base to produce the evidence for improving the quality of care for our clients."[82] But for advocates of the DNP, the existence of two distinct doctoral programs would help students better identify and select the type of doctoral education needed to meet their career goals. The University of Minnesota School of Nursing was an early adopter of the DNP. Prior to offering the DNP, the faculty had found that many of the nurses who pursued a PhD in order to teach "really didn't want to be researchers."[83] After earning their PhD, "they'd go teach and they wouldn't be researchers."[84] After a decade of offering both the DNP and the PhD, several of the faculty noted that the while the DNP degree was an option for nurses who wanted to teach but were not interested in becoming researchers, "people who are coming into our PhD program really want to be researchers. So that's a good thing."[85]

Nevertheless, by 2020, concerns about declining enrollments in nursing PhD programs—and the resulting shortage of PhD-prepared faculty, and thus nurse scientists—had grown.[86] While enrollments in DNP programs had expanded significantly since the turn of the twenty-first century, enrollments in nursing PhD programs have been declining since 2013.[87] This not only has implications for the advancement of nursing science, but it also contributes to the ongoing shortage of PhD-prepared nurse faculty and the attendant downstream effects on limiting admissions into undergraduate and graduate nursing degree programs, even as the U.S. is in the midst of a nursing shortage. Indeed, upon entering the third decade of the twenty-first century, the U.S. is in the midst of another nursing shortage. Although the country has faced cyclical nursing shortages since the turn of the twentieth century, experts warn that the early twenty-first century shortage is different from other shortages because of the compounding factors of the aging of the baby boom generation, the increasing incidence of chronic disease, and an aging nursing workforce.[88] The nursing shortage is exacerbated by the shrinking capacity of nursing schools to meet the demand for nursing students because of persistent shortages of PhD-prepared faculty. A survey conducted by the American Association of Colleges of Nursing in 2014 reported that 68,938 qualified applicants to baccalaureate, master's, and doctoral programs were not accepted because of insufficient capacity to teach them.[89]

As this book has explained, nursing has been plagued by a shortage of doctorally prepared nursing faculty since the 1960s. Nurse leaders hoped the introduction and expansion of nursing PhD programs from the 1960s onward would help solve this shortage. It did not. By preparing graduates for roles as expert clinical teachers, the DNP *could* be viewed as helping to solve the problem of a shortage of doctorally prepared faculty. Indeed, DNP-prepared nurses are increasingly providing the majority of clinical teaching in nursing schools located in AHCs. As they do so while maintaining robust practices, they are also helping to close the gap between nursing service and nursing education. Although master's-prepared advanced practice nurses had for decades provided this clinical teaching (also while often engaging in practice), their presence as non-doctorally prepared faculty ostensibly undermined nursing's academic project. Thus, as nursing schools shift to having an all-doctorate faculty, they are symbolically asserting nursing's ascendancy as an academic discipline and science-based profession, equal and parallel to other health professions schools within universities and AHCs. And yet, as Meleis and Dracup warned in 2005, the introduction of the practice doctorate actually reintroduced the potential for the marginalization of DNP-prepared faculty. So, too, the introduction of yet another rung on the educational hierarchy within nursing reflects and reinforces the historical and ongoing marginalization of nurses who—either by choice or because of structural barriers, including racism—have not reached the terminal degree of that pathway.

This very recent history of the DNP, and the longer history of nursing's academic project in which it is situated, ultimately demonstrates the intersections of disciplinary, institutional, and interprofessional politics, as well as the politics of health and higher education policymaking, in the transformation of American nursing. This history also makes clear the intersections of politics and policymaking in the making of new academic disciplines, the education of America's health care professionals, and the history of academic health centers and the ecosystem of knowledge production and application they were part of.

As the health care professions are called to reckon with the racism embedded within the health care system and the racial inequities created by it, it is critical to understand how one such health care profession chose to construct its discipline, determined which knowledge and thus which type of research had value, and decided who would be invited to that epistemological project.[90] Doing so makes clear that the epistemological, structural, and political choices made by the health professions in the past—as do their choices in the present—have profound implications not only for who gets to work as a health care professional, but also for who has access to health care and how those with access experience the care they receive. In other words, the health professions and the disciplines they construct have always been integral to the racism, sexism, ableism, and other forms of discrimination within the health care system—and for the inequities created by them. So too, the health care professions and the disciplines that underpin them are critical—as they have also been in the past—to challenging discrimination and affecting change in the health care system.

Acknowledgments

This book has its roots in my years as a graduate student at the University of Pennsylvania. It was there that my advisor, Ruth Schwartz Cowan, emphasized the importance of nurses as historical actors and introduced me to the Barbara Bates Center for the Study of the History of Nursing, where the faculty, especially Patricia D'Antonio and Julie Fairman, helped to nurture and guide my growing interest in the history of nursing. They have remained mentors ever since, for which I am immensely grateful. It was at the University of Minnesota, and during my research for the University of Minnesota Academic Health Center (AHC) Oral History Project, that the project took shape. It was in the university's archival records and in the interviews I conducted with nurses who had trained, worked, and taught at the School of Nursing and in the University Hospital and Clinics that it became clear that nursing was a critical lens through which to examine major changes that have taken place in American health care in the second half of the twentieth century, including the emergence of AHCs and their impact—and the role of the state—on health professions education and health care delivery.

The research for this book would not have been possible without the expertise and assistance of archivists, curators, and librarians. I am especially grateful to Erik Moore and Erin George at the University of Minnesota Archives; Charlotte Brown and Julie Jenkins at the UCLA Archives; Nina Stoyan-Rosenzweig at the University of Florida Health Center Archives and Peggy McBride at the University of Florida Archives; Hannah Day Cox at the Ruth Lilly Special Collections and Archives at Indiana University–Purdue University Indianapolis (IUPUI); Kevin O'Brien and Susan Glover at the Health Sciences Special Collections, University of Illinois Chicago; Helen Conger and Jill Tatam at Case Western Reserve University Archives; Tiffany Collier,

Elisa Stroh, and Jessica Clark at the Barbara Bates Center for the Study of
the History of Nursing; Kristen Lynn Chinery and colleagues at Wayne State
University's Walter Reuther Library; and the archivists at the California State
Archives, the State Archives of Florida, and the Minnesota Historical Society.
I am also grateful to the graduate research assistants who worked with me
on the University of Minnesota AHC Oral History Project, which was foundational to this project: Eli Vituli, Emily Beck, and Lauren Klaffke. Lauren
Klaffke is due extra thanks for doing double duty as my research assistant
during the early stages of research for this book. Thanks go also to Cory Ellen
Gatrall, who graciously shared archival material and insights about the nurse
educator and theorist Madeleine Leininger.

I was able to complete this research thanks to generous financial support
from two major sources. The first was the University of Minnesota McKnight
Land-Grant Professorship, which provided me with a year of research leave
and funding to support repeated research trips to California, Florida, Illinois,
Michigan, and Ohio. The second source was a Karen Buhler-Wilkerson Fellowship from the Barbara Bates Center for the Study of the History of Nursing at the University of Pennsylvania, which supported research trips to the
Bates Center archives, as well as the opportunity to present on early versions
of this work to very engaged audiences. I'm also very thankful to Ed, Suzanne,
Owen, and Toby Wagner, and to Faye Allard and Matthew Glass, who each
provided me with incredible hospitality during two of my research trips.

I have been fortunate to have benefited from very thoughtful and engaged
feedback on early versions of various chapters from Patricia D'Antonio, Daniel M.
Fox, and Beth Linker. I'm grateful to Beth Linker for once again coming up
with a compelling title for my book—this time, "Dr. Nurse." I owe a huge debt
of gratitude to Susan Craddock, who carefully read and gave wonderful feedback on all chapters of the book, as well as providing a lot of encouragement
throughout the process. I am also extraordinarily grateful to the two anony-
mous reviewers who gave me incredible feedback on the proposal and two
early chapters and then on the completed manuscript. This book is a much better one for the generosity of time, insights, and contributions of all my readers.
Karen Merikangas Darling has been a supportive and astute editor throughout.
I'm also thankful to the editorial and production team at the University of Chicago Press. This includes Mariah Gumpert, who copyedited the manuscript,
as well as Tristan Bates, Jenni Fry, Deirdre Kenney, and John Dertien at Book-
Comp, each of whom ensured the final stages of this process went smoothly.
Thanks also to Springer Publishing Company, which published a previous ver-
sion of chapter 2 under the title "'Coming to Grips with the Nursing Question':
The Politics of Nursing Education Reform in 1960s America," *Nursing History*

Review (2014) 22: 37–60. Copyright © 2014, reproduced with the permission of Springer Publishing Company, LLC.

On the way to completing this book, audiences at the American Association for the History of Nursing, the Barbara Bates Center for the Study of the History of Nursing, the University of Iowa History of Medicine group, the University of Minnesota Program in the History of Medicine, and the University of Virginia School of Nursing raised great questions and offered valuable comments on various aspects of this project. Colleagues and friends whose support was invaluable along the way include Rima Apple, Winifred Connerton, Cindy Connolly, Ruth Cowan, Chris Crenner, Patricia D'Antonio, Julie Fairman, Karen Flynn, Daniel M. Fox, Cory Ellen Gatrall, Mary Gibson, Jeremy Greene, Wendy Kline, Becky Kluchin, Sue Lederer, Debby Levine, Sandra Lewenson, Beth Linker, Amanda Mahoney, Annemarie McAllister, Susan Reverby, Naomi Rogers, Kylie Smith, Nancy Tomes, Keith Wailoo, John Harley Warner, Elizabeth Watkins, Barbra Mann Wall, and the late Jean Whelan.

In the final stages of writing this book, I left one university and joined another. Many thanks to my former colleagues at the University of Minnesota who shared support and feedback, especially Jennifer Alexander, Emily Beck, Sam Fletcher, Lois Hendrickson, Jennifer Gunn, Susan Jones, Sally Gregory Kohlstedt, and Mary Thomas. Thank you to my former and current graduate students Macey Flood, Lauren Klaffke, David Korostyshevsky, Jessica Nickrand, Lauren Ruhrold, Elizabeth Semler, and Aimee Slaughter for stimulating ideas and discussions. I am also grateful to the insights and experiences shared by Connie Delaney, Joanne Disch, MaryJo Kreitzer, and Marie Manthey, along with the many nurses I interviewed that were part of the University of Minnesota School of Nursing's history. I am fortunate to have joined terrific colleagues at the University of Virginia School of Nursing. Thanks, especially, to my colleagues at the Eleanor Crowder Bjoring Center for Nursing Historical Inquiry, Barbra Mann Wall, Mary Gibson, Arlene Keeling, Beth Hundt, Maura Singleton, and Hal Sharp, as well as to Ken White, Cathy Campbell, Susan Kools, and Pam Cipriano for the warm and supportive welcome. UVA has been a fantastic academic home from which to complete this book and embark on the next chapter of my career.

It is an understatement to say that my friends and family have sustained me throughout the long and arduous process of writing this book. Special thanks go to Don and Deborah Pierce, Jackie and Dale Klakoski, Susan Craddock, Lisa Peterson, Matt Tontonoz, and Jen and Aaron Whitcomb, who have been tireless in their love, support, and encouragement. Also due special thanks are the "Thouron Team" of Suzanne Wagner, Faye Allard, Jane Machin, and Alex Channer, who have been a brilliant source of support, encouragement, laughter, and hilarity since we all first met in a London pub in the summer of 2001, a couple of months before we made the big leap across the Atlantic to begin our graduate studies at the University of Pennsylvania. I am also incredibly grateful for the support and guidance that Jeannine Myrvik provided through the many ups and downs of researching and writing this book.

Finally, my greatest thanks go to Beth Klakoski and Lola Fugarino, who joined me in this journey midway through and helped me, in immeasurable ways, to finally get the book done! To my wife, Beth, for bringing so much love, joy, and laughter into my life and for being my biggest supporter. And to Lola, for always managing to cheer me up with laughter and hugs even on the most challenging of writing days. Together, Beth and Lola have taught me the importance of stepping away from the work and being present in the moment. And to our dogs, Keiko and Pompet, our cats Ben and Ajax, and to the late Taka, Beefy, and Turtle, who each provided endless entertainment, timely (and-not-so-timely) distractions, and the much-needed comfort of cuddles on demand.

Archives and Collections Consulted

Barbara Bates Center for the Study of the History of Nursing, University of Pennsylvania, Philadelphia, PA

- Florence Downs Papers
- Jessie May Scott Papers
- Dorothy Smith Papers

California State Archives, Sacramento, CA

- Department of Health Services
- Health Planning Council Records, Office of Statewide Health Planning and Development
- Records of the Office of Comprehensive Health Planning
- Senate Health and Human Services Committee Records

Case Western Reserve University Archives, Cleveland, OH

- Frances Payne Bolton School of Nursing Collection

Cassandra News Journal Digital Archive

- https://peggychinn.com/projects/cassandra/cassandra-newsjournal/

State Archives of Florida, Tallahassee, FL

- Bureau of Comprehensive Health Planning
- Florida Health Planning Council Records

- Florida State Board of Health, Long Range Planning
- Records of Governor Askew

Minnesota State Archives, Minnesota Historical Society, Saint Paul, MN

- Health Planning Agency
- Health Planning Section
- Legislative House Appropriations Committee, Medical Education Subcommittee
- Minnesota Board of Health, Division of Health Manpower
- Minnesota Higher Education Coordinating Board
- Minnesota Higher Education Coordinating Commission
- Minnesota Health Planning and Development Program
- Planning Agency, Human Services Division, Health Planning Section

Ruth Lilly Special Collections and Archives, IUPUI, Indianapolis, IN

- Midwest Alliance in Nursing Collection

University of California, Los Angeles Archives, Los Angeles, CA

- Collection 401
- #RS300
- Administrative Files of Stafford Warren
- Administrative Files of Chancellor Raymond Allen
- Administrative Files of Jeanne Williams
- Administrative Files of Ransom Arthur
- Administrative Files of Chancellor Charles E. Young
- Oral History Collection

University of California, Los Angeles Biomedical Library, Special Collections, Los Angeles, CA

- Lulu Wolf Hassenplug Papers

University of Florida Archives, Gainesville, FL

- Vice President for Academic Affairs
- Presidential Collections
  - J. Hillis Miller
  - John Allen
  - J. Wayne Reitz

- Samuel Proctor Oral History Program
- College of Nursing Oral History Project

University of Florida Health Science Center Archives, Gainesville, FL

- Series 4 VP for Health Affairs
  - Harrell, Martin, Ackell, Finger
- Series 5 Medical Center Study
- Series 10 College of Nursing

University of Illinois, Chicago Archives, Chicago, IL

- University Archives College of Nursing Papers
- Nurse Faculty Research Development in the Midwest Collection
- Midwest Nursing Research Society Collection

University of Minnesota Archives, Minneapolis, MN

- Katharine J. Densford Papers
- Medical School Collection
- Office of the Vice President for Academic Administration
- President's Office
- School of Nursing Collection
- Academic Health Center Oral History Project
- School of Nursing Oral History Project

Walter P. Reuther Library, University Archives, Wayne State University, Detroit, MI

- Madeleine M. Leininger Collection, Acc. No. 725
- College of Nursing, Acc. No. WSR 000148
- College of Nursing Collection, Acc. No. 728
- College of Nursing Center for Health Research Collection, Acc. No. 2167
- Nursing, Dean's Office, Acc. No. 672
- Office of the President William Rea Keast, Acc. No. 1883

Notes

Introduction

1. American Nurses Association, "What Is Nursing?" https://www.nursingworld.org/practice-policy/workforce/what-is-nursing/ (accessed July 19, 2019); Rachel Butler, Mauricio Monsalve, Geb W. Thomas, Ted Herman, Alberto M. Segre, Philip M. Polgreen, and Manish Suneja, "Estimating Time Physicians and other Health Care Workers Spend with Patients in an Intensive Care Unit Using a Sensor Network." *American Journal of Medicine* (2018) 131(8): 972.e9–972.e15; Bevin Cohen, Sandra Hyman, Lauren Rosenberg, and Elaine Larson, "Frequency of Patient Contact with Health Care Personnel and Visitors: Implications for Infection Prevention." *Joint Commission Journal on Quality and Patient Safety* (2012): 38(12): 560–565.

2. World Health Organization, "Nursing and Midwifery," January 9, 2020, https://www.who.int/news-room/fact-sheets/detail/nursing-and-midwifery (accessed May 11, 2021).

3. This observation is based on numerous oral histories and personal communications with nurse researchers. Related to this, in its 2016 report, the American Association of Colleges of Nursing noted that "despite notable advances in nursing-led research," deans of nursing "report a sense of being on the margin of enterprise research initiatives" and that, in general, nursing faculty, students, and academic programs "have been undervalued at best, and ignored at worse" within academic health centers. American Association of Colleges of Nursing and Manatt Health Project Team, *Advancing Healthcare Transformation: A New Era for Academic Nursing* (Washington, DC: American Association of Colleges of Nursing, March 2016), 13. Furthermore, in a 2014 editorial, Peggy Chinn coined the term "nursesogyny," which she defined as "the underlying disdain and discounting of nursing as it is expressed in discussions" of nursing theories and other aspects of nursing science. See Peggy Chinn, "From the Editor: Nursing Theories for the 21st Century," *Advances in Nursing Science* (2014) 37(1): 1.

4. Mary E. Kerr, "Support for Nursing Science," *Nursing Outlook* (2016) 64: 262–270.

5. Personal communication with several nurse scientists.

6. Susan M. Reverby, "A Legitimate Relationship: Nursing, Hospitals, and Science in the Twentieth Century," in Diana Elizabeth Long and Janet Golden (eds.) *The American General Hospital. Communities and Social Contexts* (Ithaca, NY: Cornell University Press, 1989), 135–156.

7. Julie Fairman, *Making Room in the Clinic: Nurse Practitioners and the Evolution of Modern Health Care* (New Brunswick, NJ: Rutgers University Press, 2008), 54–85. Daniel M. Fox, *The*

Convergence of Science and Governance: Research, Health Policy, and American States (Berkeley: University of California Press, 2010), 35–40.

8. Joel D. Howell, *Technology in the Hospital: Transforming Patient Care in the early Twentieth Century* (Baltimore: Johns Hopkins University Press, 1995); Rosemary A. Stevens, *In Sickness and in Wealth: American Hospitals in the Twentieth Century* (Baltimore: Johns Hopkins University Press, 1999).

9. Stevens (1999), 201–203; and Joan Lynaugh and Barbara Brush, *American Nursing: From Hospitals to Health Systems* (Malden, MA: Blackwell Publishers, 1996), 2.

10. Lynaugh and Brush (1996), 2.

11. Stevens (1999), 203–204.

12. Stevens (1999), 200–255.

13. Jennifer Klein, *For All These Rights: Business, Labor, and the Shaping of America's Public-Private Welfare State* (Princeton, NJ: Princeton University Press, 2003); Christy Ford Chapin, *Ensuring American's Health: The Public Creation of the Corporate Health Care System* (Cambridge: Cambridge University Press, 2015).

14. Rosemary Stevens, "History and Health Policy in the United States: The Making of a Health Care Industry, 1948–2008," *Social History of Medicine* (2008) 21(3): 461–483, 467.

15. Stevens (2008). For detailed analysis of the history of health insurance, see Chapin (2015).

16. Beatrix Hoffman, "Scientific Racism, Insurance, and Opposition to the Welfare State: Frederick L. Hoffman's Transatlantic Journey," *Journal of the Gilded Age and Progressive Era* (2003) 2: 150–190; Sharon A. Murphy, *Investing in Life: Insurance in Antebellum America* (Baltimore: Johns Hopkins University Press, 2010); Beatrix Hoffman, *Health Care for Some: Rights and Rationing in the United States since 1930* (Chicago: University of Chicago Press, 2012), 90–113; Chapin (2015); Benjamin Wiggins, *Calculating Race: Racial Discrimination in Risk Assessment* (Oxford: Oxford University Press, 2020).

17. Melissa A. Thomasson, "Racial Difference in Health Insurance Coverage and Medical Expenditures in the United States: A Historical Perspective," *Social Science History* (2006) 30(4): 529–550; Hoffman (2012), 90–113.

18. *Source Book of Health Insurance Data* (New York: Health Insurance Institute, 1960), 10.

19. *Source Book of Health Insurance Data* (New York: Health Insurance Institute, 1960), 9.

20. Stevens (1999), 204.

21. Lynaugh and Brush (1996), 1.

22. Only in the wake of civil rights legislation in the 1960s, which made racial discrimination illegal and led to a slow, uneven, and incomplete dismantling of racial segregation in hospitals, did Black nurses enter hospitals in any significant number. Prior to this, though, even "Black hospitals relied heavily on student labor and were slow to make the transition to a graduate nursing staff." Darlene Clark Hine, *Black Women in White* (Bloomington: Indiana University Press, 1989), 188. See also M. Elizabeth Carnegie, *The Path We Tread: Blacks in Nursing Worldwide, 1854–1994* (Sudbury, MA: Jones and Bartlett, 2000).

23. Lynaugh and Brush (1996), 4.

24. American Medical Association, "Report of the Committee on Nursing Problems," *JAMA* (1948) 137: 878; Eli Ginzberg, *A Program for the Nursing Profession by the Committee on the Function of Nursing* (New York: Macmillan, 1948) and Esther Lucile Brown. *Nursing for the Future: A Report Prepared for the National Nursing Council* (New York: Russell Sage Foundation, 1948). Discussed in Lynaugh and Brush (1996), 8–9.

25. Lynaugh and Brush (1996), 4–11; Jean C. Whelan, *Nursing the Nation: Building the Nursing Labor Force* (New Brunswick, NJ: Rutgers University Press, 2021).

26. Barbara Melosh, *"The Physician's Hand": Work Culture and Conflict in American Nursing* (Philadelphia: Temple University Press, 1982); Susan Reverby, *Ordered to Care: The Dilemma of American Nursing, 1850–1945* (New York: Cambridge University Press, 1987); Patricia D'Antonio, *American Nursing: A History of Knowledge, Authority, and the Meaning of Work* (Baltimore: Johns Hopkins University Press, 2010); D'Antonio, *Nursing with a Message: Public Health Demonstration Projects in New York City* (New Brunswick, NJ: Rutgers University Press, 2017).

27. Julie Fairman and Joan E. Lynaugh, *Critical Care Nursing: A History* (Philadelphia: University of Pennsylvania Press, 1998); Arlene Keeling, "Blurring the Boundaries Between Medicine and Nursing: Coronary Care Nursing, circa the 1960s," *Nursing History Review* (2005) 13: 139–164; Margarete Sandelowski, *Devices and Desires: Gender, Technology, and American Nursing* (Chapel Hill: University of North Carolina Press, 2000).

28. A selection of the literature documenting the changing nature of American universities after the war includes Rebecca S. Lowen, *Creating the Cold War University: The Transformation of Stanford* (Berkeley: University of California Press, 1997); Henry Etzkowitz, *MIT and the Rise of Entrepreneurial Science* (New York: Routledge, 2002); Daniel Lee Kleinman, *Impure Cultures: University Biology and the World of Commerce* (Madison: University of Wisconsin Press, 2003); Daniel S. Greenberg, *The Politics of Pure Science* (Chicago: University of Chicago Press, 1999); and Greenberg, *Science for Sale: The Perils, Rewards, and Delusions of Campus Capitalism* (Chicago: University of Chicago Press, 2007).

29. Hugh Davis Graham and Nancy Diamond, *The Rise of American Research Universities: Elites and Challengers in the Postwar Era* (Baltimore: Johns Hopkins University Press, 1997), 3. On a national scale, the postwar expansion of graduate education was intended to provide the highly trained scientific and engineering labor needed to ensure the U.S.'s scientific and technological leadership during the Cold War. This was all the more important following the Soviet Union's surprise launch of *Sputnik* in October 1957. Roger Geiger, *Research and Relevant Knowledge: American Research Universities since World War II* (New York: Routledge, 1993), 220.

30. Dominique A. Tobbell, " 'Coming to Grips with the Nursing Question': The Politics of Nursing Education Reform in 1960s America," *Nursing History Review* (2014) 22: 37–60.

31. Fairman and Lynaugh (1998); Fairman (2008); Kylie Smith, *Talking Therapy: Knowledge and Power in American Psychiatric Nursing* (New Brunswick, NJ: Rutgers University Press, 2020).

32. On boundary work, see Thomas Gieryn, "Boundary-Work and the Demarcation of Science from Non-Science: Strains and Interests in Professional Ideologies of Scientists," *American Sociological Review* (1983) 48(4): 781–795; and Andrew Abbott, *The System of Professions: An Essay on the Division of Expert Labor* (Chicago: University of Chicago Press, 1988).

33. Jeanne Daly, *Evidence-Based Medicine and the Search for a Science of Clinical Care* (Berkeley: University of California Press / Milbank Memorial Fund, 2005); Stefan Timmermans and Marc Berg, *The Gold Standard: The Challenge of Evidence-Based Medicine and Standardization in Health Care* (Philadelphia: Temple University Press, 2003).

34. Michael L. Millenson, *Demanding Medical Excellence: Doctors and Accountability in the Information Age* (Chicago: University of Chicago Press, 1997); Fox (2010), 22–50; and Nancy Tomes, *Remaking the American Patient: How Madison Avenue and Modern Medicine Turned Patients into Consumers* (Chapel Hill: University of North Carolina Press, 2016), 310–313.

35. Millenson (1997), 6.

36. Abbott (1988), 56.

37. Ellen D. Baer, "'A Cooperative Venture' in Pursuit of Professional Status: A Research Journal for Nursing," *Nursing Research* (1987) 36(1): 18–25.

38. Wendy Kline, *Bodies of Knowledge: Sexuality, Reproduction, and Women's Health in the Second Wave* (Chicago: University of Chicago Press, 2010); Alondra Nelson, *Body and Soul: The Black Panther Party and the Fight against Medical Discrimination* (Minneapolis: University of Minnesota Press, 2011); John Dittmer, *The Good Doctors: The Medical Committee for Human Rights and the Struggle for Social Justice in Health Care* (Jackson: University of Mississippi Press, 2009); Tomes (2016), 249–320.

39. For example, see Rita Arditti, "Feminism and Science," in Rita Arditti, Pat Brennan, and Steve Cavrak (eds.), *Science and Liberation* (Boston: South End Press, 1980); Elizabeth Fee, "A Feminist Critique of Scientific Objectivity," *Science for the People* (1982) 14(40): 5–8, 30–32; Hilary Rose, "Hand, Brain, and Heart: A Feminist Epistemology for the Natural Sciences," *Signs* (1983) 9(1): 73–90; Evelyn Fox Keller, "Women Scientists and Feminist Critics of Science," *Daedalus* (1987) 116(4): 77–91; Sandra Harding, *The Science Question in Feminism* (Ithaca, NY: Cornell University Press, 1986); Sandra Harding, *Whose Science? Whose Knowledge? Thinking from Women's Lives* (Ithaca, NY: Cornell University Press, 1991); and Londa Schiebinger, *Has Feminism Changed Science?* (Cambridge, MA: Harvard University Press, 1999).

40. Keller (1987), 79.

41. For overview, Schiebinger, (1999), 4.

42. For introduction to and overview of this literature, see Sandra Harding, *Science and Social Inequality: Feminist and Postcolonial Issues* (Urbana: University of Illinois Press, 2006); Sandra Harding, ed.) *The Postcolonial Science and Technology Studies Reader* (Durham, NC: Duke University Press, 2011); Kim TallBear, "Standing with and Speaking as Faith: A Feminist-Indigenous Approach to Inquiry," *Journal of Research Practice* (2014) 10(2): article N17; Anne Pollock and Banu Subramaniam, "Resisting Power, Retooling Justice: Promises of Feminist Postcolonial Technosciences," *Science, Technology, and Human Values* (2014) 41(6): 951–966; Moya Bailey and Whitney Peoples, "Towards a Black Feminist Health Science Studies," *Catalyst* (2017) 3(2): 1–27.

43. For example, see Margaret Rossiter, *Women Scientists in America: Struggles and Strategies to 1940* (Baltimore: Johns Hopkins University Press, 1982); Margaret Rossiter, *Women Scientists in America: Before Affirmative Action, 1940–1972* (Baltimore: Johns Hopkins University Press, 1998); and Schiebinger (1999).

44. Julie Fairman and Patricia D'Antonio, "Virtual Power: Gendering the Nurse-Technology Relationship," *Nursing Inquiry* (1999), 6: 178–186, 178.

45. See, for example, Schiebinger (1999), 190.

46. For brief summary of this literature, see Schiebinger (1999), 1–13. For examples of feminists who argue women scientists have distinctive ways of knowing, see Nel Noddings, *Caring: A Feminine Approach to Ethics and Moral Education* (Berkeley: University of California Press, 1984); Rose (1983); Sara Ruddick, *Maternal Thinking: Toward a Politics of Peace* (Boston: Beacon Press, 1989).

47. Rozella M. Schlotfeldt, "Nursing in the University Community," November 12, 1965, Case Western Reserve University Archives, Frances Payne Bolton School of Nursing Collection, Series 29DD, box 2, Papers of Dean Rozella Schlotfeldt, folder 1:1.

48. Lowen (1997); Etzkowitz (2002).

49. Janice E. Ruffin, "Issues for the Black Nurse Today: Competence and Commitment," *National League for Nursing Publications* (1974) 15–1513: 46–51.

50. Hine (1989); Karen C. Flynn, *Moving Beyond Borders: A History of Black Canadian and Caribbean Women in the Diaspora* (Toronto: University of Toronto Press, 2011); Charissa J. Threat, *Nursing Civil Rights: Gender and Race in the Army Nurse Corps* (Urbana: University of Illinois Press, 2015).

51. Christopher P. Loss, *Between Citizens and the State: The Politics of American Higher Education in the 20th Century* (Princeton, NJ: Princeton University Press, 2011).

52. Reverby (1987); Hine (1989); Flynn (2011); and Smith (2020).

53. On racial inequities among nursing faculty: https://www.nln.org/docs/default-source /uploadedfiles/default-document-library/distribtion-of-full-time-nurse-educators-by-race-2019 -pdf.pdf?sfvrsn=ca00d_0h (accessed Feburary 17, 2022). Karen C. Flynn, Susan M. Reverby, Kylie M. Smith, and Dominique Tobbell, "'The Thing behind the Thing': White Supremacy and Interdisciplinary Faculty in Schools of Nursing," *Nursing Outlook* (2021) 1–3, https://doi .org/10.1016/j.outlook.2021.03.001 (accessed February 17, 2022); National Academy of Medicine, *The Future of Nursing 2020-2030: Charting a Path to Achieve Health Equity* (Washington, DC: National Academies Press, 2021).

54. Rachel R. Hardeman, Eduardo M. Medina, and Katy B. Kozhimannil, "Dismantling Structural Racism, Supporting Black Lives and Achieving Health Equity: Our Role, *New England Journal of Medicine* (2016) 375(22): 2113–2115; Rachel R. Hardeman, Eduardo M. Medina, and Rhea W. Boyd, "Stolen Breaths," *New England Journal of Medicine* (2020) 383(3): 197–199; Mary T. Bassett and Sandro Galea, "Reparations as a Public Health Priority: A Strategy for Ending Black-White Health Disparities," *New England Journal of Medicine* (2020) 383(22): 2101–2103; Dereck W. Paul Jr., Kelly R. Knight, Andre Campbell, and Louise Aronson, "Beyond a Moment: Reckoning with Our History and Embracing Antiracism in Medicine," *New England Journal of Medicine* (2020) 383(15): 1404–1406; Calvin Moorley, Philip Darbyshire, Laura Serrant, Janine Mohamed, Parveen Ali, and Ruth De Souza, "Dismantling Structural Racism: Nursing Must Not Be Caught on the Wrong Side of History," *Journal of Advances in Nursing* (2020) 76: 2450–2453; Ayah Nuriddin, Graham Mooney, and Alexandre I. R. White, "Reckoning with Histories of Medical Racism and Violence in the USA," *Lancet* (2020) 396: 949–951.

55. Jonathan Harwood, "Engineering Education between Science and Practice: Rethinking the Historiography," *History and Technology* (2006) 22(1): 53–79, 55.

56. Jonathan Harwood, "Understanding Academic Drift: On the Institutional Dynamics of Higher Technical and Professional Education," *Minerva* (2010) 48: 413–427, 413.

57. See for example, Bruce E. Seely, "Research, Engineering, and Science in American Engineering Colleges: 1900–1960," *Technology and Culture* (1993) 34(2): 344–386; Bruce E. Seely, "The Other Re-engineering of Engineering Education, 1900–1965." *Journal of Engineering Education* (July 1999): 285–294; and Harwood (2006).

58. Nathan Ensmenger, *The Computer Boys Take Over: Computers, Programmers, and the Politics of Technical Expertise* (Cambridge, MA: MIT Press, 2013), 111–136, 116.

59. James H. Capshew, *Psychologists on the March: Science, Practice, and Professional Identity in America, 1929-1969* (Cambridge: Cambridge University Press, 1999); Andrew Hogan, "The 'Two Cultures' in Clinical Psychology: Constructing Disciplinary Divides in the Management of Mental Retardation," *ISIS* (2018) 109(4): 695–719; Wade Pickren, "Tension and Opportunity in Post–World War II American Psychology," *History of Psychology* (2007) 10(3): 279–299; Nancy Tomes, "The Development of Clinical Psychology, Social Work, and Psychiatric Nursing: 1900–1980," in Edwin R. Wallace and John Gach (eds.) *History of Psychiatry and Medical Psychology* (New York: Springer, 2008): 657–682.

60. Robert A. Buerki, "American Pharmaceutical Education, 1952–2002," *Journal of the American Pharmaceutical Association* (2002) 42(4): 542–544; Gregory J. Higby, "From compounding to caring: an abridged history of American pharmacy," in Calvin Knowlton and Richard Penna, eds., *Pharmaceutical Care: A Primer on the Pharmacist's Changing Role in Patient Care*, 2nd ed. (Bethesda, MD: American Society of Health-System Pharmacists, 2003), 19–42.

61. Don C. McLeod, "Clinical Pharmacy: The Past, Present and Future," *American Journal of Hospital Pharmacy* (1976) 33: 29–38; Dominique A. Tobbell, " 'Eroding the Physician's Control of Therapy': The Postwar Politics of the Prescription," in Jeremy A. Greene and Elizabeth Siegel Watkins (eds.), *Prescribed: Writing, Filling, Using, and Abusing the Prescription in Modern America* (Baltimore: Johns Hopkins University Press, 2012), 66–90; Elizabeth Siegel Watkins, "Deciphering the Prescription: Pharmacists and the Patient Package Insert," in Jeremy A. Greene and Elizabeth Siegel Watkins (eds.), *Prescribed: Writing, Filling, Using, and Abusing the Prescription in Modern America* (Baltimore: Johns Hopkins University Press, 2012), 91–116; and Dominique A. Tobbell, "Clinical Pharmacy: An Example of Interprofessional Education in the Late 1960s and 1970s," *Nursing History Review* (2016) 24: 98–102.

62. Robert A. Buerki, "In Search of Excellence: The First Century of the American Association of Colleges of Pharmacy," *American Journal of Pharmaceutical Education* (1999) 63(Fall supplement).

63. Melosh (1982); Reverby (1987); D'Antonio (2010); D'Antonio (2017); Smith (2020).

64. D'Antonio (2017); Baer (1987); Reverby (1989), 135–156; and on British nursing, see Anne Marie Rafferty, *The Politics of Nursing Knowledge* (London: Routledge, 1996).

65. Susan Rimby Leighow, *Nurses' Questions / Women's Questions: The Impact of the Demographic Revolution and Feminism on United States Working Women, 1946–1986* (New York: Peter Lang, 1996); and Susan Gelfand Malka, *Daring to Care: American Nursing and Second-Wave Feminism* (Chicago: University of Illinois Press, 2007).

66. Fairman and Lynaugh (1998); Fairman (2008).

67. On the history of nursing workforce shortages in the U.S. prior to the 1950s, see Whelan (2021).

68. Institute of Medicine, *The Future of Nursing: Leading Change, Advancing Health* (Washington, DC: National Academies Press, 2011).

69. Ann C. Greiner and Elisa Knebel, eds., Committee on the Health Professions Education Summit, Board on Health Care Services, Institute of Medicine, *Health Professions Education: A Bridge to Quality* (Washington, DC: The National Academies Press, 2003), 3.

70. American Association of Colleges of Nursing, "AACN Position Statement on the Practice Doctorate in Nursing," October 2004, 8.

71. In 2007, the professional doctorate in audiology became the entry-level degree for the clinical practice of audiology. See Academy of Doctors of Audiology, "Au.D. History." https://www.audiologist.org/membership/aud-history (accessed February 17, 2022). Since 2016, the Commission on Accreditation in Physical Therapy Education has mandated that all entry-level physical therapist education programs only offer the doctor of physical therapy degree. For discussion of the issues raised by the mandate, see Sunita Mathur, "Doctorate in Physical Therapy: Is It Time for a Conversation?" *Physiotherapy Canada* (2011) 63(2): 140–142. In 2013, the American Occupational Therapy Association recommended that by 2025 all occupational therapy education programs be moved to the clinical doctorate level. After four years of debate, in 2017, the Accreditation Council for Occupational Therapy Education mandated that the entry-level degree requirement for the occupational therapist move to the doctoral level by July 1,

2027. American Occupational Therapy Association, "Postprofessional Programs in OT: Doctorate Degree Level," https://www.aota.org/Education-Careers/entry-level-mandate-doctorate-bachelors.aspx (accessed July 30, 2019). See, for example, Ted Brown, Jeffrey L. Crabtree, Keli Mu, and Joe Wells, "The Entry-Level Occupational Therapy Clinical Doctorate: Advantages, Challenges, and International Issues to Consider," *Occupational Therapy in Health Care* (2015) 29(2): 240–251.

Chapter One

1. Julie Fairman, *Making Room in the Clinic: Nurse Practitioners and the Evolution of Modern Health Care* (New Brunswick, NJ: Rutgers University Press, 2008), 41.

2. Fairman (2008), 41.

3. This chapter expands upon my previously published article, Dominique Tobbell, "'Coming to Grips with the Nursing Question': The Politics of Nursing Education Reform in 1960s America," *Nursing History Review* (2014) 22: 37–60. See also Fairman (2008), and Joan Lynaugh and Barbara Brush, *American Nursing: From Hospitals to Health Systems* (Malden, MA: Blackwellt, 1996).

4. This resonates with Susan Reverby's assertion that nurses' efforts to professionalize in the first half of the twentieth century were "fractured both by patriarchal constraints from above and differences among women from within." Susan M. Reverby, *Ordered to Care: The Dilemma of American Nursing, 1850–1945* (New York: Cambridge University Press, 1987), 2.

5. Joan E. Lynaugh, "Nursing the Great Society: The Impact of the Nurse Training Act of 1964," *Nursing History Review* (2008) 16: 13–28, 16.

6. Esther Lucile Brown, *Nursing for the Future: A Report Prepared for the National Nursing Council* (New York: Russell Sage, 1948), 49.

7. Lynaugh (2008), 14.

8. Susan M. Reverby, "A Legitimate Relationship: Nursing, Hospitals, and Science in the Twentieth Century," in Diana E. Long and Janet Golden (eds.), *The American General Hospital: Communities and Social Contexts* (Ithaca, NY: Cornell University Press, 1989), 135–156.

9. Julie Fairman and Joan E. Lynaugh, *Critical Care Nursing: A History* (Philadelphia: University of Pennsylvania Press, 1998), 9–10.

10. Julie Fairman, "Context and Contingency in the History of Post-World War II Nursing Scholarship in the United States," *Journal of Nursing Scholarship* (2008) 40(1): 4–11, 5.

11. Frances Cooke Macgregor, *Social Science in Nursing: Applications for the Improvement of Patient Care* (New York: Russell Sage Foundation, 1960), 19–34, 32.

12. George Engel, "The Need for a New Medical Model: A Challenge for Biomedicine," *Science* (1977) 196(4286): 129–136.

13. Patricia D'Antonio and Julie Fairman, "Organizing Practice: Nursing, the Medical Model, and Two Case Studies in Historical Time," *Canadian Bulletin of Medical History* (2004) 21(2): 411–419, 412.

14. Preface by Esther Lucile Brown in Macgregor (1960), 5; see also Brown (1948), 33–41.

15. Macgregor (1960), 9.

16. Macgregor (1960), 27.

17. Richard Magraw, oral history interview by Dominique A. Tobbell, July 31, 2009, University of Minnesota AHC Oral History Project, p. 7, https://ahc-ohp.lib.umn.edu/2012/01/12/richard-magraw/ (accessed March 13, 2021).

18. Magraw (2009), 8.

19. Macgregor (1960), 27.

20. Macgregor (1960), 31.

21. Macgregor (1960).

22. Brown (1948), p.138.

23. Eli Ginzberg, *A Program for the Nursing Profession by the Committee on the Function of Nursing* (New York: Macmillan, 1948).

24. Virginia Henderson, "The Nature of Nursing," *American Journal of Nursing* (1964) 64(8): 62–68, quotation from p. 66.

25. Henderson (1964), 63, 64.

26. Henderson (1964), 66.

27. Henderson (1964), 67.

28. Hildegard E. Peplau, *Interpersonal Relations in Nursing* (New York: G. P. Putnam's Sons, 1952).

29. Hildegard E. Peplau, "Interpersonal Techniques: The Crux of Psychiatric Nursing," *American Journal of Nursing* (1962) 62(6): 50–54, 53.

30. Kylie Smith, *Talking Therapy: Knowledge and Power in American Psychiatric Nursing* (New Brunswick: Rutgers University Press, 2020), 90.

31. Macgregor (1960), 36; Frances Cooke Macgregor, "Social Sciences and Nursing Education," *American Journal of Nursing* (1957) 57(7): 899–902.

32. Preface by Esther Lucile Brown in Macgregor (1960), 5.

33. Preface by Esther Lucile Brown in Macgregor (1960), 7.

34. Macgregor (1960), 32.

35. Preface by Esther Lucile Brown in Macgregor (1960), 7.

36. See, for example, Margaret Bridgman, *Collegiate Education for Nursing* (New York: Russell Sage Foundation, 1953).

37. Dorothy Smith, "Reflections," July 3, 1967, University of Pennsylvania, Bates Center for the Study of Nursing History, Dorothy Smith Papers, MC 118, Series III, box 6, folder 12.

38. Dorothy Smith, "The Development of a Clinical Tool: A Guide for History Taking," undated, University of Florida, George T. Harrell Medical History Center, RS4-VPHA Records: 4c- VPHA Ackell, box 35, folder: Nursing—Report of the College of Nursing.

39. Betty Hilliard, interview by Ann Smith, February 2, 2001, University of Florida College of Nursing Project, Samuel Proctor Oral History Program, University of Florida, p. 30.

40. Smith (undated).

41. Smith (undated).

42. Henderson (1964).

43. Smith (undated).

44. Smith (1967).

45. Smith (1967).

46. Dorothy Smith, "Position Paper on Nursing Education and Practice at the University of Florida," March 22, 1967, University of Florida, George T. Harrell Medical History Center, Series 10b College of Nursing, box 8, folder: Speeches, Talks, etc. by Dorothy Smith.

47. Jennet Wilson, interview by Ann Smith, August 22, 2002. University of Florida Oral History Program, p. 30.

48. Smith (undated).

49. Fairman (2008), 62.

50. Hilliard (2001), 30.

51. Dorothy Smith, interview by Stephen Kerber, March 26, 1979, University of Florida Oral History Program, p. 32.

52. Lucille Mercadante, interview by Ann Smith, March 28, 2001, University of Florida College of Nursing Project, Samuel Proctor Oral History Program, University of Florida, p. 17.

53. Hilliard (2001) p. 30.

54. Jean C. Whelan, *Nursing the Nation: Building the Nursing Labor Force* (New Brunswick, NJ: Rutgers University Press, 2021), 123–144.

55. Surgeon General's Consultant Group on Nursing, *Toward Quality in Nursing: Needs and Goals; Report of the Surgeon General's Consultant Group on Nursing* (Washington, DC: Government Printing Office, 1963), 11.

56. Mildred L. Montag with Lassar G. Gottkin, *Community College Education for Nursing: An Experiment in Technical Education for Nursing* (New York: McGraw-Hill, 1959); Edith Lewis, "The Associate Degree Program," *American Journal of Nursing* (1964) 64(5): 78–81. On history and impact of community colleges on nursing education, see Patricia D'Antonio, *American Nursing: A History of Knowledge, Authority, and the Meaning of Work* (Baltimore: Johns Hopkins University Press, 2010), 168–170.

57. Christopher P. Loss, *Between Citizens and the State: The Politics of American Higher Education in the 20th Century* (Princeton, NJ: Princeton University Press, 2011).

58. Keith W. Olson, *The G.I. Bill, the Veterans, and the Colleges* (Lexington: University Press of Kentucky, 1974).

59. President's Commission on Higher Education, *Higher Education for American Democracy* (New York: Harper and Brothers, 1947).

60. Claire Krendl Gilbert and Donald E. Heller, "Access, Equity, and Community Colleges: The Truman Commission and Federal Higher Education Policy from 1947 to 2011," *Journal of Higher Education* (2013) 84(3): 417–443; Nicholas M. Strohl, "The Truman Commission and the Unfulfilled Promise of American Higher Education," (unpublished PhD diss., University of Wisconsin–Madison, 2018).

61. Gilbert and Heller (2013), 432.

62. Patricia D'Antonio (2010), 169.

63. Fairman (2008), 43. See also Patricia D'Antonio, "Women, Nursing, and Baccalaureate Education in 20th Century America," *Journal of Nursing Scholarship* (2004) 36(4): 379–384.

64. Marion Altenderfer, *Minorities and Women in the Health Fields: Applicants, Students, and Workers*, Department of Health, Education, and Welfare (Bethesda, MD: Government Printing Office, 1975), 43–46; M. Elizabeth Carnegie, "The Minority Practitioner in Nursing," *National League for Nursing Publications* (1974) 15–1513: 39–42.

65. "National League for Nursing 1965 Convention," *Nursing Outlook* (June 1965) 13: 36.

66. American Nurses Association, "Education for Nursing," *American Journal of Nursing* (1965) 65: 106–111. Susan Rimby Leighow, "Backrubs vs. Bach: Nursing and the Entry-into-Practice Debate, 1946–1986," *Nursing History Review* (1996) 4: 3–17.

67. Lynaugh (2008).

68. D'Antonio (2010), 169–170.

69. Lynaugh (2008), 24.

70. William K. Turner, "Financing Nursing Education," *Hospitals* (1959) 33: 40–44, 40.

71. Turner (1959), 43.

72. Turner (1959); Lynaugh and Brush (1996), 11–12; and D'Antonio (2010), 168.

73. Turner (1959), 40.

74. Lynaugh (2008).

75. Fairman, 2008, pp. 46, 48, 49; Arlene W. Keeling, Barbara Brodie, and John Kirchgess-ner, *The Voice of Professional Nursing Education: A 40-Year History of the American Association of Colleges of Nursing* (Washington, DC: American Association of Colleges of Nursing, 2010), xxiv–xxvi.

76. Lynaugh (2008).

77. Bonnie Bullough, "You Can't Get There from Here: Articulation in Nursing Educa-tion," *Journal of Nursing Education* (November 1972): 4–10, 6. Bullough's data comes from *Facts about Nursing: A Statistical Summary,* 1970–1971 edition (New York: American Nurses Associa-tion), 95.

78. D'Antonio (2010), 168.

79. Fairman and Lynaugh (1998), 97.

80. Smith (2020), 78–108.

81. Fairman (2008), 44.

82. Henry K. Silver, Loretta C. Ford, and Lewis R. Day, "The Pediatric Nurse-Practitioner Program," *JAMA* (1968) 204(4): 298–302. See also Fairman (2008), 44; and Arlene W. Keeling, *Nursing and the Privilege of Prescription, 1893–2000* (Columbus: Ohio State University Press, 2007), 121–137.

83. Dominique Tobbell, "Plow, Town, and Gown: The Politics of Family Practice in 1960s America." *Bulletin of the History of Medicine* (2013) 87(4): 648–680.

84. For examples of Russell Sage, see Macgregor (1960); on the Kellogg Foundation, see Joan E. Lynaugh, "Mildred Tuttle: Private Initiative and Public Response in Nursing Edu-cation after World War II," *Nursing History Review* (2006) 14: 203–21; on the Division of Nurs-ing, see Cynthia Connolly and Joan Lynaugh, *Fifty Years at the Division of Nursing: United States Public Health Service* (Washington, DC: U.S. Public Health Service Division of Nursing, 1997).

85. Joan Lynaugh, "Academic Nursing Practice: Looking Back," in Lois K. Evans and Norma M. Lang (eds.), *Academic Nursing Practice: Helping to Share the Future of Health Care* (New York: Springer, 2004), 20–37, 24.

86. Surgeon General's Consultant Group on Nursing (1963).

87. Lynaugh (2008).

88. Surgeon General's Consultant Group on Nursing (1963).

89. Fairman (2008), 213–214, note 66; and Lynaugh (2008).

90. Daniel M. Fox, "From Piety to Platitudes to Pork: The Changing Politics of Health Workforce Policy," *Journal of Health Politics, Policy, and Law* (1996) 21(4): 823–842.

91. Lynaugh (2008), 22.

92. Lynaugh (2008); Keeling, Brodie, and Kirchgessner (2010); and Beatrice J. Kalisch, *Poli-tics of Nursing* (Lippincott Williams & Wilkins, 1982).

93. Catherine Ceniza Choy, *Empire of Care: Nursing and Migration in Filipino American His-tory* (Durham, NC: Duke University Press, 2003), 65.

94. Choy (2003), 78.

95. Catherine Ceniza Choy, " 'Exported to Care': A Transnational History of Filipino Nurse Migration to the United States," in Nancy Foner, Rubén G. Rumbaut, and Steven J. Gold (eds.), *Immigration Research for a New Century: Multidisciplinary Perspectives* (New York: Russell Sage Foundation, 2000), 113–133, 127.

96. Fairman (2008), 54–85; Daniel M. Fox, *The Convergence of Science and Governance: Research, Health Policy, and American States* (Berkeley: University of California Press, 2010), 35–40.

97. Madeleine Leininger, "Political Nursing: Essential for Health and Educational Systems of Tomorrow," presentation at the dedication of the Health Science Building for the School of Nursing Seminar at the University of Evansville, Evansville, Indiana, 1975, Walter P. Reuther Library, University Archives, Wayne State University, Madeleine Leininger Collection, Accession 725, box 7.

98. Leininger (1975); Madeleine Leininger, "Psychopolitical and Ethnocentric Behaviors in Emerging Health Science Centers," November 1974, Walter P. Reuther Library, University Archives, Wayne State University, Madeleine Leininger Collection, Accession 725, box 7.

99. Lulu K. Wolf Hassenplug Papers, 1863–1995. Online Archive of California, https://oac.cdlib .org/findaid/ark:/13030/kt4s2021hf/entire_text/h (accessed February 17, 2022).

100. Lulu Wolf Hassenplug, *"UCLA School of Nursing's Founding Dean,"* oral history interview by Judi Goodfriend, Los Angeles: Oral History Program, University of California, Los Angeles, 1989.

101. Hassenplug (1989), 243.

102. W. Eugene Stern, memorandum to Stafford L. Warren, "The Role of the Student Nurse and the Nursing School Curriculum with Respect to Patient Care," February 8, 1957, UCLA Archives, Collection RS300, box 178, folder: Departments—Nursing 1957.

103. W. Eugene Stern, William P. Longmire, and Willard E. Goodwin, memorandum to Stafford L. Warren, June 5, 1957, UCLA Archives, Collection RS300, box 178, folder: Departments—Nursing 1957.

104. William P. Longmire, *"Creating the Department of Surgery at the UCLA School of Medicine,"* oral history interview by Bernard Galm, Los Angeles: Oral History Program, University of California, Los Angeles, 1988, 521–524.

105. Stafford L. Warren, memorandum, "Radical Suggestions for Consideration," May 31, 1957, UCLA Archives, Collection RS300, box 178, folder: Departments–Nursing 1957.

106. Hassenplug (1989), 249–250.

107. Sherman Mellinkoff to Franklin D. Murphy, February 25, 1963, UCLA Archives, Collection 401, box 11, folder: Nursing School 1960–1964.

108. Franklin D. Murphy to Foster H. Sherwood, January 1, 1967, UCLA Archives, Collection 401, box 9, folder: I-Med 1960–1968; Foster H. Sherwood, "Nursing at UCLA," June 21, 1968, UCLA Archives, Collection 401, box 11, folder: Nursing School 1967–1970.

109. Forrest H. Adams et al. to Committee on Educational Policy, Budget and Interdepartmental Relations, Graduate Council, and the Chancellor's Office, "UCLA School of Nursing: A Position Paper," August 23, 1968, UCLA Archives, Collection 401, box 11, folder: Nursing School 1967–1970.

110. Colin Young to Foster H. Sherwood, February 19, 1969, UCLA Archives, Collection 401, box 11, folder: Nursing School 1967–1970.

111. Hassenplug (1989), 337–342.

112. For a comprehensive history of the University of Minnesota School of Nursing, see Laurie K. Glass, *Leading the Way: The University of Minnesota School of Nursing, 1909–2009* (Minneapolis: University of Minnesota School of Nursing, 2009).

113. Edna L. Fritz, *Faculty Selection, Appointment, and Promotion in Collegiate Nursing Programs* (EdD diss., Teachers College, Columbia University, 1965), http://pocketknowledge.tc .columbia.edu/home.php/viewfile/12030 (accessed February 17, 2022).

114. On the demonstration project, see Edna Fritz, *Toward Better Nursing Care of Patients with Long-Term Illness* (New York: Division of Education, National League of Nursing, 1956).

115. A. Marilyn Sime, oral history interview by Dominique A. Tobbell, April 15, 2010, University of Minnesota AHC Oral History Project, 6.

116. Brown (1948); Peplau (1952); Peplau (1962); J. Arthur Myers, *Masters of Medicine: An Historical Sketch of the College of Medical Sciences, University of Minnesota 1888-1966* (St. Louis: Warren H. Green, 1968), 541-544.

117. Sime (2010), 11.

118. Florence Marks, oral history interview by Dominique A. Tobbell, April 13, 2010, University of Minnesota AHC Oral History Project, 41.

119. Marie Manthey, oral history interview by Dominique A. Tobbell, October 12, 2010, University of Minnesota AHC Oral History Project, 5-6.

120. Manthey (2010), 12-16.

121. Personal communication with several of the alumni who graduated from the University of Minnesota School of Nursing in the late 1960s.

122. Ruth Weise, oral history interview by Dominique A. Tobbell, July 28, 2010, University of Minnesota AHC Oral History Project, 15. Some of the medical faculty expressed similar concerns about the inadequate clinical preparation of nursing students; see, for example, John P. Delaney, oral history interview by Dominique A. Tobbell, March 27, 2012, University of Minnesota AHC Oral History Project, 16.

123. See, for example, "Recommendation for Establishing Consultative Support and Continuing Education Services from the U of MN for the Furtherance of Practical Nursing Education and for Development of Programs in Nursing Leading to an Associate Degree in the State of MN, Concurrent with Disestablishment of the University's Program in Practical Nursing," undated but 1966 or 1967, University of Minnesota Archives, Office of the Vice President of Academic Administration, box 22, folder: Medical Sciences—Programs 1966-1967.

124. Edna Fritz to William G. Shepherd, April 18, 1966, University of Minnesota Archives, Office of the Vice President for Academic Affairs Papers, box 23, folder: Medical Sciences Nursing Programs 1966-1967.

125. "Recommendation for Establishing Consultative Support and Continuing Education Services" (undated).

126. Eugenia Taylor, oral history interview by Dominique A. Tobbell, May 27, 2010, University of Minnesota AHC Oral History Project, 16-21, 16.

127. Edna Fritz to Robert Howard, "Memorandum: Discontinuance of the Practical Nursing Program," February 19, 1965, University of Minnesota Archives, Office of the Vice President for Academic Affairs Papers, box 23, folder: Medical Sciences Nursing Programs 1966-1967.

128. Florence Brennan, Agnes Dempster, Frances Moncure, Marilyn Sime, Dorothy Titt, and Elizabeth Whitney to Robert Howard, March 27 1963, Office of the Vice President for Academic Affairs, box 30, folder: School of Nursing Review of Program 1967-1968.

129. Fritz (1956).

130. Marks (2010); quotation from Edna Fritz to William Shepherd, March 25, 1968, Office of the Vice President for Academic Affairs, box 30, folder: School of Nursing Review of Program 1967-1968.

131. Marks (2010), 46.

132. For a summary of these studies, see Lynaugh and Brush (1996), 8-9.

133. Surgeon General's Consultant Group on Nursing (1963).

134. For a study of health workforce needs, including nurses, in Minnesota, see Osler L. Peterson and Ivan J. Fahs (Health Manpower Study Commission), *Health Manpower for the Upper Midwest: A Study of the Needs for Physicians and Dentists in Minnesota, North Dakota, South Dakota, and Montana* (St. Paul, MN: Hill Family Foundation, 1966).

135. "A Report on Nursing Education in the University of California as Related to the Needs of California and the West," January 7, 1957, UCLA Archives, #RS300, box 178, folder: Departments—Nursing 1957.

136. Lillian B. McCall, "Nursing Education in California," in *A Report to the Coordinating Council for Higher Education* (1966) (California State Archives, #R384.142.147, Department of Public Health, Office of Comprehensive Health Planning, D3762, box 48, folder 5: Health Manpower Council 1966–1967), 9, 11, 12.

137. Ivan J. Fahs and Kathryn Barchas, *Nursing in the Upper Midwest: Focus on the State of Minnesota* (Minneapolis: Upper Midwest Research and Development Council, 1969), 24.

138. "Nursing Education in the University of California" (1957).

139. Brown (1948); Ginzberg (1948); and Bridgman (1953).

140. "Nursing Education in the University of California," (1957). See also McCall (1966), 9, 11, 12, 15–16.

141. George A. Pettitt, memorandum to deans, March 23, 1949, UCLA Archives, #RS300, box 47, folder: Medical Education in California 1949–1955.

142. The Master Plan had grown out of a series of studies of California public higher education conducted in the 1940s and 1950s. *A Master Plan for Higher Education in California, 1960–1975* (Sacramento: California State Department of Education, 1960); Glenn S. Dumke, "Higher Education in California," *California Historical Society Quarterly* (1963) 42(2): 99–110.

143. Sidney Roberts et al. to Franklin D. Murphy, "Report of the Ad Hoc Committee on Nursing," April 2, 1962, UCLA Archives, Collection 401, box 11, folder: Nursing School 1960–1964.

144. Edna Fritz to Elmer Learn, September 1, 1966, University of Minnesota Archives, President's Office, Collection 841, box 231, folder: Medical School, School of Nursing, 1960–1969.

145. Edna Fritz to O. Meredith Wilson, September 30, 1966, President's Office, Collection 841, box 231, folder: Medical School, School of Nursing, 1960–1969; "Recommendation for Establishing Consultative Support" (undated). The first two associate degree programs in Minnesota were established in 1964 at Hibbing Junior College in Hibbing and St. Mary's Junior College in Minneapolis; by 1969 there were four associate degree programs in the state. See Fahs and Barchas (1969), 5.

146. Hassenplug (1989), 277–279. WICHE was enacted in 1953 by the western states of New Mexico, Montana, Arizona, Utah, Oregon, Wyoming, and Colorado as a way of efficiently coordinating and sharing resources among the states' higher education systems. WICHE was focused in particular on ensuring that the states without their own health science schools could work with their western colleagues to ensure that enough health care professionals would be produced for the entire region. California joined the compact in 1955.

147. Fahs and Barchas (1969).

148. Jerome P. Lysaught, *An Abstract for Action: National Commission for the Study of Nursing and Nursing Education* (New York: McGraw-Hill, 1970); Ruth M. Lunde to Isabel Harris, February 11, 1971, University of Minnesota Archives, School of Nursing Collection, box 31, folder: 512 Planning for Rural Nursing.

149. William G. Shepherd, Statement to the School of Nursing Faculty, March 22, 1968, Office of the Vice President for Academic Affairs, box 30, folder: School of Nursing Review of Program 1967–1968.

150. Sime (2010), 16.

151. Keeling, Brodie, and Kirchgessner (2010), xx. On the dissolution of the NACGN and integration of Black nurses into the ANA, see Darlene Clark Hine, *Black Women in White* (Bloomington: Indiana University Press, 1989), 183–186.

152. On the NBNA, see https://www.nbna.org/history (accessed July 8, 2020); Hine (1989), 192; and Gloria R. Smith, "From Invisibility to Blackness: The Story of the National Black Nurses' Association," *Nursing Outlook* (1975) 23: 225–229.

153. Keeling, Brodie, and Kirchgessner (2010), xx.

154. Keeling, Brodie, and Kirchgessner (2010), xx–xxvi.

155. On the history of the formation of what would become the American Association of Colleges of Nursing, see Keeling, Brodie, and Kirchgessner (2010), 1–30.

156. Sister Bernadette Armiger, "American Association of Colleges of Nursing and the Council of Baccalaureate and Higher Degree Programs: Purposes, Roles and Relationships," *National League for Nursing Publications* (1974) 15–1528, 37–40. Dorothy Mereness to Rozella Schlotfeldt, January 11, 1968, Case Western Reserve University Archives, 29DB, box 15, folder: Doctoral Program 1965–1981.

157. Dorothy Mereness and Rozella Schlotfeldt, correspondence, 1967–1969. On December 14, 1967, Schlotfledt noted to Mereness that clinical nurse specialist and nurse practitioner training programs were being established "outside the aegis of the university," such as in "comprehensive mental health centers," and that there was "also some move among the neurologists and cardiologists to prepare their own 'specialists.'" On February 17, 1969, Schlotfeldt noted that she was not a fan of nurse practitioner programs, seeing them as programs advocated not by nurses but by physicians. Case Western Reserve University Archives, Frances Payne Bolton School of Nursing Collection, 29DB, box 15, folder: Doctoral Program 1965–1981. On issues related to regional planning and comprehensive health planning, see Mary Kelly Mullane, response to "Questionnaire Regarding Role and Function of Ad Hoc Committee on Deans of Accredited Masters Programs," dated February 6, 1968, Case Western Reserve University Archives, Frances Payne Bolton School of Nursing Collection, 29DB, box 15, folder: Doctoral Program 1965–1981.

158. On this point, see Ada F. Most, "American Association of Colleges of Nursing and the Council on Baccalaureate and Higher Degree Programs: Purposes, Roles and Relationships," *National League for Nursing Publications* (1974) 15–1528, 45–46.

159. Schlotfeldt to Mereness, December 14, 1967, and January 11, 1968. Quotation is from Schlotfeldt to Mereness, February 17, 1969, Case Western Reserve University Archives, Frances Payne Bolton School of Nursing Collection, 29DB, box 15, folder: Doctoral Program 1965–1981.

160. Schlotfeldt to Mereness, January 11, 1968. On the federal funding threat, see Schlotfeldt to Mereness, February 17, 1969. Case Western Reserve University Archives, Frances Payne Bolton School of Nursing Collection, 29DB, box 15, folder: Doctoral Program 1965–1981.

161. Mary Kelly Mullane to Marcia A. Dake, February 27, 1968, Case Western Reserve University Archives, 29DB, box 15, folder: Doctoral Program 1965–1981.

162. Joseph Begando to Mary Kelly Mullane, February 28, 1968, Case Western Reserve University Archives, Frances Payne Bolton School of Nursing Collection, 29DB, box 15, folder: Doctoral Program 1965–1981.

163. Mullane to Dake (1968).

164. Keeling, Brodie, and Kirchgessner (2010), 4–6.

165. Armiger (1974).

166. Keeling, Brodie, and Kirchgessner (2010), 4–6.

167. Rose Marie Chioni, "American Association of Colleges of Nursing and the Council of Baccalaureate and Higher Degree Programs: Purposes, Roles and Relationships," *National League for Nursing Publications* (1974) 15–1528, pp. 41–42; Armiger (1974); Most (1974).

168. Quoted in Keeling, Brodie, and Kirchgessner (2010), 37.

169. The first iteration of these standards was titled *The Essentials of College and University Education for Professional Nursing* (Washington, DC: AACN, 1986). Keeling, Brodie, and Kirchgessner (2010), 38.

170. Patricia Brider, "Accrediting Issues Grow; AACN Debates 'Alliance,'" *American Journal of Nursing (1996)* 96(11): 69–73.

171. Keeling, Brodie, and Kirchgessner (2010), 33–43, 71–81; Suzanne Van Ort and Julie Townsend, "Community-Based Nursing Education and Nursing Accreditation by the Commission on Nursing Education," *Journal of Professional Nursing* (2000) 16(6): 330–335.

172. Weise, interview by Tobbell (2010), 21.

173. Mary Kelly Mullane, "Memo to Members Council of Baccalaureate and Higher Degree Programs, National League for Nursing: Nursing Faculty Roles and Functions in the Large University Setting," February 1969, University of Illinois, Chicago University Archives, College of Nursing Office of the Dean—Administrative Files, 1955–1989, RG 17-01-02, box 1, folder: 23 Minutes—CON Administrative Council, September 9, 1976.

Chapter Two

A version of this chapter previously appeared as "'Coming to Grips with the Nursing Question': The Politics of Nursing Education Reform in 1960s' America." *Nursing History Review* (2014) 22: 37–60. A Publication of the American Association for the History of Nursing. Author: Dominique A. Tobbell, PhD. Editor: Patricia D'Antonio, PhD, RN, FAAN. Copyright © 2014, reproduced with the permission of Springer Publishing Company, LLC. http://dx.doi.org/10.1891 /1062-8061.22.37. ISBN: 9780826122957.

1. Andrew Abbott, *The System of Professions: An Essay on the Division of Expert Labor* (Chicago: University of Chicago Press, 1988), 52, 54.

2. Julie Fairman and Joan E. Lynaugh, *Critical Care Nursing: A History* (Philadelphia: University of Pennsylvania Press, 1998), 9–10.

3. Julie Fairman, "Context and Contingency in the History of Post-World War II Nursing Scholarship in the United States," *Journal of Nursing Scholarship* (2008) 40(1): 4–11, 5.

4. Robert K. Merton, "The Search for Professional Status: Sources, Costs, and Consequences," *American Journal of Nursing* (1960) 60(5): 662–664. For discussion of the sociology literature on professionalization from the 1950s, see Nathan Ensmenger, *The Computer Boys Take Over: Computers, Programmers, and the Politics of Technical Expertise* (Cambridge, MA: MIT Press, 2013), 114.

5. Abbott (1988). On engineering, see Bruce E. Seely, "Research, Engineering, and Science in American Engineering Colleges: 1900–1960," *Technology and Culture* (1993) 34(2): 344–386; Bruce E. Seely, "The Other Re-engineering of Engineering Education, 1900–1965," *Journal of Engineering Education* (July 1999): 285–294; and Jonathon Harwood, "Engineering Education between Science and Practice: Rethinking the Historiography," *History and Technology* (2006) 22(1): 53–79. On computing, see Ensmenger (2013). On pharmacy, see Robert A. Buerki, "American Pharmaceutical Education, 1952–2002," *Journal of the American Pharmaceutical Association* (2002) 42(4): 542–544; and Robert A. Buerki, "In Search of Excellence: The First Century of the American Association of Colleges of Pharmacy," *American Journal of Pharmaceutical Education*

(1999) 63(Fall supplement). On social work, see June Axinn and Herman Levin, "Money, Politics and Education: The Case of Social Work," *History of Education Quarterly* (1978) 18(2): 143–158.

6. Frances Cooke Macgregor, *Social Science in Nursing: Applications for the Improvement of Patient Care* (New York: Russell Sage Foundation, 1960).

7. Myrtle Irene Brown, "Research in the Development of Nursing Theory: The Importance of a Theoretical Framework in Nursing Research," *Nursing Research* (1964) 13(2): 109–112, 111.

8. On boundary work, see Thomas Gieryn, "Boundary-Work and the Demarcation of Science from Non-Science: Strains and Interests in Professional Ideologies of Scientists," *American Sociological Review* (1983) 48(4): 781–795.

9. Darlene Clark Hine, *Black Women in White* (Bloomington: Indiana University Press, 1989); Patricia D'Antonio, *American Nursing: A History of Knowledge, Authority, and the Meaning of Work* (Baltimore: Johns Hopkins University Press, 2010). On racial exclusion in Canadian nursing, see Karen Flynn, *Moving Beyond Borders: A History of Black Canadian and Caribbean Women in the Diaspora* (Toronto: University of Toronto Press, 2011).

10. Charissa Threat, *Nursing Civil Rights: Gender and Race in the Army Nurse Corps* (Urbana: University of Illinois Press, 2015).

11. Michael L. Millenson, *Demanding Medical Excellence: Doctors and Accountability in the Information Age* (Chicago: University of Chicago Press, 1997), 6.

12. For example, see Rita Arditti, "Feminism and Science," in Rita Arditti, Pat Brennan, and Steve Cavrak (eds.), *Science and Liberation* (Boston: South End Press, 1980); Elizabeth Fee, "A Feminist Critique of Scientific Objectivity," *Science for the People* (1982) 14(40): 5–8, 30–32; Hilary Rose, "Hand, Brain, and Heart: A Feminist Epistemology for the Natural Sciences," *Signs* (1983) 9(1): 73–90; Evelyn Fox Keller, "Women Scientists and Feminist Critics of Science," *Daedulus* (1987) 116(4): 77–91; Sandra Harding, *The Science Question in Feminism* (Ithaca, NY: Cornell University Press, 1986); Sandra Harding, *Whose Science? Whose Knowledge? Thinking from Women's Lives* (Ithaca, NY: Cornell University Press, 1991); and Londa Schiebinger, *Has Feminism Changed Science?* (Cambridge, MA: Harvard University Press, 1999).

13. Schiebinger (1999), 4. Schiebinger explains that women seeking access to normal science was a strategy of liberal feminism, which contrasted with difference feminism, which advocated for distinctive feminist ways of knowing.

14. For a brief summary of this literature, see Schiebinger (1999), 1–13. For examples of feminists who argue that women scientists have distinctive ways of knowing, see Nel Noddings, *Caring: A Feminine Approach to Ethics and Moral Education* (Berkeley: University of California Press, 1984); Rose (1983); Sara Ruddick, *Maternal Thinking: Toward a Politics of Peace* (Boston: Beacon Press, 1989).

15. Julie Fairman (2008), 5.

16. Rozella Schlotfeldt, "Reflections on Nursing Research," *American Journal of Nursing* (1960) 60(4), 492–494, 493.

17. Schlotfeldt (1960), 494.

18. Walsh McDermott, "Absence of Indicators of the Influence of its Physicians on a Society's Health; Impact of Physician Care on Society," *American Journal of Medicine* (1981) 70: 833–843. For discussion, see Julie Fairman, *Making Room in the Clinic: Nurse Practitioners and the Evolution of Modern Health Care* (New Brunswick, NJ: Rutgers University Press, 2008), 23.

19. Macgregor (1960), p.34.

20. Schlotfeldt (1960), 493.

21. Surgeon General's Consultant Group on Nursing, *Toward Quality in Nursing: Needs and Goals; Report of the Surgeon General's Consultant Group on Nursing* (Washington, DC: Government Printing Office, 1963), 55.

22. Virginia Henderson, "The Nature of Nursing," *American Journal of Nursing* (1964) 64(8): 62–68, 67.

23. Susan M. Reverby, "A Legitimate Relationship: Nursing, Hospitals, and Science in the Twentieth Century," in Diana E. Long and Janet Golden (eds.) *The American General Hospital: Communities and Social Contexts* (Ithaca, NY: Cornell University Press, 1989), 135–156.

24. Virginia Henderson, "Research in Nursing Practice—When?" *Nursing Research* (1956) 4(3): 99; and Leo W. Simmons and Virginia Henderson, *Nursing Research: A Survey and Assessment* (New York: Appleton-Century-Crofts, 1964).

25. Florence S. Wald and Robert C. Leonard, "Towards Development of Nursing Practice Theory," *Nursing Research* (1964) 13(4): 309–313, 310.

26. Dorothy E. Johnson, "The Nature of a Science of Nursing," *Nursing Outlook* (1959) 7(5): 291–294, 291.

27. Wald and Leonard (1964), 310.

28. Abbott (1988), 56.

29. Henderson (1956). For discussion of Henderson's efforts to promote the science of nursing practice, see Reverby (1989).

30. See, for example, George Engel, "The Need for a New Medical Model: A Challenge for Biomedicine," *Science* (1977) 196(4286): 129–136; Harry Marks, *The Progress of Experiment: Science and Therapeutic Reform in the United States, 1900–1990* (New York: Cambridge University Press, 1997), 2–3.

31. Language of the 1930 Ransdell Act, which established the National Institutes of Health, quoted in Stephen P. Strickland, *Politics, Science, and Dread Disease: A Short History of United States Medical Research Policy* (Cambridge, MA: Harvard University Press, 1972), 192.

32. Strickland (1972), especially pp. 188–189.

33. Marks (1997), 3.

34. Jeanne Daly, *Evidence-Based Medicine and the Search for a Science of Clinical Care* (Berkeley: University of California Press / Milbank Memorial Fund, 2005), 1.

35. Daly (2005); Stefan Timmermans and Marc Berg, *The Gold Standard: The Challenge of Evidence-Based Medicine and Standardization in Health Care* (Philadelphia: Temple University Press, 2003).

36. Daly (2005), 4. For the history of clinical epidemiology, see Daly (2005), 20–48.

37. Marks (1997), 2, 5.

38. Daly (2005), 12.

39. Marks (1997).

40. Theodore M. Porter, *Trust in Numbers: The Pursuit of Objectivity in Science and Public Life* (Princeton, NJ: Princeton University Press, 1995); Daly (2005), 18.

41. Ellen D. Baer, "'A Cooperative Venture' in Pursuit of Professional Status: A Research Journal for Nursing," *Nursing Research* (1987) 36(1): 18–25.

42. Daly (2005), 16–17.

43. Martha Pitel and John Vian, "Analysis of Nurse-Doctorates: Data Collected for the International Directory of Nurses with Doctoral Degrees," *Nursing Research* (1975) 24(5), 340–351.

44. Faye G. Abdellah and Eugene Levine, *Better Patient Care through Nursing Research* (New York: Macmillan, 1965), 7.

45. Marie J. Bourgeois, "The Special Nurse Research Fellow: Characteristics and Recent Trends," *Nursing Research* (1975) 24(3): 184–188.

46. Cynthia Connolly and Joan E. Lynaugh, *Fifty Years at the Division of Nursing: United States Public Health Service* (Washington, DC: U.S. Public Health Service Division of Nursing, 1997).

47. Bourgeois (1975). For the percentages of nurses who earned their doctorates in different disciplines from 1927 to 1973, see Helen Grace, "The Development of Doctoral Education in Nursing: In Historical Perspective," *Journal of Nursing Education* (1978) 17(4): 17–27. Grace reports that after 1960, 60–70 percent of nurses graduated with doctoral degrees in education, 16–25 percent in the social sciences, 7–10 percent in nursing, and 3–5 percent in the natural sciences.

48. Margaret Rossiter, *Women Scientists in America: Struggles and Strategies to 1940* (Baltimore: Johns Hopkins University Press, 1982), 134–137; Margaret Rossiter, *Women Scientists in America: Before Affirmative Action, 1940–1972* (Baltimore: Johns Hopkins University Press, 1998), 97–105.

49. Schiebinger (1999), 91. On primatology, see also Linda Marie Fedigan, "The Paradox of Feminist Primatology: The Goddess's Discipline?" in Angela N. H. Creager, Elizabeth Lunbeck, and Londa Schiebinger, *Feminism in Twentieth Century Science, Technology, and Medicine* (Chicago: University of Chicago Press, 2001); and Donna Haraway, *Primate Visions: Gender, Race and Nature in the World of Modern Science* (New York: Routledge, 1989).

50. Hine (1989).

51. Oliver Osborne, a psychiatric and mental health nurse, received his PhD in anthropology from Michigan State University in 1967. See Oliver H. Osborne, "The Way of One Nurse-Anthropologist," *Western Journal of Nursing Research* (2001) 23(8): 828–835, and Bertin M. Louis Jr., "Oliver Osborne: African American Nurse-Anthropologist Pioneer," in Ira E. Harrison, Deborah Johnson-Simon, and Erica Lorraine Williams (eds.) *The Second Generation of African American Pioneers in Anthropology* (University of Illinois Press, 2018), 165–173.

52. Bourgeois (1975), 185.

53. Baer (1987), 20, 22.

54. Joanne S. Stevenson, "Forging a Research Discipline," *Nursing Research* (1987) 36(1): 60–64.

55. Helen K. Grace, Beverly M. LaBelle, and Nola J. Pender, "Study of Resources for Doctoral Education in the Midwest," February 1976, Ruth Lilly Special Collections and Archives, Indiana University–Purdue University Indianapolis, Indianapolis, Midwest Alliance in Nursing Collection, box 30.

56. Dorothy E. Johnson, "Theory in Nursing: Borrowed and Unique," *Nursing Research* (1968) 17(3): 206–209. This also reflects the broader struggle of translating the findings of biomedical research into clinical practice, and hence the push to establish a clinical science; see Daly (2005).

57. Grace, LaBelle, and Pender (1976).

58. "Panel discussion." *Nursing Forum* (1966) V(2), 85–86.

59. Faye Abdellah, "Doctoral Preparation for Nurses: A Continuation of the Dialogue," *Nursing Forum* (1966) V(3): 44–53, pp. 47–49.

60. "Future Directions of Doctoral Education for Nurses: Report of a Conference, Bethesda, MD, United States Public Health Service, National Institutes of Health, Bureau of Health Manpower Education, January 20, 1971," pp. 9–12, 26, Bates Center for the Study of the History of Nursing Archives, Florence S. Downs Papers, MC 130, Series IV, box 7, folder 12.

61. Marks (1997); Daly (2005).

62. Bourgeois (1975); Grace (1978).

63. Ada Jacox, "Competing Theories of Science," Fifth Forum on Doctoral Education, University

of Washington School of Nursing, June 25–26, 1981, Bates Center for the Study of the History of Nursing Archives, Florence S. Downs Papers, MC 130, Series IV, box 8, folder 6. In reference to the theory conferences held in 1969 and 1970, Jacox explained that of the forty nurses who participated, eight completed their doctoral degrees during that time: "Most of us who were finishing at that time got our degrees in sociology or education. We developed our notions of what science is in those disciplines and that's what we brought back to nursing in writing and teaching about theory construction."

64. Abbott (1988), 9.

65. Virginia S. Cleland, "Research: How Will Nursing Define It?" *Nursing Research* (1967) 16(2): 108–129; Jean S. Berthold, "Symposium on Theory Development in Nursing," *Nursing Research* (1968) 17(3): 196–197; Madeleine Leininger, "Introductory Comments: Conference on the Nature of Science and Nursing," *Nursing Research* (1968) 17(6): 484–486; and Madeleine Leininger, "Introduction: The Nature of Science in Nursing," *Nursing Research* (1969) 18(5): 388–389; Catherine M. Norris, Proceedings of the Nursing Theory Conference (Vols. 1–3, 1969–1970), Kansas City, KS: University of Kansas Medical Center, Department of Nursing.

66. Cleland(1967), 118–121; Dorothy E. Johnson, "The Nature of a Science of Nursing," *Nursing Outlook* (1959) 7(5): 291–294; Dorothy E. Johnson, "Theory in Nursing: Borrowed and Unique," *Nursing Research* (1968) 17(3): 206–209.

67. Lucy Conant, "A Search for Resolution of Existing Problems in Nursing," *Nursing Research* (1967) 16(2): 114–117, 115.

68. Rosemary Ellis, "Characteristics of Significant Theories," *Nursing Research* (1968) 17(3): 217–222, 220.

69. Ada Jacox and Mary Stewart, "Relation of Psychosocial Factors and Type of Pain," *Nursing Research Conference* (1973) 9: 13–31; and Ada Jacox, "Assessing Pain," *American Journal of Nursing* (1979) 79(5): 895–500.

70. Jean E. Johnson, "Contribution of Emotional and Instrumental Response Processes in Adaptation to Surgery," *Journal of Personality and Social Psychology* (1971) 20(1): 55–64; Jean E. Johnson, "Effects of Structuring Patients' Expectations on their Reactions to Threatening Events," *Nursing Research* (1972) 21(6): 499–504; Jean E. Johnson, John F. Morrissey, and Howard Leventhal, "Psychological Preparation for an Endoscopic Examination," *Gastrointestinal Endoscopy* (1973) 19(4): 180–182; Jean E. Johnson, Karin T. Kirchhoff, and M. Patricia Endress, "Easing Children's Fright During Health Care Procedures," *American Journal of Maternal Child Nursing* (July/August 1976): 206–210.

71. Barney G. Glaser and Anselm L. Strauss, *The Discovery of Grounded Theory: Strategies for Qualitative Research* (New York: Aldine de Gruyter, 1967).

72. See, for example, Jeanne C. Quint, *The Nurse and the Dying Patient* (New York: Macmillan, 1967). In her subsequent research, she investigated nursing care of cancer and terminally ill patients, as well as "the conspiracy of silence that surrounds the dying patient," and the impact of illness on caregivers. Washington State Nurses Association, "Hall of Fame 2004 Inductees: Jean Quint Benoliel," https://www.wsna.org/hall-of-fame/2004/Jeanne-Quint-Benoliel/ (accessed April 30, 2019). Quint's work is placed in historical context in Joy Buck, "Reweaving a Tapestry of Care: Religion, Nursing, and the Meaning of Hospice, 1945–1978," *Nursing History Review* (2007): 113–145; Emily K. Abel, *The Inevitable Hour: A History of Caring for Dying Patients in America* (Baltimore: Johns Hopkins University Press, 2013); and Emily K. Abel, *Prelude to Hospice: Florence Wald, Dying People, and their Families* (New Brunswick, NJ: Rutgers University Press, 2018).

73. Ada Jacox, "Theory Construction in Nursing: An Overview," *Nursing Research* (1974) 23(1): 4–12, 11.

74. Dorothy E. Johnson, "Development of Theory: A Requisite for Nursing as a Primary Health Profession," *Nursing Research* (1974) 23(5): 372–377, and Madeleine Leininger, "Creating and Maintaining a Nursing Research Support Center," (paper presentation, Project for Nursing Research Colloquium at Adelphi University School of Nursing, November 2, 1977), Walter P. Reuther Library, University Archives, Wayne State University Madeleine Leininger Collection, Accession 725, box 8.

75. Ernestine Wiedenbach, "Nurses' Wisdom in Nursing Theory," *American Journal of Nursing* (1970) 70(5): 1057–1062, 1057.

76. Imogene King, *Toward a Theory for Nursing: General Concepts of Human Behavior* (New York: John Wiley and Sons, 1971), xi–xx.

77. Abbott (1988).

78. Overviews of theoretical work developed by nurses in these decades include: Nursing Theories Conference Group, *Nursing Theories: The Base for Professional Nursing Practice* (Englewood Cliffs, NJ: Prentice-Hall, 1980); Joan Riehl-Sisca and Callista Roy, eds., *Conceptual Models for Nursing Practice*, 2nd ed. (New York: Appleton-Century-Crofts, 1980); Afaf Ibrahim Meleis, Theoretical Nursing: Development and Progress, 5th ed. (Philadelphia: Wolters Kluwer Health / Lippincott Williams & Wilkins, 2012).

79. Dorothy E. Johnson, "The Behavioral System Model for Nursing," in Joan Riehl-Sisca and Callista Roy (eds.) *Conceptual Models for Nursing Practice*, 2nd ed. (New York: Appleton-Century-Crofts, 1980), 207–216, 207. For a helpful summary, see: "Health Behavioral Theory," Nursing Theory, https://nursing-theory.org/theories-and-models/johnson-behavior-system-model.php.

80. Johnson (1980), particularly pp. 207–209. Talcott Parsons, *The Social System* (Glencoe, IL: Free Press, 1951); Ludwig von Bertalanffy, *General System Theory: Foundations, Development, Applications* (New York: G. Braziller, 1968).

81. Johnson (1980), 209.

82. Johnson (1980), 214.

83. Meleis (2012), 327; "Sister Callista Roy: Nursing Theorist," Nursing Theory, https://nursing-theory.org/nursing-theorists/Sister-Callista-Roy.php (accessed March 25, 2021).

84. Callista Roy, "The Roy Adaptation Model," in Joan Riehl-Sisca and Callista Roy (eds.), *Conceptual Models for Nursing Practice*, 2nd ed. (New York: Appleton-Century-Crofts, 1980), 179–188; Meleis (2012), 327.

85. Callista Roy, *Introduction to Nursing: An Adaptation Model* (Englewood Cliffs, NJ: Prentice-Hall, 1976), 11.

86. Roy (1976), 15.

87. Roy (1976), 18.

88. Wald and Leonard (1964), 309.

89. James Dickoff and Patricia James, "The Authors Comment." In Nicoll, L. H., ed., *Perspectives on Nursing Theory* (Boston: Little, Brown, 1986), 108–112, 108.

90. James Dickoff and Patricia James, "A Theory of Theories: A Position Paper," *Nursing Research* (1968) 17(3): 197–203.

91. Angelo Gonzalo, "Ida Jean Orlando: Deliberative Nursing Process Theory," Nurseslabs, https://nurseslabs.com/ida-jean-orlandos-deliberative-nursing-process-theory/ (accessed June 25, 2020).

92. Ida Jean Orlando, *The Dynamic Nurse-Patient Relationship: Function, Process, and Principles* (New York: Putnam, 1961), vii.

93. Ida Jean Orlando, *The Discipline and Teaching of Nursing Process: An Evaluative Study* (New York: Putnam, 1972).

94. Nursing Theories Conference Group, *Nursing Theories: The Base for Professional Nursing Practice* (Englewood Cliffs, NJ: Prentice-Hall, 1980), 127.

95. Meleis (2012), 243.

96. Meleis (2012), 242.

97. Orlando (1961), 60.

98. Dorothea E. Orem, "The Development of the Self-Care Deficit Theory of Nursing: Events and Circumstances," in Dorothea E. Orem, Kathie McLaughlin Renpenning, and Susan G. Taylor (eds.), *Self-Care Theory in Nursing: Selected Papers of Dorothea Orem* (New York: Springer, 2003), 257.

99. Dorothea E. Orem, Kathie McLaughlin Renpenning, and Susan G. Taylor, eds., *Self-Care Theory in Nursing: Selected Papers of Dorothea Orem* (New York: Springer, 2003), xx–xxiii; and Orem (2003).

100. Orem (2003), 260.

101. Orem quoted in Orem, McLaughlin Renpenning, and Taylor (2003), xxi–xxii.

102. Dorothea E. Orem, *Nursing: Concepts of Practice* (New York: McGraw-Hill, 1971), 13.

103. Dorothea E. Orem, "The Self-Care Deficit Theory of Nursing: A General Theory," in Imelda W. Clements and Florence Bright Roberts, *Family Health: A Theoretical Approach to Nursing Care* (New York: Wiley, 1983), 205–218, 210.

104. Orem (1971) and Orem (1983).

105. For detailed biography, see Lynne M. Hektor, "Martha E. Rogers: A Life History," in Martha E. Rogers, Violet M. Malinski, and Elizabeth Ann Manhart Barrett (eds.), *Martha E. Rogers: Her Life and Work* (Philadelphia: F. A. Davis, 1994), 10–28.

106. Martha E. Rogers, "Nursing: A Science of Unitary Man," in Joan Riehl-Sisca and Callista Roy (eds.), *Conceptual Models for Nursing Practice*, 2nd ed. (New York: Appleton-Century-Crofts, 1980), 329–338, 337.

107. Martha E. Rogers, *Introduction to the Theoretical Basis of Nursing* (Philadelphia: F. A. Davis, 1970), plus other major theoretical works, including Rogers (1980), 329–338.

108. Rogers (1980), 332.

109. Rogers (1980), 330.

110. Rogers (1980), 332.

111. Meleis (2012), 316.

112. Violet M. Malinski, "Highlights in the Evolution of Nursing Science: Emergence of the Science of Unitary Human Beings," in Martha E. Rogers, Violet M. Malinski, and Elizabeth Ann Manhart Barrett (eds.), *Martha E. Rogers: Her Life and Work* (Philadelphia: F. A. Davis, 1994), 197.

113. Rogers (1980), 329–330.

114. Rogers (1970), 122.

115. Rogers (1970), 124.

116. Meleis (2012), 316–317.

117. John R. Phillips, "Martha E. Rogers: Heretic and Heroine," *Nursing Science Quarterly* (2015) 28(1): 42–48, 44, and Martha E. Rogers, Violet M. Malinski, and Elizabeth Ann Manhart Barrett, eds., *Martha E. Rogers: Her Life and Work* (Philadelphia: F. A. Davis, 1994), v.

118. Hektor (1994), 23.

119. For overviews of other theoretical work developed by nurses in these decades, see: Nursing Theories Conference Group (1980); Riehl-Sisca and Roy (1980); Meleis (2012).

120. Jacqueline Fawcett, "A Framework for Analysis and Evaluation of Conceptual Models of Nursing," *Nurse Educator* (1980) 5(6): 10–14, 11.

121. Jacqueline H. Flaskerud and Edward J. Halloran, "Areas of Agreement in Nursing Theory Development," *Advances in Nursing Science* (1980) 3(1): 1–7, 3.

122. Rosemary Ellis, "Conceptual Issues in Nursing." *Nursing Outlook* (1982) 30(7): 406–410, 407.

123. Preface by Esther Lucile Brown in Frances Cooke Macgregor, *Social Science in Nursing: Applications for the Improvement of Patient Care* (New York: Russell Sage Foundation, 1960), 5; Esther Lucile Brown, *Nursing for the Future: A Report Prepared for the National Nursing Council* (New York: Russell Sage, 1948), 33–41; Barbara Melosh, *"The Physician's Hand": Work Culture and Conflict in American Nursing* (Philadelphia: Temple University Press, 1982), 203–205.

124. Karen Buhler-Wilkerson, *False Dawn: The Rise and Decline of Public Health Nursing, 1900–1930* (New York: Garland, 1989); Karen Buhler-Wilkerson, *No Place Like Home: A History of Nursing and Home Care in the United States* (Baltimore: Johns Hopkins University Press, 2001); Patricia D'Antonio, *Nursing with a Message: Public Health Demonstration Projects in New York City* (New Brunswick, NJ: Rutgers University Press, 2017).

125. Karen Buhler-Wilkerson, "Bringing Care to the People: Lillian Wald's Legacy to Public Health Nursing," *American Journal of Public Health* (1993) 83: 1778–1786, 1778.

126. Karen Buhler-Wilkerson, "No Place Like Home: A History of Nursing and Home Care in the U.S." *Home Healthcare Nurse* (2012) 30(8): 446–452, quotation from p. 448.

127. Kylie M. Smith, *Talking Therapy: Knowledge and Power in American Psychiatric Nursing* (New Brunswick, NJ: Rutgers University Press, 2020), 28–51.

128. Engel (1977).

129. Wendy Kline, *Bodies of Knowledge: Sexuality, Reproduction, and Women's Health in the Second Wave* (Chicago: University of Chicago, 2010); Sheryl B. Ruzek, *The Women's Health Movement: Feminist Alternatives to Medical Control* (New York: Praeger, 1978); Mary K. Zimmerman, "The Women's Health Movement: A Critique of Medical Enterprise and the Position of Women," in Beth B. Hess and Myra Marx Ferree (eds.) *Analyzing Gender: A Handbook of Social Science Research* (Newbury Park, CA: Sage, 1987), 442–472; Alondra Nelson, *Body and Soul: The Black Panther Party and the Fight against Medical Discrimination* (Minneapolis: University of Minnesota Press, 2011); Keith Wailoo, *Dying in the City of the Blues: Sickle Cell Anemia and the Politics of Race and Health* (Chapel Hill: University of North Carolina Press, 2001), especially pp. 137–164; John Dittmer, *The Good Doctors: The Medical Committee for Human Rights and the Struggle for Social Justice in Health Care* (Jackson: University of Mississippi Press, 2009); Nancy Tomes, *Remaking the American Patient: How Madison Avenue and Modern Medicine Turned Patients into Consumers* (Chapel Hill: University of North Carolina Press, 2016), 249–320.

130. Orlando (1972), 4–5.

131. Orlando (1972), ix.

132. Irving Kenneth Zola, "Medicine as an Institution of Social Control," *Sociological Review* (1972) 20(4): 487–504, 487.

133. For an overview of Zola's scholarly contributions, see Peter Conrad, Phil Brown, and Susan Bell, "Obituary: Irving Kenneth Zola (1935–1994)" *Social Science and Medicine* (1995) 41(2): v–vi.

134. Rogers (1970), 129, 123–124.

135. Rogers (1970), 129–130.

136. See, for example, Ruth B. Freeman, "Practice as Protest," *American Journal of Nursing* (1971) 71(5): 918–921; Thelma Schorr "Editorial: Encounter," *American Journal of Nursing* (1975)

75(11): 1979; Mary Bayer and Patty Brandner, "Nurse/Patient Peer Practice," *American Journal of Nursing* (1977) 77(1): 86–90; Nancy Milio, "Challenge of Patient Advocacy," *The Michigan Nurse* (October 1977): 4–6, 14; Mary F. Kohnke, "The Nurse's Responsibility to the Consumer," *American Journal of Nursing* (1978) 78(3): 440–442.

137. Susan R. Gortner, "Nursing Science in Transition," *Nursing Research* (1980) 29(3): 180–183, 181.

138. Leininger (1977). See also Susan R. Gortner, "Researchmanship: The Arena," *Western Journal of Nursing Research* (1979) 1(3): 262–264, quotation from pp. 262–263. As Andrew Hogan has described, in the 1960s and 1970s, leaders in clinical psychology pursued a similar strategy, promoting "a 'social-development model' for clinical psychology, which sought to identify and cultivate individual strengths, rather than highlight defects and weaknesses," which were central to psychiatry's "sickness model." Hogan, "The 'Two Cultures' in Clinical Psychology: Constructing Disciplinary Divides in the Management of Mental Retardation," *ISIS* (2018) 109(4): 695–719, 702.

139. "Panel Discussion: The Position of Pure and Applied Scientist," *Nursing Research* (1968) 17(6): 507–517, 511.

140. Helen Grace, "The Status of Research in Nursing," April 1974, University of Illinois Chicago, University Archives, College of Nursing, Dean–Faculty Papers Collection, Helen Grace Papers (acc. 017-01-20-01), box 28, folder 307.

141. Gortner (1980), p.180.

142. See, for example, Kathryn E. Barnard, "Knowledge for Practice: Directions for the Future," *Nursing Research* (1980) 29(4): 208–212; and American Nurses Association, *Research in Nursing: Toward a Science of Health Care* (Washington, DC: American Nurses Association, 1976).

143. Carol A. Lindeman, "Delphi Survey of Priorities in Clinical Nursing Research," *Nursing Research* (1975) 24(6): 434–441.

144. Millenson (1997); Daly (2005); Tomes (2016), 310–313.

145. Tomes (2016), 311.

146. Daly (2005), 10.

147. Tomes (2016), 311.

148. Tomes (2016), 312. On the history of clinical epidemiology, see Daly (2005); On the history of health services research, see Fox (2010), 22–50.

149. For a brief discussion of the potential role of nursing research within the field of outcomes research, see Florence Downs, "Relationship of Findings of Clinical Research and Development of Criteria: A Researcher's Perspective," *Nursing Research* (1980) 29(2): 94–97, 94.

150. Delores Santora, "Preventing Hospital-Acquired Urinary Infection," *American Journal of Nursing* (1966) 4: 790–794, and American Nurses Association (1976), 6–7.

151. Sue Donaldson, "Methods for Measuring Sputum Viscosity and Inspired Air Humidity in Tracheostomized Patients," *Nursing Research* (1968) 17(5): 388–395.

152. Among the nurse researchers studying stimulation and premature infants were Mary Neal, "Relationship between Vestibular Stimulation and Developmental Behavior of the Small Premature Infant," *American Nurses' Association Fifth Nursing Research Conference, New Orleans, LA, March 3–5, 1969* (New York: American Nurses Association), 43–57; Violet Katz, "Auditory Stimulation and Developmental Behavior of the Premature Infant," *Nursing Research* (1971) 20: 196–201; M. E. Segall, "Cardiac Responsivity to Auditory Stimulation in Premature Infants," *Nursing Research* (1972) 21: 15–19; and Kathryn Barnard, "The Effect of Stimulation on the Sleep Behavior of the Premature Infant," *Communicating Nursing Research* (1974) 6: 12–33.

153. Doris Schwartz, Barbara Henley, and Leonard Zeitz, *The Elderly Ambulatory Patient: Nursing and Psychosocial Needs* (New York: Macmillan, 1964). Quotation from Susan R. Gortner and Helen Nahm, "Overview of Nursing Research in the United States." *Nursing Research* (1977) 26(1): 10–33, 23.

154. Patricia M. MacElveen, "Cooperative Triad in Home Dialysis Care and Patient Outcomes," *Proceedings of the Clinical Dialysis and Transplant Forum* (1975) 5: 93–97.

155. Quint (1967); Jeanne Quint Benoliel, "Nursing Research on Death, Dying, and Terminal Illness: Development, Present State, and Prospects." *Annual Review of Nursing Research* (1983) 1: 101–130.

156. American Nurses Association (1976), 3.

157. American Nurses Association (1976), 3. See also Linda Aiken and Theodore F. Heinrichs, "Systematic Relaxation as a Nursing Intervention Technique with Open Heart Surgery Patients," *Nursing Research* (1971) 20(3): 212–217; Linda Aiken, oral history interview by Ann Smith, February 15, 2005, p. 14. University of Florida, Samuel Proctor Oral History Program, College of Nursing Project, https://ufdc.ufl.edu/UF00066608/00001 (accessed Feburary 17, 2022).

158. Jacox and Stewart (1973), 15; and Jacox (1979).

159. See Faye G. Abdellah, "Overview of Nursing Research 1955–1968, Part I," *Nursing Research* (1970) 19(1): 6–17, 7.

160. Daly (2005), 12; Timmermans and Berg (2003); David S. Jones and Scott H. Podolsky, "The History and Fate of the Gold Standard," *Lancet* (2015) 385: 1502–1503; Laura E. Bothwell and Scott H. Podolsky, "The Emergence of the Randomized, Controlled Trial," *New England Journal of Medicine* (2016) 375: 501–504.

161. Marks (1997).

162. Daly (2005), 231–232.

163. Daly (2005), 18.

164. Daly (2005), 232.

165. Daly (2005), 232.

166. Daly (2005), 13.

167. Mary Angela McBride, Donna Diers, and Ruth L. Schmidt, "Nurse-Researcher: The Crucial Hyphen," *American Journal of Nursing* (1970) 70(6): 1256–1260. Nurse researchers continued to confront difficulties carrying out clinical research that required access to patients through the 1980s and into 1990s. See, for example, Barbara Brodie's description of the gap between research and practice, Barbara Brodie, "Voices in Distant Camps: The Gap between Nursing Research and Nursing Practice," *Journal of Professional Nursing* (1988) 4(5): 320–328.

168. Madeleine Leininger, "Doctoral Programs for Nurses: A Survey of Trends, Issues, and Projected Developments," in Jessie M. Scott, J. Susan Gortner, and Marjorie Bourgeois (eds.), *The Doctorally Prepared Nurse: Report of Two Conferences on the Demand for Education of Nurses with Doctoral Degrees* (Bethesda, MD: Department of Health, Education, and Welfare, March 1976), 3–38, quotation from pp. 10–11.

169. Downs (1980), 95. See also Florence Downs, "Creativity in Science: What it's All About," *Nursing Research* (1979) 28(6): 324.

170. Madeleine Leininger to Doris Bloch, chief, Research Support Section, Division of Nursing, U.S. Public Health Service, April 13, 1982, Walter P. Reuther Library, University Archives, Wayne State University, Madeleine Leininger Collection, Accession 725, box 1, folder 10. The preference for quantitative research methods was similarly problematic for qualitative researchers in the social sciences. In the late 1970s and early 1980s, for example, sociologists who used

qualitative research methods were engaged in an effort to assert the value and rigor of their methods. See, for example, Robert Bogdan and Steven J. Taylor, *An Introduction to Qualitative Research Methods: A Phenomenological Approach to the Social Sciences* (New York: Wiley, 1975). See later editions, also.

171. Leininger 1982, and Susan R. Gortner, "Researchmanship: The Politics of Research Revisited," *Western Journal of Nursing Research* (1981) 3(3): 309–311.

172. Imogene King to Betty Pearson, November 21, 1980, University of Illinois Chicago University Archives, Midwest Nursing Research Society, Series II, box 43, folder: 298.

173. On the history of community-based demonstration projects by public health nurses, see Buhler-Wilkerson (1989) and D'Antonio (2017). In Detroit in 1966, for example, Nancy Milio was working as a public health nurse (for the Visiting Nurse Association) in the Kercheval neighborhood of Detroit, a predominantly low-income African American neighborhood, when she established the Moms and Tots Neighborhood Center with funding from the federal Office of Economic Opportunity and under the auspices of the Visiting Nurse Association. The center provided a range of services including prenatal care (in partnership with the Maternity and Infant Care Project hospital), family planning, limited day care for preschoolers, cooperative babysitting, help with transportation, and sex education for teenage girls. Milio directed the center until her departure in 1969. Nancy Milio, "Project in a Negro Ghetto," *American Journal of Nursing* (1967) 67(5): 1006–1009; Nancy Milio, *9226 Kercheval: The Storefront that Did Not Burn* (Ann Arbor: University of Michigan Press, 1971).

174. Nelson (2011); Wailoo (2001), especially pp. 137–164; Dittmer (2009).

175. Dittmer (2009). In addition to providing medical care to civil rights workers in Mississippi during the "Freedom Summer" of 1964, the Medical Committee for Human Rights led the movement to establish community health centers in underserved communities.

176. See, for example, the *American Journal of Nursing*'s series of articles on "The Sick Poor," published throughout 1968 and 1969. See, especially, Maria C. Phaneuf and Paul Lowinger, "Healers in a Sick Society," *American Journal of Nursing* (1968) 68(6): 1283–1284. Phaneuf was a faculty member in public health nursing in Wayne State University College of Nursing, and Lowinger was a faculty member in the medical school. They were both active in the Medical Committee for Human Rights in Detroit. See also, Rhetaugh G. Dumas, "This I Believe . . . about Nursing and the Poor," *Nursing Outlook* (September 1969): 47–49; and Freeman (1971).

177. Dumas (1969), 47.

178. Marie F. Branch, "New Approaches in Nursing: Ethnic Humanism Views," in Marie F. Branch and Phyllis P. Paxton (eds.), *Providing Safe Nursing Care for Ethnic People of Color* (New York: Appleton-Century-Crofts, 1976), 3–19, quotation p. 3. For more details on Branch, particularly her work to implement antiracist philosophy and practice into nurse education, see Cory Ellen Gatrall, "Marie Branch and the Power of Nursing," *Nursing Clio*, October 29, 2020, https://nursingclio.org/2020/10/29/marie-branch-and-the-power-of-nursing/ (accessed October 29, 2020).

179. Carolyn Sullivan, Janice Robinson, and Janice Ruffin, "Nursing in a Society in Crisis." *American Journal of Nursing* (1972) 72(2): 302–304. It is important to note that the committee faced a lot of backlash and harassment from nurses in their efforts to increase awareness of the impact that sociopolitical issues had on individual and population health. They wrote, "Some nurses view nurses who suggest that our society needs basic restructuring on political, economic, and social bases as 'destructive.' Society in Crisis members were accused of such destructiveness when they expressed belief that the United States was racist and was involved in an inhumane military-industrial orientation," p. 304.

180. Elizabeth Siegel Watkins, *On the Pill: A Social History of Oral Contraceptives* (Baltimore: Johns Hopkins University Press, 2001); Ruzek (1978); Zimmerman (1987); and Kline (2010).

181. Kline (2010).

182. Strickland (1972), especially pp. 188–189.

183. See, for example, Schiebinger (1999), 118–121.

184. Rosemary Ellis, "Conceptual Issues in Nursing." *Nursing Outlook* (1982) 30(7): 406–410; J. L. Engstrom, "Problems in the Development, Use, and Testing of Nursing Theory," *Journal of Nursing Education* (1984) 23(6): 245–251; Fawcett, 1980.

185. Florence Downs, "Some Critical Issues in Nursing Research," *Nursing Forum* (1969) 8(4): 393–404; Engstrom, 1984.

186. Maryann Pranuli's doctoral dissertation documented the role identity (researcher vs. teacher vs. clinician vs. administrator) of nursing faculty at university-based nursing schools, making clear that in the early 1980s, very few faculty identified as clinicians. Maryann F. Pranuli, *"Environmental Influences on Nursing Faculty Research Productivity at University Schools of Nursing"* (unpublished DNS diss., UCLA School of Nursing, 1984).

187. Abbott (1988); Seely (1993); Seely (1999); Ensmenger (2013).

188. Abbott (1988), 53.

189. Abbott (1988), 56.

190. For example, Afaf Meleis notes that "the focus on curriculum" caused nursing faculty "to lose sight of the reasons for theory, which is quality nursing practice and patient care." Rather than using the new theories to guide practice or research—or developing theories for practice—"emergent theories were used to guide teaching." Meleis (2012), 49, 75.

191. Abbott (1988), 56.

192. On the limited use of theory in nursing research, see Madeleine Leininger and JoAnn Glittenberg's "Textual Analysis of Doctoral Nursing Dissertation Abstracts" from 1981 through 1984, which found that only 10 percent of abstracts surveyed "explicitly identified a nurse theorist," and in an additional 12 percent of abstracts, Leininger and Glittenberg inferred or deduced a theorist from psychology, sociology, or physiology. In other words, "most of the dissertations (approximately 78 percent) did not mention a theory, conceptual framework nor theorist in the abstract." Madeleine Leininger and JoAnn Glittenberg, "Textual Analysis of Doctoral Dissertation Abstracts" (proceedings, Forum: Epistemological Strategies in Nursing, June 21–24, 1984), cosponsored by the Planning Committee for the National Forum on Doctoral Education in Nursing and the University of Colorado School of Nursing, Denver. Bates Center Archives, Florence S. Downs Papers MC 130, Series IV, box 8, folder 7.

193. Florence Downs "Hitching the Research Wagon to Theory," *Nursing Research* (1994) 43(4): 195.

194. Joseph Matarazzo, "Historical Perspective on Doctoral Education," in "Future Directions of Doctoral Education for Nurses: Report of a Conference, Bethesda, MD, United States Public Health Service, National Institutes of Health, Bureau of Health Manpower Education, January 20, 1971," pp. 10–11. Bates Center for the Study of the History of Nursing Archives, Florence S. Downs Papers, MC 130, Series IV, box 7, folder 12.

195. Unnamed biologist quoted in "Future Directions of Doctoral Education for Nurses: Report of a Conference, Bethesda, MD, United States Public Health Service, National Institutes of Health, Bureau of Health Manpower Education, January 20, 1971," p, 26. Bates Center for the Study of the History of Nursing Archives, Florence S. Downs Papers, MC 130, Series IV, box 7, folder 12.

196. Unnamed biologist (1971).

197. Unnamed biologist, (1971).

198. Peggy L. Chinn and Charlene Eldridge Wheeler, "Feminism and Nursing: Can Nursing Afford to Remain Aloof from the Women's Movement?" *Nursing Outlook* (1985) 33(2): 74–77, 75. On the broader topic of nursing and feminism, see Susan Rimby Leighow, *Nurses' Questions/ Women's Questions: The Impact of the Demographic Revolution and Feminism on United States Working Women, 1946–1986* (New York: Peter Lang, 1996); and Susan Gelfand Malka, *Daring to Care: American Nursing and Second-Wave Feminism* (Chicago: University of Illinois Press, 2007).

199. Chinn and Wheeler (1985), 76. For a broader feminist critique of science, see Rose (1983). For historical analysis of the relationship between feminism and science, see Angela N. H. Creager, Elizabeth Lunbeck, and Londa Schiebinger (eds.), *Feminism in Twentieth-Century Science, Technology, and Medicine* (Chicago: University of Chicago Press, 2001).

200. For a brief summary of this literature, see Schiebinger (1999), 1–13. For examples of feminists who argue that women scientists have distinctive ways of knowing, see Noddings (1984); Rose (1983); and Ruddick (1989).

201. Leighow (1996), 95–98; Peggy L. Chinn, "Cassandra: Radical Feminist Nurses Network," https://peggychinn.com/projects/cassandra/ (accessed June 8, 2019). Plus, for details, see the first newsletter, Cassandra (November 1982) 1(1), https://peggychinn.files.wordpress.com/2013/11/1 -1-nov-1982s.pdf (accessed June 8, 2019). On the history of Cassandra, see Jessica Dillard-Wright, "*Cassandra Radical Feminist Nurses Network: Feminism, Nursing, and a History for the Present*" (unpublished PhD diss., August University, 2020).

202. Gretchen LaGodna, "Cassandra: A Report of Beginnings," *Cassandra* (November 1982) 1(1):1–2, 2, https://peggychinn.files.wordpress.com/2013/11/1-1-nov-1982s.pdf (accessed July 19, 2019).

203. Ann Voda, letter to Peggy Chinn, published in *Cassandra* (November 1982) 1(1): 7–8, https://peggychinn.files.wordpress.com/2013/11/1-1-nov-1982s.pdf (accessed July 19, 2019).

204. Harding (1986); Harding (1991); Rossiter (1998); Schiebinger (1999).

205. Voda to Chinn (1982).

206. Kathleen I. MacPherson, "Feminist Methods: A New Paradigm for Nursing Research," *Advances in Nursing Research* (1983) 5(2): 17–25.

207. MacPherson (1983), 19, 22.

208. MacPherson (1983), 19.

209. MacPherson (1983), 21.

210. MacPherson (1983), 19.

211. Voda to Chinn (1982).

212. Letter from "Mary," *Cassandra* (April 1983) 1(2): 5, https://peggychinn.files.wordpress .com/2013/11/1-2-april-1983s.pdf (accessed July 19, 2019).

213. Keller (1987).

214. Rose (1983), 87.

215. Schiebinger (1999), 4.

216. Florence Downs, "New Questions and New Answers," *Nursing Research* (1989) 38 (6): 323.

217. Florence Downs, "Alternative Answers," *Nursing Research* (1993) 42(6): 323.

218. Downs (1989).

219. Florence Downs, "More than Skin Deep," *Nursing Research* (1992) 41(4): 195.

220. Downs (1989).

221. Downs (1992).

222. Elizabeth Wilson, *Gut Feminism* (Durham, NC: Duke University Press, 2015), 1.

223. Wilson (2015), 3.

224. Bourgeois (1975), 185.

225. Figures cited in M. Elizabeth Carnegie, "The Minority Practitioner in Nursing," *National League for Nursing Publications* (1974) 15-1513: 39-42; and M. Elizabeth Carnegie, "Educational Preparation of Black Nurses: A Historical Perspective," *The ABNF Journal* (Jan/Feb 2005): 6-7.

226. Lucille Davis, "The Minority Practitioner in Nursing," *National League for Nursing Publications* (1974) 15-1513: 43-45, quotation from p. 45.

227. Quotation taken from National Black Nurses Association, "History," https://www.nbna .org/history (accessed July 8, 2020) and from Gloria R. Smith, "From Invisibility to Blackness: The Story of the National Black Nurses' Association," *Nursing Outlook* (1975) 23: 225-229, 227.

228. Gloria R. Smith, "Multicultural Components of Nursing." *National League for Nursing Publications* (1976) 14-1625: 1-7, quotation from p. 2.

229. Carnegie (1974); Davis (1974); and Janice E. Ruffin, "Issues for the Black Nurse Today: Competence and Commitment," *National League for Nursing Publications* (1974) 15-1513: 46-51.

230. Jo Eleanor Elliott, Janelle C. Kruegar, and Jeanne M. Kearns, "Update of Nursing Research in the West," *Nursing Research* (1980) 29(3): 184-188, quotation from p. 184.

231. Elliott, Kruegar, and Kearns (1980), 185.

232. Elliott, Kruegar, and Kearns (1980), 185.

233. Marie F. Branch, "Faculty Development to Meet Minority Group Needs: Recruitment, Retention, and Curriculum, 1971-1974; Final Report," (Boulder, CO: Western Interstate Commission for Higher Education, 1975).

234. Gatrall (2020).

235. Marie F. Branch and Phyllis P. Paxton (eds.), *Providing Safe Nursing Care for Ethnic People of Color* (New York: Appleton-Century-Crofts, 1976). This effort should be seen as part of a much broader effort to institutionalize diversity within college and university curricula following passage of the 1965 Higher Education Act and the activism of black and women student groups. See Christopher P. Loss, *Between Citizens and the State: The Politics of American Higher Education in the 20th Century* (Princeton, NJ: Princeton University Press, 2011), 165-213.

236. Elliott, Kruegar, and Kearns (1980); Branch and Paxton (1976).

237. Eileen M. Jackson, "Whiting-Out Difference: Why U.S. Nursing Research Fails Black Families," *Medical Anthropology Quarterly* (1993) 7(4): 363-385, 369.

238. Jackson (1993), 371.

239. Jackson (1993); Evelyn L. Barbee, "Racism in U.S. Nursing." *Medical Anthropology Quarterly* (1993) 7(4): 346-362.

240. Barbee (1993), 349.

241. Jackson (1993), 365.

242. Jackson (1993), 371-372.

243. Barbee (1993), 358.

244. Rozella M. Schlotfeldt, "Nursing in the University Community," November 12, 1965, Case Western Reserve University Archives, Frances Payne Bolton School of Nursing Collection, Series 29DD, box 2, Papers of Dean Rozella Schlotfeldt, folder 1:1.

Chapter Three

1. Rozella M. Schlotfeldt, "Nursing in the University Community," November 12, 1965, Case Western Reserve University Archives, Frances Payne Bolton School of Nursing Collection, Series 29DD, box 2, Papers of Dean Rozella Schlotfeldt, folder 1:1.

2. Rebecca S. Lowen, *Creating the Cold War University: The Transformation of Stanford* (Berkeley: University of California Press, 1997); Henry Etzkowitz, *MIT and the Rise of Entrepreneurial Science* (New York: Routledge, 2002); Daniel Lee Kleinman, *Impure Cultures: University Biology and the World of Commerce* (Madison: University of Wisconsin Press, 2003); Daniel S. Greenberg, *The Politics of Pure Science* (Chicago: University of Chicago Press, 1999); and Daniel S. Greenberg, *Science for Sale: The Perils, Rewards, and Delusions of Campus Capitalism* (Chicago: University of Chicago Press, 2007).

3. Hugh Davis Graham and Nancy Diamond, *The Rise of American Research Universities: Elites and Challengers in the Postwar Era* (Baltimore: Johns Hopkins University Press, 1997), 3; Roger Geiger, *Research and Relevant Knowledge: American Research Universities since World War II* (New York: Routledge, 1993), 220.

4. For example, military and defense industry funding transformed the physical sciences and engineering, leading to an emphasis on fields like aeronautical and nuclear engineering, space science, and electronics. See, for example, Stuart W. Leslie, *The Cold War and American Science: The Military-Industrial-Academic Complex at MIT and Stanford* (New York: Columbia University Press, 1993); Paul Forman, "Behind Quantum Electronics: National Security as Basis of Physical Research in the United States, 1940–1960," *Historical Studies in the Physical Sciences* (1987) 18: 149–229; Peter Galison and Bruce Hevly, eds., *Big Science: The Growth of Large-Scale Research*, (Stanford, CA: Stanford University Press, 1992); Geiger (1993); Lowen (1997). The social sciences were also transformed by the postwar political economy as leading universities established new departments, fields, and programs that bore direct relevance to the geopolitical context of the Cold War, such as international relations, Soviet studies, and East Asian studies. Meanwhile, traditional social science disciplines like political science, psychology, and anthropology began emphasizing "quantitative approaches over normative ones and individual behavior and cultural studies over sociological ones" as these disciplinary approaches secured preference among patrons and university administrators. See Lowen (1997), 191–223, quotation from p. 3; Ellen Herman, *The Romance of American Psychology: Political Culture in the Age of Experts* (Berkeley: University of California Press, 1995); James H. Capshew, *Psychologists on the March: Science, Practice, and Professional Identity in America, 1929–1969* (Cambridge: Cambridge University Press, 1999); and Joy Rohde, *Armed with Expertise: The Militarization of American Social Research during the Cold War* (Ithaca, NY: Cornell University Press, 2013).

5. Margaret Rossiter, *Women Scientists in America: Before Affirmative Action, 1940–1972* (Baltimore: Johns Hopkins University Press, 1998); Londa Schiebinger, *Has Feminism Changed Science?* (Cambridge, MA: Harvard University Press, 1999); Margaret A. M. Murray, *Women Becoming Mathematicians: Creating a Professional Identity in Post-World War II America* (Cambridge, MA: MIT Press, 2000); Amy Sue Bix, *Girls Coming to Tech! A History of American Engineering Education for Women* (Cambridge, MA: MIT Press, 2013).

6. Schiebinger (1999), 30.

7. Graham and Diamond (1997), 47.

8. Graham and Diamond (1997), 34–35.

9. Leslie (1993); Lowen (1997); Geiger (1993); Dominique A. Tobbell, *Pills, Power, and Policy: The Struggle for Drug Reform in Cold War America and its Consequences* (Berkeley: University of California Press and Milbank Books on Health and the Public, 2012). In 1961, for example, the federal government (primarily the NIH) funded 56 percent of the nation's medical research, compared to 28 percent by industry. Figures cited in Faye G. Abdellah and Eugene Levine, *Better Patient Care through Nursing Research* (New York: Macmillan, 1965), 605.

10. Geiger (1993); Lowen (1997); Etzkowitz (2002); and Chandra Mukerji, *A Fragile Power: Scientists and the State* (Princeton, NJ: Princeton University Press, 1990).

11. Clark Kerr, *The Uses of the University* (Cambridge, MA: Harvard University Press, 1963). See also Christopher P. Loss, *Between Citizens and the State: The Politics of American Higher Education in the 20th Century* (Princeton, NJ: Princeton University Press, 2011), 165–166.

12. See note 4.

13. Lowen (1997), 68.

14. Graham and Diamond (1997), 74; Roger Geiger, *Knowledge and Money: Research Universities and the Paradox of the Marketplace* (Palo Alto, CA: Stanford University Press, 2004), 142–144; and Kenneth M. Ludmerer, *Time to Heal: American Medical Education from the Turn of the Century to the Era of Managed Care* (Oxford: Oxford University Press, 1999).

15. Stephen P. Strickland, *Politics, Science, and Dread Disease: A Short History of United States Medical Research Policy* (Cambridge, MA: Harvard University Press, 1972); Geiger (1993), 179–185.

16. Ludmerer (1999), 139–161.

17. Geiger (1993), 184.

18. Ludermer (1999).

19. Geiger (2004), 143.

20. Graham and Diamond (1997), 78.

21. President's Science Advisory Committee, *Scientific Progress, the Universities, and the Federal Government* (Washington, DC: Government Printing Office, 1960), cited in Geiger (1993), 169.

22. Graham and Diamond (1997), 43.

23. Graham and Diamond (1997), 43. See also Geiger (1993) and Loss (2011). The federal government also committed substantial support for health professions education with passage of the 1963 Health Professions Educational Assistance Act, which provided construction grants for teaching facilities and student loans to medical and dental students. A year later, Congress passed the Nurse Training Act, which provided matching federal funds for the construction of new and the expansion of existing nursing schools, as well grants and loans to nursing students (discussed in chapter 4). Joan E. Lynaugh, "Nursing the Great Society: The Impact of the Nurse Training Act of 1964," *Nursing History Review* (2008) 16: 13–28.

24. Geiger (1993), 223.

25. Geiger (1993), 218–219.

26. Rossiter (1995), xv.

27. Rossiter (1995), xvi.

28. Rossiter (1995), 165–185.

29. Rossiter (1995), 165.

30. Rossiter (1995), 166.

31. Rossiter (1995), 174.

32. Rossiter (1995), 185, 184.

33. Madeleine Leininger, "Psychopolitical and Ethnocentric Behaviors in Emerging Health Science Centers," November 1974, Walter P. Reuther Library, University Archives, Wayne State University, Madeleine Leininger Collection, Accession 725, box 7.

34. Dorothy Smith to Samuel P. Martin, "Memorandum: Material on Hospital Administration," February 19, 1965, University of Florida Health Science Center Archives, George T. Harrell Medical History Center, RS4-VPHA Records: 4b- VPHA Martin; box 38, folder: College of Nursing, through Sept 1965.

35. Mary Kelly Mullane, "Nursing Faculty Roles and Functions in the Large University Setting," Memo to members of the Council of Baccalaureate and Higher Degree Programs, National League for Nursing, September 1969. University of Illinois Chicago University Archives, College of Nursing Office of the Dean—Administrative Files, 1955–1989, RG 17-01-02, box 1, folder 23.

36. Lawrence J. Sharp and Mary S. Tschudin, "Nursing Faculty Research Development: Report of an Experience," *Nursing Research* (1967) 16(2): 161–166, quotation from p. 161.

37. Martha Pitel and John Vian, "Analysis of Nurse-Doctorates: Data Collected for the International Directory of Nurses with Doctoral Degrees," *Nursing Research* (1975) 24(5), 340–351.

38. Lowen (1997), 3

39. Mary S. Tschudin, "Doctoral Preparation in Other Disciplines with a Minor in Nursing," *Nursing Forum* (1966) V(2): 50–56, 50.

40. Rozella Schlotfeldt, "Doctoral Study in Basic Disciplines: A Choice for Nurses," *Nursing Forum* (1966) V(2): 68–74, 69.

41. Donna Diers, "Faculty Research Development at Yale," *Nursing Research*, 1970, 19(1): 64–71, 64. The stakes were particularly high at Yale given that until 1969, Yale only admitted women into its graduate and professional schools. As one faculty member reflected, the School of Nursing wasn't "considered part of the 'real' Yale," and after the enrollment of female undergraduates, "nurses continued to be half-invisible" on Yale's campus. Angela Barron McBride, "The Married Feminist," *American Journal of Nursing* (1976) 76(5): 754–757.

42. See, for example, various reports from the Committee for the Exploration of the Feasibility of a Doctorate Program for Nurses at Wayne State University School of Nursing, 1968–1973. Walter P. Reuther Library, University Archives, Wayne State University, Nursing—Dean's Office, Accession no. 672, box 1, folder 7.

43. Sharp and Tschudin (1967); Diers (1970); Lulu Wolf Hassenplug and Carole E. Bare, "An Evaluation and Study of Faculty Research Potential, Part I: Final Report to the U.S. Public Health Service Division of Nursing, Dept. Of Health, Education, and Welfare," December 1965, UCLA Biomedical Archives, MS41 Lulu Hassenplug Papers, box 2, folder 22; Doris R. Schwartz, "Faculty Research Development Grants: A Follow-Up Report," *NLN Exchange No. 125*, 1981.

44. On the FRDG program, see Abdellah and Levine (1965), 618–619, 630–632.

45. Schwartz (1981), 2–3. Included among these eighteen schools was Johns Hopkins University School of Hygiene and Public Health, which was an interdisciplinary graduate school with neither a separate curricular nor a BSN program. The Division of Nursing made two additional FRDGs—one to Teachers College and one to the New York State Department of Mental Hygiene—to develop programs for faculty from other institutions who were on sabbatical leave or who attended special courses at an institution other than their own.

46. Geiger (1993), 176–177.

47. Geiger (1993), 177.

48. Sharp and Tschudin (1967), 162.

49. Diers (1970), 67.

50. Schwartz (1981), 11, 22–24.

51. Diers (1970), 68–69.

52. Rozella Schlotfeldt, "Creating a Climate for Research. Project Supported by Division of Nursing Grant (Faculty Research Development Grant), January 1963–December 1972," p. 41, Case Western Reserve University Archives, Frances Payne Bolton School of Nursing Collection, Series 29DD, box 2, Papers of Dean Rozella Schlotfeldt, folder: Correspondence, 1960–1971.

53. Rozella Schlotfeldt, "Creating a Climate for Research."

54. Schwartz (1981), 3.

55. Susan R. Gortner and Helen Nahm, "Overview of Nursing Research in the United States," *Nursing Research* (1977) 26(1): 10–33; and Susan R. Gortner, "Nursing Research: Out of the Past and into the Future," *Nursing Research* (1980) 29(4): 204–207.

56. Jeanne S. Berthold, "Nursing Research Grant Proposals," *Nursing Research* (1973) 22(4): 292–299.

57. Madeline Leininger, "Creating and Maintaining a Nursing Research Support Center" (paper presentation, Project for Nursing Research Colloquium at Adelphi University School of Nursing, November 2, 1977), Walter P. Reuther Library, University Archives, Wayne State University, Madeleine Leininger Collection, Accession 725, box 8.

58. Leininger, "Creating and Maintaining a Nursing Research Support Center," (1977).

59. Madeleine Leininger, "Highlights of the Progress of and Achievements in the College of Nursing under Dean M. Leininger's Administration from July 1, 1974 to Present," October 1, 1977, Florida Atlantic University Archives, Madeleine Leininger Collection, ARC-008, series 4, subsection 4, box 45.

60. Beryl Peters to Madeleine Leininger, September 19, 1977, Florida Atlantic University Archives, Madeleine Leininger Collection, ARC-008, series 4, box 45.

61. Leininger, "Creating and Maintaining a Nursing Research Support Center," (1977).

62. Leininger, "Creating and Maintaining a Nursing Research Support Center," (1977).

63. Rozella Schlotfeldt, "Creating a Climate for Nursing Research. Project Supported by Division of Nursing Grant (Faculty Research Development Grant), January 1963–December 1972), February 1973. Case Western Research Archives, Frances Payne Bolton School of Nursing Collection, Series 29DD, Box 2, Folder: p. 26.

64. Schlotfeldt (1973), 42.

65. Harriet H. Werley, "Nursing and Research," (presentation, National Commission for the Study of Nursing and Nursing Education, January 14, 1972), Walter P. Reuther Library, University Archives, Wayne State University, College of Nursing Center for Health Research, Accession no. 2167, box 1, folder 1; Virginia Cleland, "Developing a Doctoral Program," *Nursing Outlook* (1976) 24(10): 631–635.

66. All of these studies are cited in Gortner and Nahm (1977), 21–22.

67. Harriet H. Werley and Fredericka P. Shea, "The First Center for Research in Nursing: Its Development, Accomplishments, and Problems," *Nursing Research* (1973) 22(3): 217–231, 218.

68. Werley (1972).

69. Mabel A. Wandelt, "Research Development—Center for Nursing Research," application for research grant, Public Health Service, June 11, 1969, Walter P. Reuther Library, University Archives, Wayne State University, College of Nursing Center for Health Research, Accession no. 2167, box 1, folder 1.

70. Judy G. Ozbolt, "Harriet Helen Werley," *Journal of the American Medical Informatics Association* (2003) 10(2): 224–225.

71. Harriet W. Werley, "Center for Health Research, College of Nursing, Wayne State University," December 11, 1972, Walter P. Reuther Library, University Archives, Wayne State University, Nursing—Dean's Office, Accession no. 2167, box 1, folder 1.

72. Michael L. Millenson, *Demanding Medical Excellence: Doctors and Accountability in the Information Age* (Chicago: University of Chicago Press, 1997); Jeanne Daly, *Evidence-Based Medicine and the Search for a Science of Clinical Care* (Berkeley: University of California Press / Milbank Memorial Fund, 2005); Daniel M. Fox, *The Convergence of Science and Governance: Research, Health Policy, and American States* (Berkeley: University of California Press, 2010), 22–50; and Nancy Tomes, *Remaking the American Patient: How Madison Avenue and Modern Medicine Turned Patients into Consumers* (Chapel Hill: University of North Carolina Press, 2016), 310–313.

73. Harriet H. Werley, Fredericka Shea, and Jean E. Johnson, "Research Development—Center for Nursing Research, Terminal Progress Report, Grant NU00361, Division of Nursing, U.S. Department of Health, Education, and Welfare, May 1, 1970–September 30, 1975," Walter P. Reuther Library, University Archives, Wayne State University, College of Nursing Center for Health Research, Accession no. 2167, box 1, folder 1.

74. Werley, Shea, and Johnson (1975).

75. Werley, Shea, and Johnson (1975).

76. Harriet H. Werley, Joel W. Ager, R. A. Hudson Rosen, and Fredericka P. Shea, "Medicine, Nursing, Social Work: Professionals and Birth Control: Student and Faculty Attitudes," *Family Planning Perspectives* (1973) 5(1): 42–49.

77. Doris V. Allen, Fredericka P. Shea, Paul A. Reichelt, Norma McHugh, and Harriet H. Werley, "Factors to Consider in Staffing an Abortion Service Facility," *Journal of Nursing Administration* (July/August 1974): 22–27.

78. Werley, Shea, and Johnson (1975); Paul A. Reichelt and Harriet H. Werley, "Contraception, Abortion and Venereal Disease: Teenagers' Knowledge and the Effect of Education," *Family Planning Perspectives* (1975) 7(2): 83–88.

79. See, for example, Joel W. Ager, Harriet H. Werley, and Fredericka P. Shea, "Correlates of Continuance in a Family Planning Program," *Journal of Obstetrical and Gynecological Nursing* (November/December 1973): 15–23; Reichelt and Werley (1975); and Paul A. Reichelt and Harriet H. Werley, "A Sex Information Program for Sexually Active Teenagers," *Journal of School Health* (1976) XLV(2): 100–107.

80. Leininger, "Creating and Maintaining a Nursing Research Support Center," (1977).

81. Graham and Diamond (1997), 84. On the financial crisis at universities in the late 1960s and 1970s, see Geiger (1993), 243–252, and Geiger (2004), 22–27. See Geiger (1993), 267 for data on enrollment and funding changes in ten states between 1968 and 1978.

82. Graham and Diamond (1997), 84.

83. Graham and Diamond (1997), 88. According to one estimate, cited by Graham and Diamond, the number of federal fellowships and traineeships fell from 57,000 in 1968 to 41,000 in 1970.

84. Harriet H. Werley, "Report to the Graduate Faculty November 29, 1972 about Center for Health Research," Walter P. Reuther Library, University Archives, Wayne State University, College of Nursing Center for Health Research, Accession no. 2167, box 1, folder 1.

85. Margaret Shetland to Harriet H. Werley, "Memo: Budgetary Planning for 1972–1973," August 23, 1971, and Harriet H. Werley, "Health Sciences Professions Instruction, Center for Health Research, WSU College of Nursing," June 1973, Walter P. Reuther Library, University Archives,

Wayne State University, College of Nursing Center for Health Research, Accession no. 2167, box 1, folder 1.

86. Werley and Shea (1973), 229.

87. Werley, Shea, and Johnson (1975).

88. Werley and Shea (1973), 229.

89. Werley, Shea, and Johnson (1975).

90. Hassenplug and Bare (1965); Diers (1970); Sharp and Tshudin (1967); Marjorie Batey, "Research Developing in University Schools of Nursing: Organizational Structure and Process Variables Related to Research Goal Attainment," Division of Nursing, 1978; Schwartz (1981); Marjorie Batey, "Programmatic Structure for Research Productivity," Fifth Forum on Doctoral Education, University of Washington School of Nursing, June 25–26, 1981, Bates Center for the Study of the History of Nursing Archives, Florence S. Downs Papers, MC 130, series IV, box 8, folder 6.

91. Faye G. Abdellah, "Overview of Nursing Research 1955–1968, Part I," *Nursing Research* (1970) 19(1): 6–17; Faye G. Abdellah, "Overview of Nursing Research 1955–1968, Part II," *Nursing Research* (1970) 19(2): 151–162; Faye G. Abdellah, "Overview of Nursing Research 1955–1968, Part III," *Nursing Research* (1970) 19(3): 239–252.

92. Joanne S. Stevenson, "Forging a Research Discipline," *Nursing Research* (1987) 36(1): 60–64.

93. Cynthia Connolly and Joan E. Lynaugh, *Fifty Years at the Division of Nursing: United States Public Health Service* (Washington, DC: U.S. Public Health Service Division of Nursing, 1997).

94. Madeleine Leininger, "Doctoral Programs for Nursing: Trends, Questions, and Projected Plans," *Nursing Research* (1976) 25(3): 201–210.

95. Abdellah and Levine, 1965, pp. 633–635. Rozella Schlotfeldt, "The Nurse Scientist Program at Case Western Reserve University," (paper presentation, meeting of the Council of Baccalaureate and Higher Degree Programs, National League for Nursing, March 27, 1968, Cleveland, Ohio), Case Western Reserve Archives, Frances Payne Bolton School of Nursing Collection, Series 29DD, box 2, folder 1:1.

96. Rozella Schlotfeldt to Florence Wald, Yale University, March 10, 1968, Case Western Reserve University Archives, Frances Payne Bolton School of Nursing Collection, Series 29DB, box 5, folder: Nurse Scientist Program, General Info and Recruiting, 1963–1974.

97. Cleland (1976), 631. On discrimination against women in the sciences, see Rossiter (1995) and Schiebinger (1999).

98. Katherine Hoffman, "An Overview of the Nurse Scientist Program at the University of Washington," *National League for Nursing Publications* (1968) 15–1342: 30–34, 32.

99. Helen Grace, "The Research Doctorate in Nursing," August 4, 1978, University of Illinois Chicago, University Archives, College of Nursing, Dean–Faculty Papers Collection, Helen Grace Papers (acc. 017-01-20-01), box 4, folder 49.

100. On the history of sociology within UCSF's School of Nursing, see University of California, San Francisco, "A History of UCSF: Helen Nahm," https://history.library.ucsf.edu/nahm .html (accessed December 4, 2020), and University of California, San Francisco, "Sociology Doctoral Program: History of the Department," https://sociology.ucsf.edu/history-department (accessed December 4, 2020). On Strauss's role in the UCSF School of Nursing, see Sociological Research Online, "Anselm L. Strauss Obituary," https://www.socresonline.org.uk/1/4/strauss .html (accessed December 4, 2020).

101. On the gendering of science, see Schiebinger (1999), particularly pp. 67–91. See also Rossiter (1995).

102. Rozella Schlotfeldt to Faye Abdellah, June 20, 1967, Case Western Reserve University Archives, Frances Payne Bolton School of Nursing Collection, 29DB, box 5.

103. Grace (1978).

104. Marian Olsen, "Doctoral Preparation for Nurses: A Continuation of the Dialogue," *Nursing Forum* (1966) V(3): 57.

105. Grace (1978).

106. "Interdisciplinary-Physiology Research Interest Group," (1st Annual Midwest Nursing Research Society Conference, Indiana University, June 20–21, 1977), University of Illinois Chicago, University Archives, Midwest Nursing Research Society, series 1, box 1, folder 1.

107. Grace (1978).

108. Harry Marks, *The Progress of Experiment: Science and Therapeutic Reform in the United States, 1900–1990* (New York: Cambridge University Press, 1997); Daly (2005).

109. Graham and Diamond (1997), 88.

110. Graham and Diamond (1997), 122–123.

111. Lynaugh (2008), 22.

112. Susan R. Gortner, "Researchmanship: The Politics of Research Revisited," *Western Journal of Nursing Research* (1981) 3(3): 309–311.

113. Data from National Institutes of Health, https://officeofbudget.od.nih.gov/pdfs/spending_history/Mechanism%20Detail%20for%20Total%20NIH%20FY%201983%20-%20FY%201999.pdf (accessed July 1, 2019).

114. Marie J. Bourgeois, "The Special Nurse Research Fellow: Characteristics and Recent Trends," *Nursing Research* (1975) 24(3): 184–188, 185.

115. "Panel discussion," *Nursing Forum* (1966) V(2): 83–104, pp. 85–86.

116. Geiger (1993), pp 217–229.

117. Rozella Schlotfeldt, "The Nurse with the Doctorate," (presentation, Upsilon chapter of Sigma Theta Tau, New York University, March 21, 1969), Case Western Reserve University Archives, Frances Payne Bolton School of Nursing Collection, Series 29DD, box 2, folder 1.

118. Joanne S. Jamann, "Proceedings of Doctoral Programs in Nursing: Consensus for Quality," American Association of Colleges of Nursing and Division of Nursing, Department of Health and Human Services, August 13–15, 1985.

119. See, for example, Lulu Wolf Hassenplug, "Doctoral Preparation for Nurses: A Continuation of the Dialogue," *Nursing Forum* (1966) V(3): 53–56. Hassenplug thought "we may find some answers by studying what other disciplines have done." (p. 55). Nursing reformers had long looked to engineering as a potential model for nursing education reform. See, for example, Esther Lucile Brown, *Nursing for the Future: A Report Prepared for the National Nursing Council* (New York: Russell Sage Foundation, 1948), 138–173. For discussion of this, see Joan Lynaugh and Barbara Brush, *American Nursing: From Hospitals to Health Systems* (Malden, MA: Blackwell, 1996), 5–11.

120. Bruce E. Seely, "Research, Engineering, and Science in American Engineering Colleges: 1900–1960," *Technology and Culture* (1993) 34(2): 344–386; Bruce E. Seely, "The Other Re-engineering of Engineering Education, 1900–1965," *Journal of Engineering Education* (July 1999): 285–294; and Jonathon Harwood, "Engineering Education between Science and Practice: Rethinking the Historiography," *History and Technology* (2006) 22(1): 53–79.

121. For distinction between the two, see: "Future Directions of Doctoral Education for Nurses: Report of a Conference, Bethesda, MD, United States Public Health Service, National Institutes of Health, Bureau of Health Manpower Education, January 20, 1971," p. 34, Bates

Center for the Study of the History of Nursing Archives, Florence S. Downs Papers, MC 130, Series IV, box 7, folder 12.

122. Rozella Schlotfeldt to Roy E. Bolz, Dean of Engineering, Case Western Reserve University, March 21, 1969, Case Western Reserve University Archives, Frances Payne Bolton School of Nursing Collection, Series 29DB, box 15, folder: Graduate Curriculum 1970–1972.

123. Wade Pickren, "Tension and Opportunity in Post–World War II American Psychology," *History of Psychology* (2007) 10(3): 279–299; Nancy Tomes, "The Development of Clinical Psychology, Social Work, and Psychiatric Nursing: 1900–1980," in Edwin R. Wallace and John Gach (eds.), *History of Psychiatry and Medical Psychology* (New York: Springer, 2008): 657–682; Capshew (1999), 171–174.

124. Andrew Hogan, "The 'Two Cultures' in Clinical psychology: Constructing Disciplinary Divides in the Management of Mental Retardation," *ISIS* (2018) 109(4): 695–719, 701.

125. Capshew (1999), 246–247; Pickren (2007).

126. Pickren (2007), 288.

127. Discussion, Midwest Invitation Conference on Resources for Doctoral Education in Nursing, June 29, 1976, Ruth Lilly Special Collections and Archives, Indiana University–Purdue University Indianapolis, Indianapolis, Midwest Alliance in Nursing Collection, box 3.

128. Scott, Gortner, and Bourgeois (1976), 98.

129. Jamann (1985), 9; Rita Snyder-Halpern, "Doctoral Programs in Nursing: An Examination of Curriculum Similarities and Differences," *Journal of Nursing Education* (1986) 25(9): 358–365; Margretta Styles, "Doctoral Education in Nursing: The Current Situation in Historical Perspective," (First National Conference on Doctoral Education," June 23–24, 1977), Bates Center for the Study of the History of Nursing Archives, Florence S. Downs Papers, MC 130, Series II, box 4, folder 10.

130. Helen Grace, "Doctoral Education in Nursing: An Overview," 1973, University of Illinois Chicago University Archives, College of Nursing, Dean–Faculty Papers Collection, Helen Grace Papers, Accession no. 017-01-20-01, box 4, folder 47. See also Reva Rubin and Florence Erickson, "Clinical Doctorate," in "Future Directions of Doctoral Education for Nurses: Report of a Conference, Bethesda, MD, United States Public Health Service, National Institutes of Health, Bureau of Health Manpower Education, January 20, 1971," pp. 144–157.

131. Grace (1973).

132. Barbara Schneider quoted in Michael J. Pelczar, "The Nature of the Doctorate and Criteria for Quality," in Joanne S. Jamann, "Proceedings of Doctoral Programs in Nursing: Consensus for Quality," American Association of Colleges of Nursing and Division of Nursing, Department of Health and Human Services, August 13–15, 1985.

133. Pelczar (1985).

134. Virginia Cleland to Margretta Styles, November 7, 1973. See also, Minutes, Doctoral Program Committee, Wayne State University College of Nursing, October 30, 1973, Walter P. Reuther Library, University Archives, Wayne State University, Nursing—Dean's Office, Accession no. 672, box 1, folder 8.

135. Helen Grace, "Program Design," (First National Conference on Doctoral Education, June 23–24, 1977), Bates Center for the Study of the History of Nursing Archives, Florence S. Downs Papers, MC 130, Series II, box 4, folder 10. On UCSF, see Susan Gortner, "The Clinical Doctorate" in *Proceedings. Forum: Epistemological Strategies in Nursing*, June 21–24, 1984, Bates Center for the Study of the History of Nursing Archives, Florence S. Downs Papers, MC 130, Series IV, box 8, folder 7. Gortner explains the DNS at UCSF "began as a research degree, because

it was impossible at that time (i.e., 1965) to get a PhD program in nursing approved through the Graduate Division of our campus." Gortner continued that "the research base in 1965 at the U of Ca-San Fran was provided mainly from the sociology faculty in the Department of Social and Behavioral Sciences, and, as many of you are aware, the dominant mode of inquiry was field research. Today [c. 1984], the research base is provided by the nurse scientist faculty and uses multiple modes of inquiry." On the University of Pennsylvania, see Claire M. Fagin to Madeleine Leininger, October 28, 1976, Walter P. Reuther Library, University Archives, Wayne State University, Madeleine Leininger Collection, Accession 725, box 1.

136. Claire Fagin, "Introduction," (First National Conference on Doctoral Education, June 23–24, 1977), Bates Center for the Study of the History of Nursing Archives, Florence S. Downs Papers, MC 130, Series II, box 4, folder 10.

137. Grace (1977).

138. Grace (1977). See also Leininger (1976); and Florence Downs, "Doctoral Education in Nursing: Future Directions," *Nursing Outlook* (1978) 26(11): 56–61.

139. Fagin to Leininger (1976); Styles (1977); and Dorothy Crowley, "Theoretical and Pragmatic Issues Related to the Goals of Doctoral Education in Nursing," (First National Conference on Doctoral Education, June 23–24, 1977), Bates Center for the Study of the History of Nursing Archives, Florence S. Downs Papers, MC 130, Series II, box 4, folder 10.

140. Scott, Gortner, and Bourgeois (1976), p.4.

141. This was the case at the University of Minnesota where the nursing faculty did not have any difficulties with the other health professions but with the basic scientists. Mariah Snyder, oral history interview by Dominique Tobbell on June 13, 2012, p. 17, https://editions.lib.umn.edu/ahc-ohp/2013/08/04/snyder-mariah/ (accessed July 19, 2019).

142. Snyder (2012), 17.

143. Marilyn Sime, oral history interview by Dominique Tobbell, April 15, 2010, p. 24, https://editions.lib.umn.edu/ahc-ohp/2012/03/29/a-marilyn-sime/ (accessed July 19, 2019). "To Health Sciences Policy and Review Council," June 17, 1981, University of Minnesota Archives, School of Nursing Collection, box 55, folder: H.S. Policy and Review Council, Program Review Committee 1981.

144. Helen Grace, "The Research Doctorate in Nursing," August 4, 1978, University of Illinois Chicago University Archives, College of Nursing, Dean–Faculty Papers Collection, Helen Grace Papers, Accession no. 017-01-20-01, box 4, folder 49.

145. Graham and Diamond (1997), 86–88.

146. Scott, Gortner, and Bourgeois (1976), 10–11.

147. Madeleine Leininger, "Annual Report of the School of Nursing University of Washington, 1972–1973," Walter P. Reuther Library, University Archives, Wayne State University Madeleine Leininger Collection, Accession 725, box 3, folder 34.

148. Scott, Gortner, and Bourgeois (1976), 40.

149. See, for example, Cleland (1976), 633.

150. Mary Lohr, "To Joseph S. Begando, Chancellor: A Proposal for the Degree Doctor of Philosophy," July 29, 1974, University of Illinois Chicago University Archives, College of Nursing, Dean–Faculty Papers Collection, Helen Grace Papers, Accession no. 017-01-20-01, box 38, folder 309. See also "Minutes of University of Illinois Chicago College of Nursing Faculty Meeting, Oct 8, 1975," University of Illinois Chicago University Archives, College of Nursing, Administration—Faculty Meeting Minutes 1963–1983, Accession no. 017-01-20-01, box 1, folder 1974–1983.

151. Lois Malasanos, oral history interview by Ann Smith, June 20, 2005, p. 12, University of Florida Digital Collections, https://ufdc.ufl.edu/UF00066610/00001 (accessed July 25, 2019). See also Ida Martinson, oral history interview by Dominique A. Tobbell, July 7, 2010, University of Minnesota Academic Health Center Oral History Project, https://editions.lib.umn.edu/ahc -ohp/2012/01/12/ida-m-martinson/ (accessed July 25, 2019). Martinson also earned her PhD in physiology at the University of Illinois Chicago during the late 1960s and early 1970s, working with a different stress physiologist.

152. Minutes, Committee on Institutional Cooperation, Meeting of Nursing Deans, November 26, 1974, University of Illinois Chicago University Archives, College of Nursing, Dean− Faculty Papers Collection, Helen Grace Papers, Accession no. 017-01-20-01, box 22, folder 256.

153. Lohr (1974). Minutes, University of Illinois Chicago College of Nursing Faculty Meeting, October 8, 1975, University of Illinois Chicago University Archives, College of Nursing, Administration—Faculty Meeting Minutes 1963–1983, box 1, folder 1974–1983.

154. Lohr (1974).

155. See, for example, Cleland (1976); and Helen K. Grace, Beverly M. LaBelle, and Nola J. Pender, "Study of Resources for Doctoral Education in the Midwest," February 1976, Ruth Lilly Special Collections and Archives, Indiana University–Purdue University Indianapolis, Indianapolis, Midwest Alliance in Nursing Collection, box 30.

156. Leininger and Glittenberg, "Textual Analysis of Doctoral Dissertation Abstracts," (proceedings, Forum: Epistemological Strategies in Nursing, June 21–24, 1984, cosponsored by the Planning Committee for the National Forum on Doctoral Education in Nursing and the University of Colorado School of Nursing, Denver. Bates Center Archives, Florence S. Downs Papers MC 130, Series IV, box 8, folder 7.

157. Helen Grace, "Program Design," (First National Conference on Doctoral Education in Nursing, University of Pennsylvania, June 23–24, 1977), 54–56, quotation from p. 56. Bates Center for the Study of the History of Nursing Archives, Florence S. Downs Papers MC 130, Series II, box 4, folder 10.

158. New York University, University of Pittsburgh, Case Western Reserve University, University of Texas System at Austin and at San Antonio, University of Illinois Chicago, Texas Women's University, University of Arizona, and Wayne State University.

159. University of California, San Francisco, Catholic University of America, Boston University, and the University of Alabama-Birmingham.

160. Teachers College, Columbia University, and New York University. Leininger (1976).

161. Rozella Schlotfeldt, "Nursing Research: Reflection of Values," Nursing Research (1977) 26(1): 4–9, 8.

162. Malasanos (2005), 23.

163. Eva Clark, "Educators Are No Help," American Journal of Nursing (1969) 69(9): 1878.

164. Patricia Duick, "Nursing's No Science," American Journal of Nursing (1968) 68(1): 52, 54.

165. Andrew Abbott, The System of Professions: An Essay on the Division of Expert Labor (Chicago: University of Chicago Press, 1988), 56.

166. Alice M. Chait, ". . . Teach Nursing Students to Meet Real Needs . . ." American Journal of Nursing (1973) 73(3): 430.

167. Abbott (1988).

168. Seely, "The Other Re-engineering of Engineering Education," (1999), 291–292.

169. Seely (1993), 383.

170. Eric A. Walker, *Now It's My Turn: Engineering My Way* (New York: Vantage Press, 1989), 106, xii. Cited in Seely, "The Other Re-engineering of Engineering Education," (1999), 292.

171. Seely, "The 'Imbalance' of Theory and Practice," (1999), 57.

172. Florence Downs, "Doctoral Education in Nursing: Future Directions from Current Experiences," (First National Conference on Doctoral Education, June 23-24, 1977), Bates Center for the Study of the History of Nursing Archives, Florence S. Downs Papers, MC 130, Series II, box 4, folder 10.

173. Pauline F. Brimmer, Martha M. Skoner, Nola J. Pender, Carolyn A. Williams, Juanita W. Fleming, and Harriet H. Werley, "Nurses with Doctoral Degrees: Education and Employment Characteristics," *Research in Nursing and Health* (1983) 6: 157-165. On the difficulties doctorally prepared faculty faced as they sought to craft a research career but were overwhelmed by undergraduate teaching, see Frances Taira, "Is That Doctorate Necessary?" *Nursing Outlook* (1983) 31(1): 12-15.

174. Ellen D. Baer, "'A Cooperative Venture' in Pursuit of Professional Status: A Research Journal for Nursing," *Nursing Research* (1987) 36(1): 18-25; Susan M. Reverby, "A Legitimate Relationship: Nursing, Hospitals, and Science in the Twentieth Century," in Diana Elizabeth Long and Janet Golden (eds.) *The American General Hospital: Communities and Social Contexts* (Ithaca, NY: Cornell University Press, 1989), 135-156.

175. Lowen (1997), 236-237.

176. Jessie M. Scott, "Midwest Contributions to the National Nursing Scene," in Rozella Schlotfeldt and Judith Wood (eds.), "Midwest Alliance in Nursing: Final Report to Division of Nursing," 1979, Ruth Lilly Special Collections and Archives, Indiana University Purdue University Indianapolis, Indianapolis, Midwest Alliance in Nursing Collection, box 4.

177. Virginia Henderson, "Research in Nursing Practice—When?" *Nursing Research* (1956) 4(3): 99; Reverby (1989).

178. Virginia Henderson, "We've 'Come a Long Way' but What of the Direction?" *Nursing Research* (1977) 26(3): 163-164.

179. Carolyn Sullivan, Janice Robinson, and Janice Ruffin, "Nursing in a Society in Crisis." *American Journal of Nursing* (1972) 72(2): 302-304.

180. Jane Kennedy, "Begin with Education," *American Journal of Nursing* (1969) 69(11): 2445-2447, 2447.

181. Janice E. Ruffin, "Issues for the Black Nurse Today: Competence and Commitment," *National League for Nursing Publications* (1974) 15-1513: 46-51.

182. Lucie Young Kelly, "Open Curriculum: What and Why," *American Journal of Nursing* (1974) 74(12): 2232-2238; Bonnie Bullough, "Public, Legal, and Social Pressures for a Career Ladder in Nursing," *National League for Nursing Publications* (1972) 15-1473: 32-36.

Chapter Four

1. Jessie M. Scott, Susan R. Gortner, and Marie J Bourgeois, "The Doctorally Prepared Nurse," in *Report of Two Conferences on the Demand for Education of Nurses with Doctoral Degrees* (Florence S. Downs Papers MC 130, Series IV, box 8, folder 21976). p. 4.

2. Surgeon General's Consultant Group on Nursing, *Toward Quality in Nursing: Needs and Goals; Report of the Surgeon General's Consultant Group on Nursing* (Washington, DC: Government Printing Office, 1963).

3. See, for example, Rosemary Stevens, *In Sickness and in Wealth: American Hospitals in the Twentieth Century* (Baltimore: Johns Hopkins University Press, 1999); Daniel M. Fox, *The*

Convergence of Science and Governance (Berkeley: University of California Press, 2010); Joan E. Lynaugh and Barbara L. Brush, *American Nursing: From Hospitals to Health Systems* (Malden, MA: Blackwell, 1996).

4. Rosemary A. Stevens, "Health Care in the Early 1960s," *Health Care Financing Review* (1996) 18(2): 11–22, 16. See also Julie Fairman and Joan Lynaugh, *Critical Care Nursing: A History* (Philadelphia: University of Pennsylvania Press, 1998).

5. Julie Fairman, "Context and Contingency in the History of Post-World War II Nursing Scholarship in the United States," *Journal of Nursing Scholarship* (2008) 40(1): 4–11, 5. See also Lynaugh and Brush (1996), 33–37.

6. Julie Fairman, *Making Room in the Clinic: Nurse Practitioners and the Evolution of Modern Health Care* (New Brunswick, NJ: Rutgers University Press, 2008), 23.

7. Fairman (2008).

8. Avedis Donabedian, "Evaluating the Quality of Medical Care," *Milbank Memorial Fund Quarterly* (1966) 66(3): 166–206; John E. Wennberg and Alan Gittelsohn, "Small Area Variations in Health Care Delivery," *Science* (1973) 182: 1102–1108; John P. Bunker and John E. Wennberg, "Operation Rates, Mortality Statistics, and Quality of Life," *New England Journal of Medicine* (1973) 289(23): 1249–150; John E. Wennberg, John P. Bunker, and Benjamin Barnes, "The Need for Assessing the Outcomes of Common Medical Practices," *Annual Review of Public Health* (1980) 1: 1168–1173. For discussion, see Fox (2010), 22–50; Nancy Tomes, *Remaking the American Patient* (Chapel Hill: University of North Carolina Press, 2016), 310–313; Jeanne Daly, *Evidence-Based Medicine and the Search for a Science of Clinical Care* (Berkeley: University of California Press / Milbank Memorial Fund, 2005); Michael L. Millenson, *Demanding Medical Excellence: Doctors and Accountability in the Information Age* (Chicago: University of Chicago Press, 1997).

9. Tomes (2016), 311.

10. Jerome Lysaught, "National Commission for the Study of Nursing and Nursing Education: Summary Report and Recommendations," *American Journal of Nursing* (1970) 70(2): 285–286.

11. Surgeon General's Consultant Group on Nursing, *Toward Quality in Nursing. Needs and Goals; Report of the Surgeon General's Consultant Group on Nursing* (Washington, DC: Government Printing Office, 1963), 36.

12. Hugh Davis Graham and Nancy Diamond, *The Rise of American Research Universities: Elites and Challengers in the Postwar Era* (Baltimore: Johns Hopkins University Press, 1997), 91.

13. Christopher P. Loss, *Between Citizens and the State: The Politics of American Higher Education in the 20th Century* (Princeton, NJ: Princeton University, 2012), 165–213.

14. Loss (2012), 15.

15. John D. Millett, *Conflict in Higher Education: State Government Coordination Versus Institutional Independence* (San Francisco: Jossey-Bass Publishers, 1984), 75.

16. Loss (2012), 168.

17. Loss (2012), 168.

18. Loss (2012), 210–211.

19. Loss (2012), 211, plus Graham and Diamond (1997), 89. Graham and Diamond note that ratification of the Twenty-Sixth Amendment "made 98% of the nation's college students eligible to vote."

20. Frank Newman, et al., *Report on Higher Education: March 1971* (Washington, DC: U.S. Government Printing Office, 1971)

21. Carnegie Commission on Higher Education, *Less Time, More Options: Education Beyond*

the High School; Special Report and Recommendations (New York: McGraw-Hill, 1971), 14. Cited in and quoting Lucie Young Kelly, "Open Curriculum: What and Why." *American Journal of Nursing* (1974) 74(12): 2232–2238. See also Carnegie Commission on Higher Education, *Higher Education and the Nation's Health: Policies for Medical and Dental Education; Special Report and Recommendations* (New York: McGraw-Hill, 1970).

22. Loss (2012), 211.

23. Graham and Diamond (1997), 90.

24. Millett (1984), 76–77.

25. See Rozella Schlotfeldt, "The Health Manpower Shortage in Nursing," December 30, 1966, Case Western Reserve University Archives, 29DD, box 2 (29DD7), Papers of Dean Rozella Schlotfeldt, folder 1:2; and Schlotfeldt, "The ANA Position Paper on Education," May 5, 1965, Case Western Reserve University Archives, 29DD, box 2 (29DD7), Papers of Dean Rozella Schlotfeldt, folder 1:1; National League for Nursing, 1979; and Mullane (1968).

26. Lynaugh and Brush (1996), 5.

27. Virginia Cleland, "Sex Discrimination: Nursing's Most Pervasive Problem," *American Journal of Nursing* (1972) 71(8): 1542–1547, 1542.

28. Ellen Baer, "The Feminist Disdain for Nursing," *New York Times*, February 23, 1991. See also Susan Rimby Leighow, *Nurses' Questions / Women's Questions: The Impact of the Demographic Revolution and Feminism on United States Working Women, 1946–1986* (New York: Peter Lang, 1996); and Susan Gelfand Malka, *Daring to Care: American Nursing and Second-Wave Feminism* (Chicago: University of Illinois Press, 2007), 65.

29. Baer (1991).

30. M. Elizabeth Carnegie, "The Minority Practitioner in Nursing," *National League for Nursing Publications* (1974) 15–1513: 39–42; Lucille Davis, "The Minority Practitioner in Nursing," *National League for Nursing Publications* (1974) 15–1513: 43–45; Janice E. Ruffin, "Issues for the Black Nurse Today: Competence and Commitment," *National League for Nursing Publications* (1974) 15–1513: 46–51; Alice M. Robinson, "Black Nurses Tell You: Why So Few Blacks in Nursing," *RN Magazine*, July 1972, pp. 35–41.

31. Marion Altenderfer, *Minorities and Women in the Health Fields: Applicants, Students, and Workers*, Department of Health, Education, and Welfare (Bethesda, MD: Government Printing Office, 1975).

32. Carnegie (1974), 42.

33. Bonnie Bullough and Vern Bullough, "A Career Ladder in Nursing: Problems and Prospects," *American Journal of Nursing* (October 1971) 71(10): 1938–1943.

34. Bullough and Bullough (October 1971), 1938–1939. See Department of Health, Education, and Welfare (1975), 47 for numbers of minorities in various allied health fields: in academic year 1973–1974, 13 percent of LPNs were minorities, 35 percent of nurse aides were minorities, and 34 percent of orderlies were minorities.

35. Darlene Clark Hine, *Black Women in White* (Bloomington: Indiana University Press, 1989), 191.

36. Janice E. Ruffin, "Issues for the Black Nurse Today: Competence and Commitment," *National League for Nursing Publications* (1974) 15–1513: 46–51, 47–48.

37. Lucille Davis, "The Minority practitioner in nursing." *National League for Nursing Publications* (1974) 15–1513: 43–45, 45.

38. Hine (1989), 190–193, 192.

39. Davis (1974), 45.

40. Quotation taken from National Black Nurses Association, "History," https://www.nbna
.org/history (accessed July 8, 2020) and from Hine (1989), 192. On the history of the NBNA, see
Gloria R. Smith, "From Invisibility to Blackness: The Story of the National Black Nurses' Association," *Nursing Outlook* (1975) 23: 225–229.

41. Robinson (1972), 37–39.

42. On this point, see Evelyn L. Barbee, "Racism in U.S. Nursing," *Medical Anthropology
Quarterly* (1993) 7(4): 346–362.

43. Rebecca S. Lowen, *Creating the Cold War University: The Transformation of Stanford*
(Berkeley: University of California Press, 1997); Henry Etzkowitz, *MIT and the Rise of Entrepre-
neurial Science* (New York: Routledge, 2002); Daniel Lee Kleinman, *Impure Cultures: University
Biology and the World of Commerce* (Madison: University of Wisconsin Press, 2003); Daniel S.
Greenberg, *The Politics of Pure Science* (Chicago: University of Chicago Press, 1999); and Daniel S.
Greenberg, *Science for Sale: The Perils, Rewards, and Delusions of Campus Capitalism* (Chicago:
University of Chicago Press, 2007).

44. See, for example, Elizabeth Tandy Shermer, *Sunbelt Capitalism: Phoenix and the Trans-
formation of American Politics* (Philadelphia: University of Pennsylvania Press, 2013); Margaret
Pugh O'Mara, *Cities of Knowledge: Cold War Science and the Search for the Next Silicon Valley*
(Princeton, NJ: Princeton University Press, 2005).

45. Millett (1984), 81.

46. Daniel M. Fox, *Health Policies, Health Politics: The British and American Experience,
1911–1965* (Princeton, NJ: Princeton University Press, 1986), 191. See also Daniel M. Fox, "From
Piety to Platitudes to Pork: The Changing Politics of Health Workforce Policy," *Journal of Health
Politics, Policy and Law* (1996) 21(4): 823–842; and Fox (2010), 51–76.

47. Evan Melhado, "Health Planning in the United States and the Decline of Public-Interest
Policymaking," *Milbank Quarterly* (2006) 84(2): 359–440, 359.

48. Melhado (2006).

49. Stevens (1999); Stevens (1996).

50. Section 900, Public Law 89-239 quoted in National Library of Medicine, "Regional
Medical Programs: History," https://profiles.nlm.nih.gov/ps/retrieve/Narrative/RM/p-nid/94 (ac-
cessed July 6, 2019). See also Stephen P. Strickland, *The History of Regional Medical Programs:
The Life and Death of a Small Initiative of the Great Society* (Lanham, MD, University Press of
America, 2000).

51. Daniel M. Fox, "The History of Regional Medical Programs: The Life and Death of a
Small Initiative of the Great Society (Review)," *Bulletin of the History of Medicine* (2003) 77(1):
220–221, 220.

52. National Library of Medicine, "Regional Medical Programs: History," https://profiles
.nlm.nih.gov/ps/retrieve/Narrative/RM/p-nid/94 and National Library of Medicine, "Regional
Medical Programs: History," https://profiles.nlm.nih.gov/ps/retrieve/Narrative/RM/p-nid/99 (accessed July 6, 2019).

53. Melhado (2006).

54. Stevens (1996); Fox (2010); Melhado (2006).

55. Carl F. Ameringer, *The Health Care Revolution: From Medical Monopoly to Market Competition* (Berkeley: University of California Press and Milbank Books on Health and the Public,
2008); Beatrix Hoffman, *Health Care for Some: Rights and Rationing in the United States Since
1930* (Chicago: University of Chicago Press 2012), 175–176; Tomes (2016), 323–331.

56. Ameringer (2008), 4, Hoffman (2012), 191–195.

57. Tomes (2016), 326–327.

58. Mary Kelly Mullane used this term in her 1968 untitled presentation to the Chicago Council on Community Nursing. University of Illinois Chicago University Archives, College of Nursing Dean–Faculty Papers Collection, Mary Kelly Mullane Papers, RG 17-01-20-02, Box 2, Folder: Speeches—Mary Kelly Mullane (1964–1980). See also Joyce M. Schowalter and Lynda F. Cole, *Nursepower in Minnesota, 1970* (Northlands Regional Medical Program, 1971).

59. Schowalter and Cole (1971).

60. For more detailed discussion of the Lysaught Report, see Lynaugh and Brush (1996), 44–45 and Fairman (2008), pp 47–51. The impetus for the Lysaught Commission was the 1963 Surgeon General's Consultant Group on Nursing's report, *Toward Quality in Nursing*, and the concerns raised by that report. In particular, the Lysaught Commission focused on "the continuing disparity between supply and demand; the changing roles and functions of nursing practice; the patterns and institutions for nursing education; and the difficulties of making nursing a satisfying lifetime career." The Commission was established at the urging of the ANA and NLN, and was funded by both organizations along with the W. K. Kellogg Foundation, the Avalon Foundation, the American Nurses Foundation, and a private donor. It issued a series of recommendations addressing nursing roles, education, and careers, that were oriented around three basic priorities. The first was to increase "research into both the practice of nursing and the education of nurses." The second was to establish "enhanced educational systems and curricula based on the results of that research," and the third was to increase "financial support for nurses and for nursing to ensure adequate career opportunities that will attract and retain" adequate numbers of nurses within the health care system. Jerome Lysaught, "National Commission for the Study of Nursing and Nursing Education," *American Journal of Nursing* (1970) 70(2): 279–294, 1970, 285.

61. Jerome P. Lysaught, *An Abstract for Action: National Commission for the Study of Nursing and Nursing Education* (New York: McGraw-Hill, 1970).

62. Jessie M Scott, Susan R Gortner, and Marie J Bourgeois, "The Doctorally Prepared Nurse," in *Report of Two Conferences on the Demand for Education of Nurses with Doctoral Degrees*, Florence S. Downs Papers MC 130, Series IV, box 8, folder 21976, pp. 39–40.

63. On the importance, more broadly, of AHCs to state health policy during the 1970s, see Fox (2010), 63–72.

64. Joan E. Lynaugh, "Nursing in the Great Society: The Impact of the Nurse Training Act of 1964," *Nursing History Review* (2008) 16: 13–28, 20.

65. Patricia D'Antonio, "Women, Nursing, and Baccalaureate Education in 20th Century America," *Journal of Nursing Scholarship* (2004) 4 Quarter: 379–384.

66. Lucie Young Kelly, "Open Curriculum: What and Why," *American Journal of Nursing* (1974) 74(12): 2232–2238, 2232.

67. Kelly (1974), 2233. On the development of the physician assistant program in response to skills and needs of medical corpsmen, see Fairman (2008), 95–108.

68. Grace and Spitzer, "Nursing and Nursing Education Issues and Projected Responses," Presented to the Board of Trustees, University of Illinois, May 2, 1981, University of Illinios Chicago University Archives College of Nursing, Dean—Faculty Papers Collection, Helen Grace Papers, Acc 017-01-20-01, box 14, folder: 166—Nursing and Nursing Education Issues and Projected Responses, 1981.

69. Bonnie Bullough, "You Can't Get There from Here: Articulation in Nursing Education," *Journal of Nursing Education* (November 1972): 4–10, 6.

70. Bullough (1972), 7

71. Lysaught (1970), 291.

72. Eva Clark, "Educators Are No Help," *American Journal of Nursing* (1969) 69(9): 1878.

73. "Letter to Editor," *American Journal of Nursing* (1977) 77(11): 1784.

74. Patricia Ann Brake, "Letter to Editor," *American Journal of Nursing* (1973) 73(1): 50.

75. Linda Kuhn, "Letter to Editor," *American Journal of Nursing* (1976) 76(10): 1578–1579.

76. Nancy Divistea, "Letter to Editor," *American Journal of Nursing* (1976) 76(8): 1246.

77. Elizabeth Barker, "Letter to Editor," *American Journal of Nursing* (1979) 79(4): 630.

78. Linda Robinson, "Letter to Editor," *American Journal of Nursing* (1974) 74(5): 835.

79. Sharon Lower, "Letter to Editor," *American Journal of Nursing* (1976) 76(9): 1418, 1421.

80. Clare Kuch, "Letter to Editor," *American Journal of Nursing* (1977) 77(11): 1782, 1784.

81. Patricia Staes Brown, "Letter to Editor," *American Journal of Nursing* (1976) 76(2): 208.

82. Jean McNeil, "Letter to Editor," *American Journal of Nursing* (1976) 76(1): 44, 46.

83. American Nurses Association, "Education for Nursing," *American Journal of Nursing* (1965) 65: 106–111. Susan Rimby Leighow, "Backrubs vs. Bach: Nursing and the Entry-into-Practice Debate, 1946–1986," *Nursing History Review* (1996) 4: 3–17.

84. See, for example, "New York's '1985 Plan' Goes to Legislature, Controversy over It Deepens among Nurses," *American Journal of Nursing* (June 1976), 76(6): 878.

85. Deborah Woods, "Letter to Editor," *American Journal of Nursing* (1979) 79(10): 1710.

86. Patricia Carolan, "Letter to Editor," *American Journal of Nursing* (1978) 78(9): 1462.

87. See, for example, Carnegie (1974), Ruffin (1974).

88. See Illinois Board of Higher Education, "An Assessment of Progress in Education for the Health Professions since 1968," September 12, 1979, University of Illinios Chicago University Archives College of Nursing, Dean–Faculty Papers Collection, Helen Grace Papers, Acc 017-01-20-01, box 14, folder: 155—Illinois Board of Higher Education: "The 1985 Resolution," 1978.

89. Bullough and Bullough (1971); Bullough (1972), and Kelly (1974). On NLN's Open Curriculum Project, see Carrie Lenburg and Walter Johnson, "Career Mobility through Nursing Education: A Report on the NLN's Open Curriculum Project," *Nursing Outlook* (1974) 22(4): 265–269.

90. Bullough (1972), 34.

91. Rosalyn Koffman and Olga Andruskiw, "From Diploma or Associate Degree to Bachelor's Degree," *American Journal of Nursing* (1971) 71(11): 2184–2186.

92. Bullough describes such proposals in New York, North Carolina, and California. Bullough (1972), 34–35.

93. Dorothy F. Corona, "College Education Tailor-Made for Registered Nurses," *American Journal of Nursing* (1973) 73(2): 294–297, 295.

94. Corona (1973).

95. Adrian Schoenmaker, "An Articulated Nursing Program: Five Years Later," *Nursing Outlook* (1975) 23(2): 110–113, 110. See also Laura Dustan, "Needed: Articulation between Nursing Education Programs and Institutions of Higher Learning," *Nursing Outlook* (December 1970) 18: 34–37.

96. Schoenmaker (1975), 113.

97. Schoenmaker (1975), 111.

98. Joan Cobin, Wilma Traber, and Bonnie Bullough, "A Five-Level Articulated Program," *Nursing Outlook* (1976) 24(5): 309–312.

99. Lenburg and Johnson (1974).

100. As quoted in Kelly (1974), 2232.

101. National League for Nursing, Research Division, *Proceedings: Open Curriculum Conference 1*. A project of the NLN study of the open curriculum in nursing education, held in St. Louis, November 1973, cited in Cobin, Traber, and Bullough (1976), 310.

102. Comprehensive Health Planning Advisory Council, Subcommittee on Nursing, *Subcommittee on Nursing Report*, 1970, Minnesota Historical Society, State Planning Agency, Health Planning Section, 128.E.8.4F, folder: Comprehensive Health Planning Advisory Council Minutes, Nov 1970–Mar 1971.

103. Minnesota Higher Education Coordinating Commission, "Nursing Education in Minnesota: Report to the Commission for Action on Planning Policies," Minnesota State Archives, State Planning Agency, Health Planning Subject Files 1965–1977, 117.I.10.10F, folder: Higher Education Coordinating Commission 1973.

104. Kelly (1974); Bullough (1972); Cobin, Traber, and Bullough (1976).

105. Verne E. Long to Stanley J. Wenberg, April 29, 1971, University of Minnesota Archives, President's Office, Collection 841, box 231, folder: Medical School, School of Nursing, 1971–1980.

106. Long to Wenberg (1971).

107. Stanley J. Wenberg to Lyle French, Isabel Harris, Stanley Kegler, George Robb, William G. Shepherd, and Donald Smith, May 7, 1971, University of Minnesota Archives, President's Office, Collection 841, box 262, folder: Planning Nursing.

108. Testimony of Isabel Harris before Medical Education Subcommittee, January 20, 1972, Minnesota State Archives, Legislative House Appropriations Committee, 129.C.3.7B, folder: Medical Education Subcommittee.

109. School of Nursing, "Legislative Special Proposal: Career Mobility-Nursing," School of Nursing Collection, box 23, folder: NW.A. Negotiations 1972.

110. Mariah Snyder, oral history interview by Dominique Tobbell, June 13, 2012, p. 15, https://editions.lib.umn.edu/ahc-ohp/2013/08/04/snyder-mariah/ (accessed July 19, 2019).

111. Snyder (2012), 16.

112. Fairman (2008); and Arlene W. Keeling, *Nursing and the Privilege of Prescription, 1893–2000* (Columbus: The Ohio State University Press, 2007), 121–137.

113. Henry K. Silver, Loretta C. Ford, and Lewis R. Day, "The Pediatric Nurse Practitioner Program," *JAMA* (1968) 204(4): 298–302.

114. Silver, Ford, and Day, (1968), 298.

115. Fairman (2008).

116. Dominique A. Tobbell, "Plow, Town, and Gown: The Politics of Family Practice in 1960s America," *Bulletin of the History of Medicine* (2013) 87(4): 648–680.

117. Stevens (1996); Tobbell (2013).

118. See, for example, The Secretary's Committee to Study Extended Roles for Nurses, *Extending the Scope of Nursing Practice* (Washington, DC: Government Printing Office, 1971); Gary L. Appel and Aaron Loivin, *Physician Extenders: An Evaluation of Policy-Related Research* (Washington, DC: National Science Foundation, 1975); Congressional Budget Office, *Physician Extenders: Their Current and Future Role in Medical Care Delivery* (Washington, DC: Government Printing Office, 1979).

119. Osler L. Peterson and Ivan J. Fahs (Health Manpower Study Commission), *Health Manpower for the Upper Midwest: A Study of the Needs for Physicians and Dentists in Minnesota, North Dakota, South Dakota, and Montana* (St. Paul, MN: Hill Family Foundation, 1966).

120. Comprehensive Health Planning Advisory Council, "Health Manpower Policy for Minnesota," November 17, 1970, Minnesota State Archives, State Planning Agency, Health Planning Section, 128.E.8.4F, folder: Comprehensive Health Planning Advisory Council Minutes, Nov 1970–Mar 1971. For additional support from the legislature for nurse practitioners, see John Milton, "Opening Statement: Hearing on Allied Health Personnel," September 26, 1974, University of Minnesota Archives, School of Nursing Collection, Box 32, Folder: Legislation 1974–1975. See also Comprehensive Health Planning Advisory Council, "Nurse Practitioner Program," November 17, 1973, Minnesota State Archives, State Planning Agency, Health Planning Section, 128.E.8.4F, folder: Comprehensive Health Planning Advisory Council Minutes Jun–Dec 1973.

121. "Minutes: Advisory Committee Meeting for Midwest Regional Workshop on Health Manpower Distribution," Minnesota State Archives, Health Department, Manpower Division Records, 104.C.5.1 (B), folder: Director's Correspondence 1974–1975.

122. Schowalter and Cole (1970), 25.

123. In 1991, the division of public health nursing and the majority of its faculty and programs were transferred to the School of Nursing. For information on the complicated history of public health nursing at the University of Minnesota, see Laurie K. Glass, *Leading the Way: The University of Minnesota School of Nursing, 1909–2009* (Minneapolis: University of Minnesota School of Nursing, 2009), 24–28.

124. Comprehensive Health Planning Advisory Council, "The Nurse Practitioner Program," 1973. See also Barbara Leonard, oral history interview by Dominique Tobbell, October 20, 2011, University of Minnesota Academic Health Center Oral History Project; and University of Minnesota School of Nursing, "Pediatric Primary Care Nurse Practitioner," https://www.nursing.umn.edu/about/history/program-histories/Pediatric-Primary-Care-Nurse-Practitioner (accessed July 9, 2019).

125. Comprehensive Health Planning Agency (1973). See also Elaine Richard and Sharon K. Ostwald, "A Model for Development of an Off-Campus Rural Nurse Practitioner Program," *Journal of Nursing Education* (1983) 22(2): 87–92, and University of Minnesota School of Nursing, "Adult-Gero Nurse Practitioner Programs," https://www.nursing.umn.edu/about/history/program-histories/adult-gero-nurse-practitioner-programs (accessed July 9, 2019).

126. Richard and Ostwald (1983), 87. See also, Eva Anderson, Elaine Cooley, and Alma Sparrow, "Role and Preparation of the Adult and Geriatric Nurse Associate," *Minnesota Medicine* (October 1973), 69–72; and Comprehensive Health Planning Advisory Council, "Nurse Practitioner Program," November 17, 1973, Minnesota State Archives, State Planning Agency, Health Planning Section, 128.E.8.4F , folder: Comprehensive Health Planning Advisory Council Minutes Jun–Dec 1973.

127. Richard and Ostwald (1983), 88.

128. Richard and Ostwald (1983), 87.

129. Alma Sparrow, "To Senator Al Kowalczyk: Proposal to Provide Primary Health Care to Citizens in Minnesota through Utilization of Nurses Prepared as Family Health Practitioners," December 3, 1973, Minnesota State Archives, State Planning Agency, Health Planning Subject Files 1965–1977, 117.I.11.2F, folder: Nurse Practitioner 1973–1974. By 1979, ninety graduates from rural areas had completed the adult and geriatric nurse practitioner program, 88 percent of whom remained employed in rural communities. Of those remaining in rural communities, 73 percent reported that they were working in a nurse practitioner role, while the remainder were serving in administrative and educational roles in their rural communities. Richard and Ostwald (1983), 91.

130. Richard and Ostwald (1983), 91.

131. In 1971, Congress had established the Area Health Education Center program to recruit, train, and retain health care providers committing to working in underserved communities. A network of federally funded Area Health Education Centers was established throughout the country, often located on academic health center campuses, to coordinate the supply and distribution of health care professionals within a region. https://www.nationalahec.org/page/Copy ofMissionHistoryBoard (accessed February 17, 2022).

132. Sparrow (1973); Letter from William Fifer, MD (UMN AHEC) to Al Kowalcyzk, April 23, 1973, Minnesota State Archives, State Planning Agency, Health Planning Subject Files 1965–1977, 117.I.11.2F, folder: Nurse Practitioner 1973–1974. Kowalcyzk represented Hennepin County (location of UMN) and served on the state senate committee on Health, Welfare, and Corrections: Health, within which Milton's subcommittee on medical care was situated. Minnesota Legislative Reference Library, "Kowalczyk, Al," Minnesota Legislature, https://www.leg.state .mn.us/legdb/fulldetail?id=10341 (accessed July 15, 2020)

133. Fifer (1973).

134. Alma Sparrow, "Letter to Senator John Milton Re Legislative Support for Nurse Practitioner Programs through the School of Public Health," January 18, 1974, Minnesota State Archives, State Planning Agency, Health Planning Subject Files 1965–1977, 117.I.11.2F, folder: Nurse Practitioner 1973–1974.

135. John Milton, "Opening Statement, Hearing on Allied Health Personnel," September 26, 1974, University of Minnesota Archives, School of Nursing Collection, box 32, folder: Legislation 1974–1975.

136. Milton (1974).

137. Richard and Ostwald (1983).

138. On the role of nurse practitioners in the U.S. health care system since the late 1970s, see Fairman (2008), 184–195.

139. Surgeon General's Consultant Group on Nursing (1963), 36.

140. Division of Nursing, "Legislation Program for 1968," 1968, Justification Materials, University of Pennsylvania, Bates Center for the Study of the History of Nursing, Jessie Scott Papers, MC 129, box JMST.0015.

141. Division of Nursing (1968).

142. See Abbott's discussion of the role of a profession's academic knowledge system to that profession's legitimacy, research, and instruction. Andrew Abbott, *The System of Professions: An Essay on the Division of Expert Labor* (Chicago: University of Chicago Press, 1988), especially pp. 52–57.

143. Roger Geiger, *Research and Relevant Knowledge: American Research Universities since World War II* (New York: Routledge, 1993), 218.

144. Geiger (1993), 219.

145. Helen Grace, "A History of Doctoral Program Planning," March 1974, University of Illinois Chicago University Archives, College of Nursing, Dean–Faculty Papers Collection, Helen Grace Papers, Acc 017-01-20-01, box 4, folder: 48—A History of Doctoral Program Planning, 1974.

146. Illinois Study Commission on Nursing, "Nursing in Illinois: An Assessment, 1968, and a Plan, 1980." January 1968, University of Illinois Chicago University Archives, College of Nursing Dean–Faculty Papers Collection, Mary Kelly Mullane Papers, RG 17-01-20-02, box 1, folder: Nursing in Illinois: An Assessment, 1968.

147. Mullane (1968).

148. Mullane (1968).

149. Illinois Study Commission on Nursing (1968).

150. "The proposed doctoral program in nursing—draft." 1974. University of Illinois Chicago University Archives College of Nursing, Dean–Faculty Papers Collection, Helen Grace Papers, Acc 017-01-20-01, box 28, folder: 308–Drafts–proposed doctoral program in nursing c. 1974.

151. Mary Lohr to Joseph S. Begando, chancellor, "A Proposal for the Degree Doctor of Philosophy," July 29, 1974, University of Illinois Chicago University Archives College of Nursing, Dean–Faculty Papers Collection, Helen Grace Papers, Acc 017-01-20-01, box 28, folder: 309–Proposal materials and Proposal Analysis Format Report, 1974.

152. See also Graham and Diamond (1997), 84–88.

153. As Eli Ginzburg wrote in 1975, "In Illinois, the major state institutes requested approval of 280 new PhD programs; the state board approved 6!" Eli Ginzburg, *The Manpower Connection: Education and Work* (Cambridge, MA: Harvard University Press, 1975), p.115.

154. Discussed by Mary Lohr in "Doctoral Program Site Visit October 15, 1975," to University of Utah School of Nursing, 1976, in Madeleine Leininger, "Excerpts from the Proposal of the Program of Study Leading to the PhD in Nursing, University of Utah College of Nursing," Developed by the Committee on Doctoral (PhD) Program in Nursing of the College of Nursing, Walter P. Reuther Library, University Archives, Wayne State University, Madeleine Leininger Collection, Accession 725, box 3, folder 58.

155. Minutes of University of Illinois Chicago College of Nursing Faculty Meeting, October 8, 1975, University of Illinois Chicago University Archives College of Nursing Administration: Faculty Meeting Minutes 1963–1983, box 1, folder 1974–1983.

156. Minutes, Doctoral Program Committee, Wayne State University College of Nursing, December 4, 1973, Walter P. Reuther Library, University Archives, Wayne State University, Nursing–Dean's Office, Accession no. 672, box 1, folder 8.

157. Minutes, Doctoral Program Committee, Wayne State University College of Nursing, December 12, 1973, Walter P. Reuther Library, University Archives, Wayne State University, Nursing–Dean's Office, Accession no. 672, box 1, folder 8; Minutes, Doctoral Program Committee, Wayne State University College of Nursing, December 10, 1973, Walter P. Reuther Library, University Archives, Wayne State University, Nursing–Dean's Office, Accession no. 672, box 1, folder 8; Minutes, Doctoral Program Committee, Wayne State University College of Nursing, November 30, 1973, Walter P. Reuther Library, University Archives, Wayne State University, Nursing–Dean's Office, Accession no. 672, box 1, folder 8.

158. "Research development: Center for Nursing Research, Terminal Progress Report for Grant NU00361, Division of Nursing, U.S. Department of Health, Education, and Welfare, May 1, 1970–September 30, 1972," Center for Health Research, College of Nursing, Wayne State Archives, p. 7, College of Nursing Center for Health Research Acc # 2167, box 1, folder: 1 CHR: Accumulation of Papers, Documents Related to the Center 1969–1973. For some details on the curriculum / program of study, see 104–341, 357.

159. Sandra Edwardson quoted in Glass (2009), 30–31.

160. Floris King, "PhD in Nursing Proposal," University of Minnesota Archives, School of Nursing Collection, box 21, folder: Doctoral Committee 1978.

161. During 1976 and 1977, the university had graduated 115 from its two master's degree programs in nursing. "At this rate," the committee noted, "these programs cannot meet the needs of the State." Minutes of meeting for Advisory Committee on Nursing Education, October 26,

1978, Minnesota State Archives, Minnesota Higher Education Coordinating Board, Committee / Task Force Files, 120.I.3.5B, folder: Advisory Committee on Nursing Education, 1978–1980. See also "Planning Report Number 12," cited in minutes of meeting for Advisory Committee on Nursing Education, October 26, 1978, Minnesota State Archives, Minnesota Higher Education Coordinating Board, Committee / Task Force Files, 120.I.3.5B, folder: Advisory Committee on Nursing Education, 1978–1980.

162. Minutes of meeting for Advisory Committee on Nursing Education, October 26, 1978. See also, for example, Karen L. Mokros, chair, Department of Nursing, College of St. Scholastica, February 10, 1977; Marguerite Hessian, chair, Department of Nursing, College of St. Catherine, February 11, 1977. Both in "Series of Letters Offering to Floris King or Dean Ramey Support for Development of Phd in Nursing Program," University of Minnesota Archives, School of Nursing Collection, box 21, folder: Doctoral Grant Committee Dr. King 1977–1980.

163. Edna Thayer to Floris King, February 2, 1977, in "Series of Letters Offering to Floris King or Dean Ramey Support for Development of Phd in Nursing Program," Univesity of Minnesota Archives, School of Nursing Collection, box 21, folder: Doctoral Grant Committee Dr. King 1977–1980.

164. Hazel Johnson to Floris King, February 9, 1977, in "Series of Letters Offering to Floris King or Dean Ramey Support for Development of Phd in Nursing Program."

165. King (1978).

166. Marilyn Sime, oral history interview by Dominique A. Tobbell, April 15, 2010, University of Minnesota AHC Oral History Project, p. 24. See also "Minutes of Doctoral Committee Meeting, February 11, 1982," and "Minutes of Doctoral Committee Meeting, April 12, 1982," University of Minnesota Archives, School of Nursing Collection, box 51, folder: School of Nursing Doctoral Committee, 1979 (Oct)–1981 (June); Glass (2009) p. 32.

167. Joyce Fitzpatrick, "The Case for the Clinical Doctorate in Nursing," *Reflections of Nursing Leadership* (2003) 29(1): 8–9, 37, 8.

168. Patricia D'Antonio, *American Nursing: A History of Knowledge, Authority, and the Meaning of Work* (Baltimore: Johns Hopkins University Press, 2010), 178–179. See also D'Antonio (2004).

169. Institute of Medicine, *The Future of Nursing: Leading Change, Advancing Health.* (Washington, DC, National Academies Press, 2011), 73.

170. See American Association of Colleges of Nursing, "The Essentials of Doctoral Education for Advanced Nursing Practice," October 2006; and A. L. O'Sullivan, M. Carter, L. Marion, J. M. Pohl, and K. E. Werner, "Moving Forward Together: The Practice Doctorate in Nursing," *Online Journal of Issues in Nursing* (2005) 10(3).

Chapter Five

1. The education-service gap is not unique to nursing; rather, it is common within other practice professions with an academic base. See Andrew Abbott, *The System of Professions: An Essay on the Division of Expert Labor* (Chicago: University of Chicago Press, 1988); Bruce E. Seely, "Research, Engineering, and Science in American Engineering Colleges: 1900–1960," *Technology and Culture* (1993) 34(2): 344–386; and Nathan Ensmenger, *The Computer Boys Take Over: Computers, Programmers, and the Politics of Technical Expertise* (Cambridge, MA: MIT Press, 2013), 111–136.

2. Rozella M. Schlotfeldt, "Academic Leadership for Nursing," Annual Lectureship, School of Nursing, Medical College of Georgia, May 3, 1969, Case Western Reserve University Archives,

Frances Payne Bolton School of Nursing Collection, Series 29DD, box 2, Papers of Dean Rozella Schlotfeldt, folder 1:2.

3. Lois K. Evans and Norma M. Lang, eds., *Academic Nursing Practice: Helping to Share the Future of Health Care* (New York: Springer, 2004).

4. Jerome P. Lysaught, *An Abstract for Action: National Commission for the Study of Nursing and Nursing Education* (New York: McGraw Hill, 1970), 94–96, 95.

5. See, for example, "Minutes of American Association of Deans of College and University Schools of Nursing Meeting, October 4–5, 1971," Wayne State University Archives, Madeleine Leininger Collection, Accession 725, box 13, 33.

6. Loretta C. Ford, "Response to 'Institutionalizing Practice: Historical and Future Perspectives,'" *Annual Symposium on Nursing Faculty Practice* (1985) 2: 17–23, 18. See also Claire M. Fagin, "Institutionalizing Practice: Historical and Future Perspectives," *Annual Symposium on Nursing Faculty Practice* (1985) 2: 1–17, 7.

7. Ford (1985), 18.

8. See, for example, Kenneth M. Ludmerer, *Time to Heal: American Medical Education from the Turn of the Century to the Era of Managed Care* (Oxford: Oxford University Press, 1999).

9. Terrance Keenan, Linda Aiken, and Leighton E. Cluff, eds., *Nurses and Doctors: Their Education and Practice* (Cambridge, MA: Oelgeschlager, Gunn, and Hain, 1981), 15–16, 107; Evans and Lang (2004), 8, 158–161.

10. Carol Taylor, "Operation Phoenix or the Perilous Experiment: An Interim Report about the Unit Manager System," March 1968, University of Florida, George T. Harrell Medical History Center, RS4-VPHA Records: 4c- VPHA Ackell, box 35, folder: Nursing: Report of the College of Nursing. See also Dorothy Smith to Donald R. Olley, September 23, 1964, University of Florida, George T. Harrell Medical History Center, Series 10a College of Nursing, 1956–1965, box 4, folder: Correspondence, Miscellaneous 1964.

11. Frances Reiter, "The Nurse-Clinician," *American Journal of Nursing*, (1966) 66(2): 274–280, 276.

12. Reiter (1966), 276–277.

13. Laura L. Simms, "The Clinical Nursing Specialist: An Approach to Nursing Practice in the Hospital," *JAMA* (1966) 198(6): 207–209, 207. See also Laura L. Simms, "The Clinical Nursing Specialist," *Nursing Outlook* (1965) 13: 26–28.

14. Simms (1966), 209; Simms (1965); Nancy Rae Scully, "The Clinical Nursing Specialist: Practicing Nurse," *Nursing Outlook* (1965) 13: 28–30.

15. Reiter (1966), 277.

16. Julie Fairman, *Making Room in the Clinic: Nurse Practitioners and the Evolution of Modern Health Care* (New Brunswick, NJ: Rutgers University Press, 2008), 44; Joan E. Lynaugh, "Mildred Tuttle: Private Initiative and Public Response in Nursing Education after World War II," *Nursing History Review* (2006) 14: 203–211; Julie Fairman and Joan E. Lynaugh, *Critical Care Nursing: A History* (Philadelphia: University of Pennsylvania Press, 1998), 97, 99.

17. Helen K. Grace, "The Development of Doctoral Education in Nursing: In Historical Perspective," *Journal of Nursing Education* (1978) 17(4): 17–27, 26.

18. Dorothy Smith, oral History Interview, by Stephen Kerber, March 26, 1979, p. 19, University of Florida, Samuel Proctor Oral History Program, University of Florida Digital Collections https://ufdc.ufl.edu/UF00006286/00001 (accessed May 5, 2021).

19. Mary Kelly Mullane, "Nursing Faculty Roles and Function in the Large University Setting," Memorandum to Members: Council of Baccalaureate and Higher Degree Programs, Na-

tional League for Nursing, February 1969, University of Illinois Chicago, University Archives, College of Nursing, Office of the Dean–Administrative Files, 1955–1989, RG 17-01-02, box 1, folder: 23 Minutes–CON administrative council, September 9, 1976.

20. Myrtle K. Aydelotte, "Nursing Education and Practice: Putting it all Together," *Journal of Nursing Education* (1972) 11(4): 21–28, 22. See also on this point Smith (1979), 19–21. On the history of academic nursing practice, see Joan E. Lynaugh, "Academic Nursing Practice: Looking Back," in Lois K. Evans and Norma M. Lang (eds.), *Academic Nursing Practice: Helping to Shape the Future of Health Care* (New York: Springer, 2004), 20–37.

21. Lynaugh (2004), 28.

22. Schlotfeldt (1969).

23. Thelma Ingles, "The University Medical Center as a Setting for Nursing Education," *Journal of Medical Education* (1962) 37(5): 411–420, 413.

24. Ingles (1962), 413.

25. Ingles (1962), 414.

26. Ingles (1962), 413.

27. Mullane (1969).

28. Dorothy Smith, "Statement as to the Relationship between the Department of Nursing of the Teaching Hospital and the College of Nursing," September 17, 1958, University of Florida, George T. Harrell Medical History Center, RS4-VPHA Records: 4b- VPHA Martin, box 39, folder: College of Nursing–Curriculum and Philosophy.

29. Fairman (2008), 59.

30. Smith (1979), 24

31. Smith (1979), 22; and Dorothy Smith, "The Relationship between Nursing Education and Nursing Service: A Dual or Separate Administrative Responsibility," 1963, George T. Harrell Medical History Center, RS4-VPHA Records: 4b- VPHA Martin; box 38, folder: College of Nursing, through Sept 1965.

32. "Purposes, Philosophy, and Organization, College of Nursing, University of Florida, March 1965," University of Florida, George T. Harrell Medical History Center, Series 4b, VPHA-Martin Records, box 15.

33. Taylor (1968).

34. Smith (1979), 28. On this point, see also Barbra Mann Wall and Billye J. Brown, *Through the Eyes of Nursing: Educational Reform at the University of Texas School of Nursing, 1890–1989* (Austin, TX: Austin Books Consortium, 2017), 98.

35. Smith (1979), 28.

36. Dorothy Smith to Carol Hayes, 1970, University of Pennsylvania, Bates Center for the Study of Nursing History, Dorothy Smith Papers, MC 118, Series III, as cited in Fairman (2008), 59, 218.

37. See, for example, Virginia Henderson, "Editorial: Research in Nursing Practice—When?" *Nursing Research* (1956) 4(3): 99; Faye G. Abdellah, *Patient-Centered Approaches to Nursing* (New York: Macmillan, 1960), 40.

38. Smith typically referred to the nurse in this role as the "clinical specialist." This was at a moment when the terms "clinical specialist," "clinical nurse specialist," "nurse clinician," and "nurse practitioner" were being worked out and often used interchangeably.

39. Taylor (1968). See also Smith to Olley (1964).

40. "Job Specifications for the Unit Manager," c. 1958. University of Florida, George T. Harrell Medical History Center, Series 10a College of Nursing, 1956–1965, box 1, folder: Correspondence, Articles, Memos 1958.

41. Smith (1979), 24; Lucille Mercandante, interview by Ann Smith, March 28, 2001, p. 13, University of Florida, Samuel Proctor Oral History Program, College of Nursing Project. http:// ufdc.ufl.edu//UF00066387/00001 (accessed May 5, 2021).

42. On the unit manager system, see Taylor (1968).

43. Smith (1963).

44. Dorothy Smith to Muriel Uprichard, December 6, 1962, University of Florida, George T. Harrell Medical History Center, Series 10a College of Nursing, 1956–1965, box 2, folder: Correspondence, Memos 1963; Dorothy Smith "Memorandum to Faculty," July 3, 1962, University of Florida, George T. Harrell Medical History Center, Series 10b College of Nursing, box 5, folder: Faculty, Memoranda: Smith gives example of a patient refusing to take her medication. In this situation, a nurse would normally chart that the patient refused medication or call in the doctor. Smith says, however, that "this is a nursing problem" and rather than charting or calling in the doctor, the "nurse should call a faculty member to help her with this nursing problem." See also, Carol Christiansen, oral history interview by Ann Smith, October 18, 2001, p. 14, University of Florida, Samuel Proctor Oral History Program, College of Nursing Project, https://ufdc.ufl .edu/UF00066595/00001 (accessed May 5, 2021); and Edna Mae Jones, oral history interview by Ann Smith, October 30, 2002, pp. 15–16, University of Florida, Samuel Proctor Oral History Program, College of Nursing Project, https://ufdc.ufl.edu/UF00066602/00001 (accessed February 17, 2022).

45. For example, Edna Mae Jones, Jane Kordana, and Ann Smith, all of whom held master's degrees in medical-surgical nursing, were all hired as faculty, holding a dual position of teacher-practitioner in medical-surgical nursing. They each had twenty-four-hour responsibility, seven days a week, for the nursing care provided on one of the medical-surgical floors at Shands Hospital, while also sharing responsibility for teaching medical-surgical nursing to students in the BSN program. See, for example, Edna Mae Jones, who was hired as faculty in 1957, along with Jane Kordana, in 1958. See Jones (2002), 9–15. Ann Smith was hired in 1966 and assumed the teacher-practitioner role in one of the orthopedic wings of the Medical-Surgery Nursing Section, see Ann Smith, oral history interview by Julian Pleasants, June 3, 2005, p. 23, University of Florida, Samuel Proctor Oral History Program, College of Nursing Project, https://ufdc.ufl.edu /UF00066611/00001 (accessed February 17, 2022). See also Fairman (2008), 60.

46. See, for example, Ann Smith (2005), 31: "I, for example, had A service, and when I made rounds in the morning with the physicians and the kit and caboodle of them, the team leader for that group of patients would be there and both of us would work together on what the students should be doing or what we would be doing the rest of the time. So, there was a very close working relationship."

47. Mercadante (2001), 11–12; Betty Hilliard, oral history interview by Ann Smith, February 2, 2001, p. 28, University of Florida, Samuel Proctor Oral History Program, College of Nursing Project, http://ufdc.ufl.edu/UF00066386/00001 (accessed May 5, 2021). See also Pauline Barton, oral history interview by Ann Smith, June 21, 2001, pp. 12–13, University of Florida, Samuel Proctor Oral History Program, College of Nursing Project, https://ufdc.ufl.edu/UF00066388/00001 (accessed May 5, 2021).

48. Mercadante (2001), 12.

49. Mercadante (2001), 24. On this point, see also Christiansen (2001), 17 and Jones (2002), 20.

50. Jones (2002), 20.

51. Mercadante (2001), 24.

52. Mercadante (2001), 10, see also p. 26.

53. Fairman (2008), 64.

54. See, for example, Smith, "Memo to Faculty: Graduate Program in the College of Nursing," November 20, 1962, University of Florida, George T. Harrell Medical History Center, RS4-VPHA Records: 4b- VPHA Martin, box 40, folder: College of Nursing–Nursing College. A broader range of clinical master's programs were established during the 1970s.

55. Fairman (2008), 58. See, for example, Virginia Strozier, oral history interview by Ann Smith, October 22, 2001, p. 6, University of Florida, Samuel Proctor Oral History Program, College of Nursing Project, https://ufdc.ufl.edu/UF00066596/00001 (accessed February 17, 2022): "We began to look at medicine, at patient care units, and our jobs and our patients more than I had experienced thus far. We began to see them as potentially one larger, bigger unit in which the chief concern was the patient. The idea was to surround patients with the people who had special gifts to give but who, for the most part, wanted to share them for the good of the patient." See also Smith to Uprichard (1962); Smith to Olley (1964); Taylor (1968).

56. Jennet Wilson, oral history interview by Ann Smith, August 2002, pp. 22–23, University of Florida, Samuel Proctor Oral History Program, College of Nursing Project, https://ufdc.ufl.edu/UF00066599/00001 (accessed May 5, 2021).

57. Barton (2001), 16–17.

58. See, for example, Myron W. Wheat to L. R. Jordan, June 10, 1963, and Wheat to Jordan, June 17, 1963; see also Lucille Mercadante to L. R. Jordan, June 14, 1963, and Dorothy Smith to George Harrell, June 21, 1963, University of Florida, George T. Harrell Medical History Center, RS4-VPHA Records: 4b- VPHA Martin; box 30, folder: Hospital-General-Nursing Services. Carol (Hayes) Christiansen, who was a faculty member on the surgical unit and who worked with Wheat, noted, "His bark was a lot worse than his bite, but just the same, he was hard to get along with." Christiansen (2001), 14.

59. Hilliard (2001), 30.

60. This included visitors from South Africa and Israel (Barton [2001], 3) and Australia (Fairman [2008], 61).

61. E.g., see Hilliard (2001), 29.

62. Fairman (2008), 61, and Dorothy Smith to Edmund F. Ackell, March 11, 1970, University of Pennsylvania, Bates Center for the Study of Nursing History, Dorothy Smith Papers, MC 118, Series III, box 6, folder 5.

63. Taylor (1968).

64. Dorothy M. Smith, "Response: Faculty Practice from a 25-Year Perspective," *Annual Symposium on Nursing Faculty Practice* (1985) 2: 30–32, 32.

65. Hilliard (2001), 29–30.

66. Mercadante (2001), 25.

67. Dorothy Smith to Edmund F. Ackell, December 23, 1969, University of Florida, George T. Harrell Medical History Center, RS4-VPHA Records: 4c- VPHA Ackell, box 34, folder: Nursing–Dean 1969–1970; Fairman (2008), 66.

68. Myron W. Wheat to Lamar E. Cervasse, March 25, 1969, University of Florida, George T. Harrell Medical History Center, RS4-VPHA Records: 4c- VPHA Ackell, box 34, folder: Nursing 1969–1970.

69. Dorothy Smith to Samuel Martin, Edmund F. Ackell, and Stu Westbury, April 2, 1969, University of Florida, George T. Harrell Medical History Center, RS4-VPHA Records: 4c- VPHA Ackell, box 34, folder: Nursing 1969–1970.

70. Smith to Martin, Ackell, and Westbury (1969).

71. Fairman (2008), 67.

72. Christiansen (2001), 21–22.

73. Dorothy Smith to Edmund Ackell, October 28, 1969, University of Florida, George T. Harrell Medical History Center, RS4-VPHA Records: 4c- VPHA Ackell, box 34, folder: Nursing-Faculty and Staff 1969–1970.

74. Smith to Ackell, March 11, 1970.

75. Dorothy Smith to Edmund F. Ackell, "Memorandum: Nursing Organization," July 13, 1970, University of Pennsylvania, Bates Center for the Study of Nursing History, Dorothy Smith Papers, MC 118, Series III, box 6, folder 5.

76. Dorothy Smith to Edmund F. Ackell, January 15, 1971, University of Florida, George T. Harrell Medical History Center, RS4-VPHA Records: 4c- VPHA Ackell, box 34, folder: Nursing-Dean 1969–1970.

77. Lynaugh (2004); Ann Broussard, Carolyn P. Delahoussaye, and Gail P. Poirrier, "The Practice Role in the Academic Nursing Community," *Journal of Nursing Education* 35, no. 2 (1996): 82–87.

78. Fairman (2008), 55.

79. On Case Western Reserve University, see John S. Millis, "The University," *Journal of Medical Education* (1961) 37: 264–269, and Schlotfeldt (1969). On the University of Rochester, see Fairman (2008), 68–85; Loretta C. Ford, "Unification of Nursing Practice, Education and Research," *International Nursing Review* (1980) 27(6): 178–192; and Margaret D. Sovie, "University Education and Practice: One Medical Center's Design: Part 1," *Journal of Nursing Administration* (January 1981): 41–49—hereafter, Sovie (1981a), and Margaret D. Sovie, "University Education and Practice: One Medical Center's Design: Part 2," *Journal of Nursing Administration* (February 1981): 30–33—hereafter, Sovie (1981b). On Rush University, see Luther Christman, "The Practitioner-Teacher," *Nurse Educator* (March–April 1979): 8–11; and Luther Christman, "Response to 'Institutionalizing Practice: Historical and Future Perspectives,'" *Annual Symposium on Nursing Faculty Practice* (1985) 2: 24–30.

80. Jannetta MacPhail, "Organizational Structure Appropriate for Nursing: Now and in the Future," Address given at 3rd Progress Report: Program on Experiment in Nursing, November 4–5, 1971. Case Western Reserve University (CWRU) Archives, 29DD, box 2 (29DD8 Papers of Dean Jannetta MacPhail), Professional Paper Presented, 1971–1980.

81. Rozella M. Schlotfeldt, "The Development of a Model for Unifying Nursing Practice and Nursing Education," in Linda H. Aiken (ed.), *Health Policy and Nursing Practice* (New York: McGraw Hill, 1981), 218–228.

82. Schlotfeldt (1969).

83. MacPhail (1971).

84. Rozella Schlotfeldt and Jannetta MacPhail, "An Experiment in Nursing: Rational and Characteristics," *American Journal of Nursing* (1969) 69(5): 1018–1023. Hereafter, Schlotfeldt and MacPhail (1969a).

85. MacPhail (1971).

86. Jannetta MacPhail, "Promoting Collaboration Between Nursing Education and Nursing Service: Case Western Reserve University Model," Workshop sponsored by RWJ Foundation and American Nurses Foundation, October 3–5, 1979, CWRU Archives, 29DD, box 2 (29DD8 Papers of Dean Jannetta MacPhail), Professional Paper Presented, 1971–1980; and Janetta MacPhail, "Promoting Collaboration/Unification Models for Nursing Education and Service," *National League for Nursing Publications* (1980) 15–1831: 33–36, 35.

87. Rozella Schlotfeldt and Jannetta MacPhail, "An Experiment in Nursing: Introducing Planned Change," *American Journal of Nursing* (1969) 69(6): 1247–1251. Hereafter, Schlotfeldt and MacPhail (1969b).

88. Schlotfeldt and MacPhail (1969a), (1969b), and Rozella Schlotfeldt and Jannetta MacPhail, "An Experiment in Nursing: Implementing Planned Change," *American Journal of Nursing* (1969) 69(7): 1475–1480. Hereafter, Schlotfeldt and MacPhail (1969c).

89. MacPhail (1979).

90. Marjorie D. Powers and S. Shumway, "The Joint Appointee: Role Development and Clinical Impact," in *Defining Patient Care Outcomes and Evaluating Nursing Care: Development of Tools and Approaches,* Proceedings of Fourth Annual Clinical Nursing Specialist Symposium, Bloomington, Indiana, Indiana University, 1974, 16, quoted in Marjorie J. Powers, "A Unification Model in Nursing," *Nursing Outlook* (1976) 24(8): 482–487, 484.

91. MacPhail (1979).

92. For an evaluation of the demonstration project, see Ruth M. Anderson, "A Study of Planned Change in Nursing," *Nursing Research Conference* (1972) 8: 289–313; Jannetta MacPhail, *An Experiment in Nursing: Planning, Implementing, and Assessing Planned Change* (Cleveland, OH: Case Western Reserve University, 1972).

93. Christman (1985) says that Rush Medical Center and Rush University were reorganizing in the early 1970s, instilling all components within the medical center and university with "parity."

94. Fairman (2008), 68. For extensive discussion of the integrated model of nursing at the University of Rochester, see pp. 68–85. On the origins and early years of the unified model at the University of Rochester, see also Ford (1980) and Sovie (1981).

95. Fairman (2008), 68.

96. Sovie (1981a), 42.

97. Sovie (1981a), 41.

98. Hilliard (2001), 29.

99. Christman (1979), 9–10. See also Dorothy D. Nayer, "Bringing Nursing Service and Nursing Education Together," *American Journal of Nursing* (1980) 80(6): 1110–1114, 1112–1113.

100. MacPhail (1979).

101. Schlotfeldt and MacPhail (1969c) and MacPhail (1979). For the University of Rochester, see Loretta Ford Oral History by Lucretia M. McClure in October 1994, https://urresearch.rochester.edu/institutionalPublicationPublicView.action?institutionalItemVersionId=27770 (accessed May 5, 2021).

102. Sovie (1981a) and (1981b).

103. At the University of Rochester, for example, the specialties included pediatrics, OB/GYN, psychiatric / mental health, medical/surgical, community health, and gerontological. When Ford arrived at the University of Rochester as dean, there had been eleven students in the master's in medical-surgical nursing program. By the time Ford left the University of Rochester in 1985, the school had over 150 master's students in the hospital's seven clinical nurse specialty areas. Ford Oral History (1994).

104. Ford Oral History (1994).

105. Joan Lynaugh and Barbara Brush, *American Nursing: From Hospitals to Health Systems* (Malden, MA: Blackwell, 1996), 37–38; Marie Manthey, Karen Ciske, Patricia Robertson, and Isabel Harris, "Primary Nursing," *Nursing Forum* (1970) IX(1): 65–84; Marie Manthey, oral history interview by Dominique A. Tobbell, October 12, 2010, University of Minnesota AHC Oral

History Project. Lucille Mercadante credits Dorothy Smith with establishing "the vision" for the "whole concept of primary nursing" in Mercadante (2001), 23.

106. Ford (1980), 181.

107. Christman (1979), 9.

108. Christman (1985), 26.

109. Christman (1979), 9.

110. Schlotfeldt (1981); Christman (1985), 26.

111. Schlotfeldt (1981).

112. Christman (1979), 9.

113. Ford (1985), 21.

114. See, for example, Mary Angela McBride, Donna Diers, and Ruth L. Schmidt, "Nurse-Researcher: The Crucial Hyphen," *American Journal of Nursing* (1970) 70(6): 1256–1260; Barbara Brodie, "Voices in Distant Camps: The Gap between Nursing Research and Nursing Practice," *Journal of Professional Nursing* (1988) 4(5): 320–328.

115. Christman (1979), 9.

116. Ford Oral History (1994). See also Christman (1979).

117. Schlotfeldt (1981), 222. See also Christman (1979), 9.

118. Sovie (1981b) and Ford (1980).

119. MacPhail (1971). See also Ford Oral History (1994).

120. Joyce J. Fitzpatrick, Edward J. Halloran, and Donna L. Algase, "An Experiment in Nursing Revisited," *Nursing Outlook* (1987) 25(1): 29–33, 31.

121. Schlotfeldt and MacPhail (1969c).

122. MacPhail (1971).

123. MacPhail (1971).

124. Ford (1980), p.183.

125. MacPhail (1979).

126. MacPhail (1979).

127. MacPhail (1979).

128. MacPhail noted, however, that some collaborative research had taken place between medicine and nursing "in the field of maternal and child care, where both physicians and nurses are interested in such investigations as maternal-infant bonding." MacPhail (1979).

129. MacPhail (1979).

130. MacPhail (1979).

131. MacPhail (1979).

132. Smith (1985), 32.

133. Christman (1985), 26–27.

134. Lynaugh and Brush (1996), 50.

135. Luther Christman, Donna Diers, Ellen T. Fahy, and Claire M. Fagin, et al., "Statement of Belief Regarding Faculty Practice," January 12, 1979. Printed in *Nurse Educator* (1979) 4(3): 5.

136. American Association of Colleges of Nursing, "Responsibilities of Nursing Education for the Quality of Nursing Care in Clinical Setting," 1981; the 1980 AAN resolution and 1981 ANA statement are discussed in Broussard, Delahoussaye, and Poirrier (1996), 83.

137. Fairman (2008), 185.

138. Fagin (1985). See also Lynaugh (2004).

139. Claire M. Fagin, "Faculty Practice Clinical Specialties," *Nursing Outlook* (1987) 35(4): 167–169, 168.

140. Claire M. Fagin, "Institutionalizing Faculty Practice," *Nursing Outlook* (1986) 34(3): 140–144, 143. For examples of CE roles at Penn in the 1980s and 1990s, see Jane Barnsteiner, Lenore H. Kurlowicz, Terri H. Lipman, Diane L. Spatz, and Marilyn Stringer, "Establishing an Evidence Base in Academic Practice: The Role of the Clinician-Educator Faculty," in Lois K. Evans and Norma M. Lang (eds.), *Academic Nursing Practice: Helping to Shape the Future of Health Care* (New York: Springer, 2004), 205–218.

141. Fagin (1986), 143.

142. Fagin (1986), 143.

143. Lynaugh (2004), 34.

144. Lynaugh (2004), 29.

145. Lydia E. Hall, "A Center for Nursing," *Nursing Outlook* (November 1963): 805–807; Lydia E. Hall, "The Loeb Center for Nursing and Rehabilitation, Montefiore Hospital and Medical Center, Bronx, New York," *International Journal of Nursing* Studies (1969) 6: 81–97; Lynaugh (2004), 29.

146. Hilliard (2001), 40.

147. Wilson (2002), 26.

148. For details of the Carver Clinic, see Wilson (2002), 25–27 and Hilliard (2001), 38–41.

149. Hilliard (2001), 38.

150. Hilliard (2001), 38–41. See also Wilson (2002), 26.

151. Lois K. Evans, Joanne M. Pohl, and Nancy L. Rothman, "Building Alliances: A Survival Strategy," in Lois K. Evans and Norma M. Lang (eds.), *Academic Nursing Practice: Helping to Shape the Future of Health Care* (New York: Springer, 2004), 236–257.

152. Norma M. Lang, "Nurse-Managed Centers: Will They Thrive?" *American Journal of Nursing* (1983) 83(9): 1290–1296, 1295.

153. Lang (1983), 1296.

154. Juliann G. Sebastian, Marcia Stanhope, and Carolyn A. Williams, "Academic Nursing Practice Models and Related Strategic Issues," in Lois K. Evans and Norma M. Lang (eds.), *Academic Nursing Practice: Helping to Shape the Future of Health Care* (New York: Springer, 2004), 38–65.

155. Evans, Pohl, and Rothman (2004), 236–257.

156. Zana Rae Higgs, "The Academic Nurse-Managed Center Movement: A Survey Report," *Journal of Professional Nursing* (1988) 4(6): 422–429, 422.

157. Mathy D. Mezey, "Securing a Financial Base," *American Journal of Nursing* (1983) 83(9): 1297–1298. For a survey of the status, key characteristics, and operational challenges of more than sixty ANMCs in the late 1980s, see Higgs (1988).

158. Higgs (1988), 425.

159. Mezey (1983), 1297.

160. Lynaugh (2004), 28.

161. MacPhail (1979).

162. Beth Ann Swann, Betty S. Adler, Melinda Jenkins, and Eileen Sullivan-Marx, "Infrastructure to Support Academic Nursing Practice," in Lois K. Evans and Norma M. Lang (eds.), *Academic Nursing Practice: Helping to Shape the Future of Health Care* (New York: Springer, 2004), 144–163.

163. Swann et al. (2004), 158. Arlene W. Keeling, *Nursing and the Privilege of Prescription, 1893–2000* (Columbus: The Ohio State University Press, 2007), 138–155; and Julie Fairman, "The Right to Write: Prescription and Nurse Practitioners," in Jeremy A. Greene and Elizabeth S. Watkins (eds.), *Prescribed: Writing, Filling, Using, and Abusing the Prescription in Modern America* (Baltimore: Johns Hopkins University Press, 2012), 117–133.

164. American Association of Colleges of Nursing and Manatt Health Project Team, *Advancing Healthcare Transformation: A New Era for Academic Nursing* (Washington, DC: American Association of Colleges of Nursing, March 2016).

Conclusion

1. Philip L. Cantelon, *NINR: Bringing Science to Life* (Bethesda, MD: National Institutes of Health, 2010).

2. Rachel Butler, Mauricio Monsalve, Geb W. Thomas, Ted Herman, Alberto M. Segre, Philip M. Polgreed, and Manish Suneja, "Estimating Time Physicians and Other Health Care Workers Spend with Patients in an Intensive Care Unit Using a Sensor Network," *American Journal of Medicine* (2018) 131(8): 972.e9–972.e15.

3. See, for example, Eileen T. Lake, "How Effective Response to COVID-19 Relies on Nursing Research," *Research in Nursing and Health* (2020) 43: 213–214; Patricia D'Antonio, Mary Naylor, and Linda Aiken, "Nursing Research is Coronavirus Research," *Research in Nursing and Health* (2020) 43: 215; Fiona Maxton, Philip Darbyshire, and David R. Thompson, "Research Nurses Rising to the Challenges of COVID-19," *Journal of Clinical Nursing* (2021) 30: e13–e15; Kelly L. Wierenga, Scott Emory Moore, Susan J. Pressler, Eileen Danaher Hacker, and Susan M. Perkins, "Associations between COVID-19 Perceptions, Anxiety, and Depressive Symptoms among Adults Living in the United States," *Nursing Outlook* (2021) 69(5): 755–766; and Kristen Choi and Anna Dermenchyan, "The Nursing Science Behind Nurses as Coronavirus Hospital Heroes," *STAT*, July 30, 2020, https://www.statnews.com/2020/07/30/science-behind-nurses-as-coronavirus-hospital-heroes/ (accessed October 1, 2021).

4. Joyce Fitzpatrick, "The Case for the Clinical Doctorate in Nursing," *Reflections on Nursing Leadership* (2003): 8, 9, 37; p. 8. For historical perspective on multiple educational pathways, social mobility in nursing, and diversity within the nursing workforce see Patricia D'Antonio, *American Nursing: A History of Knowledge, Authority, and the Meaning of Work* (Baltimore: Johns Hopkins University Press, 2010), 168–180.

5. Institute of Medicine, *The Future of Nursing: Leading Change, Advancing Health* (Washington, DC: National Academies Press, 2011).

6. Jordan M. Harrison, Linda H. Aiken, Douglas M. Sloane, J. Margo Brooks Carthon, Raina M. Merchant, Robert A. Berg, and Matthew D. McHugh, "In Hospitals with More Nurses Who Have Baccalaureate Degrees, Better Outcomes for Patients after Cardiac Affairs," *Health Affairs* (2019) 38(7): 1087–1094, 1087; Linda H. Aiken, "Baccalaureate Nurses and Hospital Outcomes: More Evidence," *Medical Care* (2014) 52(10): 861–863; Linda H. Aiken, Sean P. Clarke, Robyn B. Cheung, Douglas M. Sloane, and Jeffrey H. Silber, "Educational Levels of Hospital Nurses and Surgical Patient Mortality," *JAMA* (2003) 290(12): 1617–1623.

7. Institute of Medicine (2011).

8. Institute of Medicine, *Assessing Progress on the Institute of Medicine Report: The Future of Nursing* (Washington, DC: National Academies Press, 2015), 73, 130.

9. On nurse faculty: https://www.nln.org/docs/default-source/uploadedfiles/default-document -library/distribtion-of-full-time-nurse-educators-by-race-2019-pdf.pdf?sfvrsn=ca00d_0h (accessed Feburary 17, 2022)

10. Health Resources and Services Administration, "Review Health Workforce Research," https://bhw.hrsa.gov/data-research/review-health-workforce-research (accessed March 12, 2021).

11. Table 2, *Sex, Race, and Ethnic Diversity of U.S. Health Occupations (2011–2015)*, HRSA,

U.S. Department of Health and Human Services, https://bhw.hrsa.gov/sites/default/files/bureau-health-workforce/data-research/diversity-us-health-occupations.pdf (accessed May 11, 2021); Janette Dill, Odichinma Akosionu, J'Mag Karbeah, Carrie Henning-Smith, "Addressing Systemic Racial Inequity in the Health Care Workforce," *Health Affairs Blog*, September 10, 2020.

12. National Nurses United, "Sins of Omission: How Government Failures to Track Covid-19 Data Have Led to More Than 1,700 Health Care Worker Deaths and Jeopardize Public Health," September 2020, https://www.nationalnursesunited.org/sites/default/files/nnu/documents/0920_Covid19_SinsOfOmission_Data_Report.pdf (accessed October 28, 2021). See also Samantha Artiga, Matthew Rae, Olivia Pham, Liz Hamel, and Cailey Muñana, "COVID-19 Risks and Impacts among Health Care Workers by Race/Ethnicity," Kaiser Family Foundation, November 11, 2020, https://www.kff.org/report-section/covid-19-risks-and-impacts-among-health-care-workers-by-race-ethnicity-issue-brief/ (accessed October 28, 2021).

13. Dill, Akosionu, Karbeah, and Henning-Smith (2020).

14. For example, Institute of Medicine, *In the Nation's Compelling Interest: Ensuring Diversity in the Health-Care Workforce* (Washington, DC: National Academies Press, 2004); National Academy of Medicine, *The Future of Nursing 2020–2030: Charting a Path to Achieve Health Equity* (Washington DC: National Academies Press, 2021).

15. Brad N. Greenwood, Rachel R. Hardeman, Laura Huang, and Aaron Sojourner, "Physician-Patient Racial Concordance and Disparities in Birthing Mortality for Newborns," *Proceedings of the National Academy of Sciences* 117 (September 1, 2020), https://doi.org/10.1073/pnas.1913405117 (accessed May 10, 2021).

16. J'Mag Karbeah, Rachel Hardeman, Jennifer Almanza, and Katy Kozhimannil, "Identifying the Key Elements of Racially Concordant Care in a Freestanding Birth Center," *Journal of Midwifery and Women's Health* (2019) 64: 592–597.

17. Deirdre Cooper Owens and Sharla M. Fett, "Black Maternal and Infant Health: Historical Legacies of Slavery," *American Journal of Public Health* (2019) 109(1): 1342–1345.

18. CDC Newsroom, "Racial and Ethnic Disparities Continue in Pregnancy-Related Deaths," https://www.cdc.gov/media/releases/2019/p0905-racial-ethnic-disparities-pregnancy-deaths.html (accessed May 14, 2021).

19. U.S. Department of Health and Human Services Office of Minority Health, "Infant Mortality and African Americans," https://minorityhealth.hhs.gov/omh/browse.aspx?lvl=4&lvlid=23 (accessed May 14, 2021).

20. Yvette P. Conley, Margaret Heitkemper, and Donna McCarthy et al., "Educating Future Nurse Scientists: Recommendations for Integrating Omics Content in PhD Programs," *Nursing Outlook* (2015) 63: 417–427; Pamela June Grace, Danny G. Willis, Sr. Callista Roy, and Dorothy Jones, "Profession at the Crossroads: A Dialog Concerning the Preparation of Nursing Scholars and Leaders," *Nursing Outlook* (2016) 64: 61–70; Patricia A. Grady, "National Institute of Nursing Research Commentary on the Idea Festival for Nursing Science Education," *Nursing Outlook* (2015) 63: 432–435; Susan J. Henly, Donna O. McCarthy, Jean F. Wyman, and Patricia W. Stone, et al., "Integrating Emerging Areas of Nursing Science into PhD Programs," *Nursing Outlook* (2015) 63: 408–416; Sally Thorne, "What Constitutes Core Disciplinary Knowledge," *Nursing Inquiry* (2014) 21(1): 1–2; Antonia M. Villarruel and Julie A. Fairman, "The Council for the Advancement of Nursing Science, Idea Festival Advisory Committee: Good Ideas that Need to go Further," *Nursing Outlook* (2015) 63: 536–438.

21. Adela Yarcheski and Noreen Mahon, "Characteristics of Quantitative Nursing Research from 1990 to 2010," *Journal of Nursing Scholarship* (2013) 45(4): 405–411; Grace et al., (2016);

Susan J. Henly, Donna O. McCarthy, Jean F. Wyman, and Margaret M. Heitkemper, et al., "Emerging Areas of Science: Recommendations for Nursing Science Education from the Council for the Advancement of Nursing Science Idea Festival," *Nursing Outlook* (2015) 63: 398–407; Jean F. Wyman and Susan J. Henly, "PhD Programs in Nursing in the United States: Visibility of American Association of Colleges of Nursing Core Curricular Elements and Emerging Areas of Science," *Nursing Outlook* (2015) 63: 390–397.

22. Donna Algase, Karen Stein, Cynthia Arslanian-Engoren, Colleen Corte, Marilyn Sawyer Sommers, and Mary G. Carey, "An Eye Toward the Future: Pressing Questions for Our Discipline in Today's Academic and Research Climate," *Nursing Outlook* (2021) 69: 57–64; Karen C. Flynn, Susan M. Reverby, Kylie M. Smith, and Dominique Tobbell, "'The Thing behind the Thing': White Supremacy and Interdisciplinary Faculty in Schools of Nursing," Nursing Outlook (2021) 1–3, https://doi.org/10.1016/j.outlook.2021.03.001 (accessed February 17, 2022); Wendy B. Bostwick, Julienne N. Rutherford, Crystal L. Patil, Robert J. Ploutz-Snyder, Joanne Spetz, Rob Stephenson, and Olga Yakusheva, "Envisioning a More Expansive Future for Multidisciplinary Nursing Scholarship and Education," Nursing Outlook (2021) 1–3, https://doi.org /10.1016/j.outlook.2021.03.003 (accessed May 11, 2021); Patricia D'Antonio and Cynthia A. Connolly "Turning a Historical Eye to the Future," Nursing Outlook (2021) 1–3, https://doi .org/10.1016/j.outlook.2021.03.010(accessed February 17, 2022); and Antonio M. Villarruel and Julie F. Fairman, "An Eye toward a More Inclusive Future," Nursing Outlook (2021) 1–3, https:// doi.org/10.1016/j.outlook.2021.03.004 (accessed May 11, 2021).

23. Sheria Robinson-Lane, "Letter to the Editor: Interdisciplinary Nursing Faculty and the Advancement of Nursing Knowledge," *Nursing Outlook* (2021) 1–2, https://doi.org/10.1016/j.out look.2021.02.003 (accessed May 6, 2021).

24. Mary E. Kerr, "Support for Nursing Science," *Nursing Outlook* (2016) 64: 262–270.

25. A selection of the literature documenting the changing nature of American universities after the war includes Rebecca S. Lowen, *Creating the Cold War University: The Transformation of Stanford* (Berkeley: University of California Press, 1997); Henry Etzkowitz, *MIT and the Rise of Entrepreneurial Science* (New York: Routledge, 2002); Daniel Lee Kleinman, *Impure Cultures: University Biology and the World of Commerce* (Madison: University of Wisconsin Press, 2003); Daniel S. Greenberg, *The Politics of Pure Science* (Chicago: University of Chicago Press, 1999); and Daniel S. Greenberg, *Science for Sale: The Perils, Rewards, and Delusions of Campus Capitalism* (Chicago: University of Chicago Press, 2007).

26. Grace et al., (2016).

27. American Association of Colleges of Nursing and Manatt Health Project Team, *Advancing Healthcare Transformation: A New Era for Academic Nursing* (Washington, DC: American Association of Colleges of Nursing, March 2016), 2.

28. For examples of this literature, see Harrison et al. (2019); and Aiken et al. (2003).

29. Kenneth M. Ludmerer, *Time to Heal: American Medical Education from the Turn of the Century to the Era of Managed Care* (Oxford: Oxford University Press, 1999). On this point, see also Roger Geiger, *Knowledge and Money: Research Universities and the Paradox of the Marketplace* (Palo Alto, CA: Stanford University Press, 2004), 142–144. Ludmerer has also documented the history of graduate medical education in *Let Me Heal: The Opportunity to Preserve Excellence in American Medicine* (New York: Oxford University Press, 2014).

30. On the influence of the Cold War on the development of the physical sciences and engineering see, for example, Stuart W. Leslie, *The Cold War and American Science: The Military-Industrial-Academic Complex at MIT and Stanford*; Paul Forman, "Behind Quantum Electron-

ics: National Security as Basis of Physical Research in the United States, 1940–1960," *Historical Studies in the Physical Sciences* (1987) 18: 149–229; Peter Galison and Bruce Hevly, eds., *Big Science: The Growth of Large-Scale Research*, (Stanford, CA: Stanford University Press, 1992); Lowen (1997). On changes in the social sciences, see Lowen (1997), 191–223; Ellen Herman, *The Romance of American Psychology: Political Culture in the Age of Experts* (Berkeley: University of California Press, 1995); James H. Capshew, *Psychologists on the March: Science, Practice, and Professional Identity in America, 1929–1969* (Cambridge: Cambridge University Press, 1999); and Joy Rohde, *Armed with Expertise: The Militarization of American Social Research during the Cold War* (Ithaca, NY: Cornell University Press, 2013).

31. On engineering, see Bruce E. Seely, "Research, Engineering, and Science in American Engineering Colleges: 1900–1960," *Technology and Culture* (1993) 34(2): 344–386; Bruce E. Seely, "The Other Re-engineering of Engineering Education, 1900–1965," *Journal of Engineering Education* (July 1999): 285–294; and Jonathon Harwood, "Engineering Education between Science and Practice: Rethinking the Historiography," *History and Technology* (2006) 22(1): 53–79. On computing, see Nathan Ensmenger, *The Computer Boys Take Over: Computers, Programmers, and the Politics of Technical Expertise* (Cambridge, MA: MIT Press, 2013). On pharmacy, see Robert A. Buerki, "American Pharmaceutical Education, 1952–2002," *Journal of the American Pharmaceutical Association* (2002) 42(4): 542–544; and Robert A. Buerki, "In Search of Excellence: The First Century of the American Association of Colleges of Pharmacy," *American Journal of Pharmaceutical Education* (1999) 63(Fall supplement). On social work, see June Axinn and Herman Levin, "Money, Politics and Education: The Case of Social Work," *History of Education Quarterly* (1978) 18(2): 143–158.

32. Margaret Rossiter, *Women Scientists in America: Before Affirmative Action, 1940–1972* (Baltimore: Johns Hopkins University Press, 1995).

33. Rossiter (1995); Margaret Rossiter, *Women Scientists in America: Forging a New World since 1972* (Baltimore: Johns Hopkins University Press, 2012); Amy Sue Bix, *Girls Coming to Tech! A History of American Engineering Education for Women* (Cambridge, MA: MIT Press, 2013); Laura Micheletti Puaca, *Searching for Scientific Womanpower: Technocratic Feminism and the Politics of National Security* (Chapel Hill: University of North Carolina Press, 2014); Margaret A. M. Murray, *Women Becoming Mathematicians: Creating a Professional Identity in Post-World War II America* (Cambridge, MA: MIT Press, 2000); Londa Schiebinger, *Has Feminism Changed Science?* (Cambridge, MA: Harvard University Press, 1999); Regina Morantz Sanchez, *Sympathy and Science: Women Physicians in American Medicine* (New York: Oxford University Press, 1985); Ellen S. More, Elizabeth Fee, and Manon Parry, eds., *Women Physicians and the Cultures of Medicine* (Baltimore: Johns Hopkins University Press, 2009).

34. Thomas Gieryn, "Boundary-Work and the Demarcation of Science from Non-Science: Strains and Interests in Professional Ideologies of Scientists," *American Sociological Review* (1983) 48(4): 781–795; and Andrew Abbott, *The System of Professions: An Essay on the Division of Expert Labor* (Chicago: University of Chicago Press, 1988).

35. Abbott (1988), 56.

36. Abbott (1988), 54. See also Ensmenger (2013), 234.

37. Reverby (1987); Hine (1989); and Flynn (2011).

38. Algase et al. (2021); Robinson-Lane (2021).

39. On women seeking access to normal science, see Schiebinger (1999), 4. Examples from the extensive literature on the history of racism in Western science that focus on the impacts of "race science" on health and disease include: Warwick Anderson, *The Cultivation of Whiteness:*

Science, Health, and Racial Destiny in Australia (Durham, NC: Duke University Press, 2006); Warwick Anderson, *Colonial Pathologies: American Tropical Medicine, Race, and Hygiene in the Philippines* (Manila: Ateneo de Manila University Press, 2007); Alison Bashford, *Imperial Hygiene: A Critical History of Colonialism, Nationalism, and Public Health* (London: Palgrave Macmillan, 2004); Lundy Braun, *Breathing Race into the Machine: The Surprising Career of the Spirometer from Plantation to Genetics* (Minneapolis: University of Minnesota Press, 2014); Laurie B. Greene, John McKiernan-González, and Martin Summers, eds., *Precarious Prescriptions: Contested Histories of Race and Health in North America* (Minneapolis: University of Minnesota Press, 2014); Evelynn M. Hammonds and Rebecca Herzig, eds., *The Nature of Difference: Sciences of Race in the United States from Jefferson to Genomics* (Cambridge, MA: MIT Press, 2008); Rana A. Hogarth, *Medicalizing Blackness: Making Racial Difference in the Atlantic World, 1780–1840* (Chapel Hill: University of North Carolina Press, 2017); Deirdre Cooper Owens, *Medical Bondage: Race, Gender, and the Origins of American Gynecology* (Athens: University of Georgia Press, 2017); Dorothy Roberts, *Fatal Invention: How Science, Politics, and Big Business Re-Create Race in the Twenty-First Century* (New York: New Press, 2011); Suman Seth, *Difference and Disease: Medicine, Race, and the Eighteenth-Century British Empire* (Cambridge: Cambridge University Press); Kim Tallbear, *Native American DNA: Tribal Belonging and the False Promise of Genetic Science* (Minneapolis: University of Minnesota Press, 2013); Keith Wailoo, *Dying in the City of the Blues: Sickle Cell Anemia and the Politics of Race and Health* (Chapel Hill: University of North Carolina Press, 2001).

40. For an excellent example of scholarship on the history of American health policy, see Rosemary A. Stevens, Charles E. Rosenberg, and Lawton R. Burns, eds., *History and Health Policy in the United States: Putting the Past Back In* (New Brunswick, NJ: Rutgers University Press, 2006). For a survey of the history of post–World War II federal health policy, see Rosemary A. Stevens, "History and Health Policy in the United States: The Making of a Health Care Industry, 1948–2008," *Social History of Medicine* (2008) 21(3): 461–483. Daniel M. Fox has emphasized the intersections of state and federal health policy in Daniel M. Fox, *The Convergence of Science and Governance: Research, Health Policy, and American States* (Berkeley: University of California Press, 2010). My previous scholarship has also highlighted the importance of attending to the history of state health policy and politics. See Dominique A. Tobbell, *Pills, Power, and Policy: The Struggle for Drug Reform in Cold War America and its Consequences* (Berkeley: University of California Press and Milbank Books on Health and the Public, 2011), 163–192; Dominique A. Tobbell, "Plow, Town, and Gown: The Politics of Family Practice in 1960s America," *Bulletin of the History of Medicine* (2013) 87(4): 648–680; and Dominique A. Tobbell, "'Coming to Grips with the Nursing Question': The Politics of Nursing Education Reform in 1960s America." *Nursing History Review* (2014) 22: 37–60.

41. On the history of nursing workforce shortages in the U.S. prior to the 1950s, see Jean C. Whelan, *Nursing the Nation: Building the Nursing Labor Force* (New Brunswick, NJ: Rutgers University Press, 2021).

42. Linda T. Kohn, Janet M. Corrigan, and Molla S. Donaldson, eds., Committee on Quality of Health Care in America, Institute of Medicine, *To Err is Human: Building a Safer Health System* (Washington, DC: National Academies Press, 1999).

43. Committee on Quality of Health Care in America, Institute of Medicine, *Crossing the Quality Chasm: New Health System for the 21ˢᵗ Century* (Washington, DC: National Academies Press, 2003), 20.

44. Ann C. Greiner and Elisa Knebel, eds., *Health Professions Education: A Bridge to Quality* (Washington, DC: National Academies Press, 2003), 1.

45. Greiner and Knebel (2003), 3.

46. Michael L. Millenson, *Demanding Medical Excellence: Doctors and Accountability in the Information Age* (Chicago: University of Chicago Press, 1997); Fox (2010), 22–50; and Nancy Tomes, *Remaking the American Patient: How Madison Avenue and Modern Medicine Turned Patients into Consumers* (Chapel Hill: University of North Carolina Press, 2016), 310–313.

47. American Association of Colleges of Nursing, "AACN Position Statement on the Practice Doctorate in Nursing," October 2004, p. 8.

48. E. R. Lenz, "The Practice Doctorate in Nursing: An Idea Whose Time Has Come," *Online Journal of Issues in Nursing* (2005) 10(3).

49. Janetta MacPhail, "People and Ideas: The Professional Doctorate in Nursing," paper presentation, University of Western Ontario, October 17, 1980, Case Western Reserve University Archives, 29DD, box 2 (29DD8 Papers of Dean Jannetta MacPhail), folder: 1971–1980.

50. Janetta MacPhail, "Implementation of the Doctor of Nursing (ND) Program: A Blueprint for the Future of Nursing Education," March 1980, Case Western Reserve University Archives, A98–035, box 7, folder: Materials for Implementation of the Doctor of Nursing Program.

51. Joyce J. Fitzpatrick, "The Professional Doctorate as an Entry Level into Clinical Practice," *National League for Nursing Publications* (1987) 41–2199: 53–56, 55.

52. MacPhail, "Implementation of the Doctor of Nursing (ND) Program," (1980).

53. "Evaluation of ND Program by Cleveland Area Hospitals," 1981, Case Western Reserve University Archives, A98–035, box 7, folder: Materials for Implementation of the Doctor of Nursing Program.

54. Case Western Reserve University and the University of Colorado also offered the ND as an advanced practice option.

55. Geraldine E. Edens and Georgie C. Labadie, "Opinions about the Professional Doctorate in Nursing," *Nursing Outlook* (1987) 35(3): 136–140, 140.

56. American Association of Colleges of Nursing, "Indicators of Quality in Research-Focused Doctoral Programs in Nursing," (2001) Reprinted in *Journal of Professional Nursing* 18(5) (September–October 2002): 289–294.

57. American Association of Colleges of Nursing (2004), 4.

58. Sandra R. Edwardson, oral history interview by Dominique A. Tobbell, May 30, 2012, University of Minnesota Academic Health Center Oral History Project, p. 43.

59. American Association of Colleges of Nursing (2004), 4.

60. Edwardson (2012), 43.

61. American Association of Colleges of Nursing (2004), 6.

62. American Association of Colleges of Nursing (2004), 1, 8, 11.

63. American Association of Colleges of Nursing (2004), 13.

64. Lenz (2005).

65. Janet S. Fulton and Brenda L. Lyon, "The Need for Some Sense Making: Doctor of Nursing Practice," *Online Journal of Issues in Nursing (2005)* 10(3).

66. Michael Arnone, "State Spending on Colleges Drops over All for the First Time in 11 Years," *Chronicle of Higher Education*, January 8, 2004, https://www.chronicle.com/article/state-spending-on-colleges-drops-over-all-for-first-time-in-11-years/ (accessed August 10, 2021); Sara Hebel, "State Spending on Higher Education up Slightly, a Reversal from Previous Years," *Chronicle of Higher Education*, December 17, 2004, https://www.chronicle.com/article/state-spending-on-higher-education-up-slightly-a-reversal-from-previous-year/ (accessed August 10, 2021).

67. Peter Zetterberg, "University of Minnesota Funding: FY 1978–FY 2008," January 2009, University of Minnesota School of Nursing, Dean Connie W. Delaney Files.

68. Phyllis N. Horns and Phyllis S. Turner, "Funding in Higher Education: Where Does Nursing Fit?" *Journal of Professional Nursing* (2006) 22(4): 221–225; Patricia L. Starck, "The Cost of Doing Business in Nursing Education," *Journal of Professional Nursing* (2005) 21(3): 183–190; Phyllis N. Horns, "Surviving the Enrollment Growth Funding Formula," *Nursing Leadership Forum* (2005) 9(4): 137–141.

69. Zetterberg (2009).

70. Amy J. Barton, Patricia Moritz, Jerry Griffin, Marlaine Smith, Kathy Magilvy, Gayle Preheim, Lauren Clark, Gene Marsh, Joann Congdon, Mary Blegen, Roxie Foster, and Sue Hagedorn, "A Model to Identify Direct Costs of Nursing Education: The Colorado Experience," *Nursing Leadership Forum* (2005) 9(4): 155–162.

71. Jean Wyman, oral history interview by Dominique Tobbell, June 6, 2017, University of Minnesota School of Nursing Oral History Project, p. 14.

72. Kathleen Dracup and Christopher W. Bryan-Brown, "Doctor of Nursing Practice: MRI or Total Body Scan?" *American Journal of Critical Care* (July 2005) 14(4): 278–281.

73. Ellen Olshansky, "Are Nurses at the Table? A New Nursing Degree Could Help," *Journal of Professional Nursing* (July–August 2004) 20(4): 211–212. See also A. L. O'Sullivan, M. Carter, L. Marion, J. M. Pohl, and K. E. Werner, "Moving Forward Together: The Practice Doctorate in Nursing," *Online Journal of Issues in Nursing* (2005) 10(3).

74. Gardiner Harris, "Calling the Nurse 'Doctor,' a Title that Physicians Oppose," *New York Times,* October 2, 2011.

75. John K. Inglehart, "Expanding the Role of Advanced Nurse Practitioners: Risks and Rewards," *New England Journal of Medicine* (May 16, 2013) 368(20), and AMA Advocac Resource Center, "Truth in Advertising Campaign." (AMA, 2018), https://www.ama-assn.org/system/files/2020–10/truth-in-advertising-campaign-booklet.pdf (accessed February 17, 2022).

76. Linda L. Lindeke, oral history interview by Dominique Tobbell, July 12, 2017, University of Minnesota School of Nursing Oral History Project, p. 14.

77. Janice E. Ruffin, "Issues for the Black Nurse Today: Competence and Commitment," *National League for Nursing Publications* (1974) 15–1513: 46–51.

78. Afaf I. Meleis and Kathleen Dracup, "The Case against the DNP: History, Timing, Substance, and Marginalization," *Online Journal of Issues in Nursing* (2005) 10(3).

79. Lenz (2005). At the University of Minnesota, Sandra Edwardson recalled laying "out all of the credits that our students would have taken from the time they graduated high school until they got a master's degree. I did the same thing with PharmD students. The number of credits was the same. I thought, *oh,* my goodness, it's time that we recognize what we're doing with the appropriate degree." Edwardson (2012), 46.

80. For example, Dracup and Meleis (2005); Susan K. Chase and Rosanne H. Pruitt, "The Practice Doctorate: Innovation or Disruption?" *Journal of Nursing Education* (2006) 45(5): 155–161; Linda Cronenwett, Kathleen Dracup, Margaret Grey, Linda McCauley, Afaf Meleis, and Marla Salmon, "The Doctor of Nursing Practice: A National Workforce Perspective," *Nursing Outlook* (2011) 59: 9–17.

81. Meleis and Dracup (2005).

82. Meleis and Dracup (2005).

83. Christine Mueller, oral history interview by Dominique Tobbell, July 7, 2017, University of Minnesota School of Nursing Oral History Project, pp. 24–25. See also Mary M. Rowan, oral

history interview by Dominique Tobbell, June 15, 2017, University of Minnesota School of Nursing Oral History Project; Joanne Disch, oral history interview by Dominique Tobbell, July 6, 2017, University of Minnesota School of Nursing Oral History Project.

84. Mueller (2017), 24–25. See also Rowan (2017).

85. Mueller (2017), 24–25. See also Rowan (2017).

86. See, for example, Marion E. Broome and Julie Fairman, "Changing the Conversation about Doctoral Education in Nursing," *Nursing Outlook* (2018) 66: 217–218; Maureen E. Groer and John M. Clochesy, "Conflicts within the Discipline of Nursing: Is There a Looming Paradigm War?" *Journal of Professional Nursing* (2020) 36: 53–55.

87. On recent PhD program statistics, see American Association of Colleges of Nursing, "PhD in Nursing," https://www.aacnnursing.org/News-Information/Research-Data-Center/PhD (accessed May 11, 2021). On recent DNP program statistics, see American Association of Colleges of Nursing, "Fact Sheet: DNP," updated October 2020, https://www.aacnnursing.org/News -Information/Fact-Sheets/DNP-Fact-Sheet (accessed May 11, 2021).

88. Rebecca Grant, "The U.S. is Running out of Nurses," *Atlantic*, February 3, 2016.

89. American Association of Colleges of Nursing, "Nursing Faculty Shortage Fact Sheet," March 16, 2015.

90. See, for example, Rachel R. Hardeman, Eduardo M. Medina, and Katy B. Kozhimannil, "Dismantling Structural Racism, Supporting Black Lives and Achieving Health Equity: Our Role," *New England Journal of Medicine* (2016) 375(22): 2113–2115; Rachel R. Hardeman, Eduardo M. Medina, and Rhea W. Boyd, "Stolen Breaths," *New England Journal of Medicine* (2020) 383(3): 197–199; Mary T. Bassett and Sandro Galea, "Reparations as a Public Health Priority: A Strategy for Ending Black-White Health Disparities," *New England Journal of Medicine* (2020) 383(22): 2101–2103; Dereck W. Paul Jr., Kelly R. Knight, Andre Campbell, and Louise Aronson, "Beyond a Moment: Reckoning with our History and Embracing Antiracism in Medicine," *New England Journal of Medicine* (2020) 383(15): 1404–1406; Calvin Moorley, Philip Darbyshire, Laura Serrant, Janine Mohamed, Parveen Ali, and Ruth De Souza, "Dismantling Structural Racism: Nursing Must Not Be Caught on the Wrong Side of History,a" *Journal of Advances in Nursing* (2020) 76: 2450–2453; Ayah Nuriddin, Graham Mooney, and Alexandre I. R. White, "Reckoning with Histories of Medical Racism and Violence in the USA" *Lancet* (2020) 396: 949–951.

Selected Bibliography

Abbott, Andrew. *The System of Professions: An Essay on the Division of Expert Labor* (Chicago: University of Chicago Press, 1988).

Arditti, Rita. "Feminism and Science." In Rita Arditti, Pat Brennan, and Steve Cavrak (eds.), *Science and Liberation* (Boston: South End Press, 1980).

Baer, Ellen D. "'A Cooperative Venture' in Pursuit of Professional Status: A Research Journal for Nursing." *Nursing Research* (1987) 36(1): 18–25.

———. "The Feminist Disdain for Nursing," *New York Times,* February 23, 1991.

Bix, Amy Sue. *Girls Coming to Tech! A History of American Engineering Education for Women* (Cambridge, MA: MIT Press, 2013).

Bothwell, Laura E., and Scott H. Podolsky. "The Emergence of the Randomized, Controlled Trial." *New England Journal of Medicine* (2016) 375: 501–504.

Brodie, Barbara. "Voices in Distant Camps: The Gap between Nursing Research and Nursing Practice." *Journal of Professional Nursing* (1988) 4(5): 320–328.

Buck, Joy. "Reweaving a Tapestry of Care: Religion, Nursing, and the Meaning of Hospice, 1945–1978." *Nursing History Review* (2007) 15(1): 113–145.

Buerki, Robert A. "In Search of Excellence: The First Century of the American Association of Colleges of Pharmacy." *American Journal of Pharmaceutical Education* (1999) 63 (Fall supplement).

———. "American Pharmaceutical Education, 1952–2002." *Journal of the American Pharmaceutical Association* (2002) 42(4): 542–544.

Buhler-Wilkerson, Karen. *False Dawn: The Rise and Decline of Public Health Nursing, 1900–1930* (New York: Garland, 1989).

———. "Bringing Care to the People: Lillian Wald's Legacy to Public Health Nursing." *American Journal of Public Health* (1993) 83: 1778–1786.

———. *No Place Like Home: A History of Nursing and Home Care in the United States* (Baltimore: Johns Hopkins University Press, 2001).

———. "No Place Like Home: A History of Nursing and Home Care in the U.S." *Home Healthcare Nurse* (2012) 30(8): 446–452.

Capshew, James H. *Psychologists on the March: Science, Practice, and Professional Identity in America, 1929–1969* (Cambridge: Cambridge University Press, 1999).

Chapin, Christy Ford. *Ensuring America's Health: The Public Creation of the Corporate Health Care System* (Cambridge: Cambridge University Press, 2015).

Choy, Catherine Ceniza. "'Exported to Care': A Transnational History of Filipino Nurse Migration to the United States." In Nancy Foner, Rubén G. Rumbaut, and Steven J. Gold (eds.), *Immigration Research for a New Century: Multidisciplinary Perspectives* (New York: Russell Sage Foundation, 2000), pp. 113–133.

———. *Empire of Care: Nursing and Migration in Filipino American History* (Durham, NC: Duke University Press, 2003).

Connolly, Cynthia, and Joan Lynaugh. *Fifty Years at the Division of Nursing: United States Public Health Service* (Washington, DC: U.S. Public Health Service Division of Nursing, 1997).

Creager, Angela N. H., Elizabeth Lunbeck, and Londa Schiebinger, eds. *Feminism in Twentieth-Century Science, Technology, and Medicine* (Chicago: University of Chicago Press, 2001).

Daly, Jeanne. *Evidence-Based Medicine and the Search for a Science of Clinical Care* (Berkeley: University of California Press / Milbank Memorial Fund, 2005).

D'Antonio, Patricia. "Women, Nursing, and Baccalaureate Education in 20th Century America." *Journal of Nursing Scholarship* (2004) 36(4): 379–384.

———. *American Nursing: A History of Knowledge, Authority, and the Meaning of Work* (Baltimore: Johns Hopkins University Press, 2010).

———. *Nursing with a Message: Public Health Demonstration Projects in New York City* (New Brunswick, NJ: Rutgers University Press, 2017).

D'Antonio, Patricia, and Julie Fairman. "Organizing Practice: Nursing, the Medical Model, and Two Case Studies in Historical Time." *Canadian Bulletin of Medical History* (2004) 21(2): 411–419.

D'Antonio, Patricia, and Cynthia A. Connolly. "Turning an Historical Eye to the Future." *Nursing Outlook* (2021) 1–3, https://doi.org/10.1016/j.outlook.2021.03.010.

Dittmer, John. *The Good Doctors: The Medical Committee for Human Rights and the Struggle for Social Justice in Health Care* (Jackson: University of Mississippi Press, 2009).

Dumke, Glenn S. "Higher Education in California," *California Historical Society Quarterly* (1963) 42(2): 99–110.

Ensmenger, Nathan. *The Computer Boys Take Over: Computers, Programmers, and the Politics of Technical Expertise* (Cambridge, MA: MIT Press, 2013).

Etzkowitz, Henry. *MIT and the Rise of Entrepreneurial Science* (New York: Routledge, 2002).

Fairman, Julie, "The roots of collaborative practice: nurse practitioner pioneers' stories." *Nursing History Review* (2002) 10: 159–174.

———. "Context and Contingency in the History of Post-World War II Nursing Scholarship in the United States." *Journal of Nursing Scholarship* (2008) 40(1): 4–11.

———. *Making Room in the Clinic: Nurse Practitioners and the Evolution of Modern Health Care* (New Brunswick, NJ: Rutgers University Press, 2008).

———. "The Right to Write: Prescription and Nurse Practitioners." In Jeremy A. Greene and Elizabeth S. Watkins (eds.), *Prescribed: Writing, Filling, Using, and Abusing the Prescription Modern America* (Baltimore: Johns Hopkins University Press, 2012), pp. 117–133.

Fairman, Julie, and Joan E. Lynaugh. *Critical Care Nursing: A History* (Philadelphia: University of Pennsylvania Press, 1998).

Fairman, Julie, and Patricia D'Antonio. "Virtual Power: Gendering the Nurse-Technology Relationship." *Nursing Inquiry* (1999) 6: 178–186.

Fee, Elizabeth. "A Feminist Critique of Scientific Objectivity." *Science for the People* (1982) 14(40): 5–8, 30–32.

Flynn, Karen C. *Moving Beyond Borders: A History of Black Canadian and Caribbean Women in the Diaspora* (Toronto: University of Toronto Press, 2011).

Flynn, Karen C., Susan M. Reverby, Kylie M. Smith, and Dominique Tobbell. "'The Thing behind the Thing': White Supremacy and Interdisciplinary Faculty in Schools of Nursing." *Nursing Outlook* (2021) 1–3, https://doi.org/10.1016/j.outlook.2021.03.00.

Fox, Daniel M. *Health Policies, Health Politics: The British and American Experience, 1911–1965* (Princeton, NJ: Princeton University Press, 1986).

———. "From Piety to Platitudes to Pork: The Changing Politics of Health Workforce Policy." *Journal of Health Politics, Policy, and Law* (1996) 21(4): 823–842.

———. *The Convergence of Science and Governance: Research, Health Policy, and American States* (Berkeley: University of California Press, 2010).

Gatrall, Cory Ellen. "Marie Branch and the Power of Nursing," *Nursing Clio*, October 29, 2020, https://nursingclio.org/2020/10/29/marie-branch-and-the-power-of-nursing/.

Geiger, Roger. *Research and Relevant Knowledge: American Research Universities since World War II* (New York: Routledge, 1993).

———. *Knowledge and Money: Research Universities and the Paradox of the Marketplace* (Palo Alto, CA: Stanford University Press, 2004).

Gieryn, Thomas. "Boundary-Work and the Demarcation of Science from Non-Science: Strains and Interests in Professional Ideologies of Scientists." *American Sociological Review* (1983) 48(4): 781–795.

Gilbert, Claire Krendl, and Donald E. Heller. "Access, Equity, and Community Colleges: The Truman Commission and Federal Higher Education Policy from 1947 to 2011." *Journal of Higher Education* (2013) 84(3): 417–443.

Graham, Hugh Davis, and Nancy Diamond. *The Rise of American Research Universities: Elites and Challengers in the Postwar Era* (Baltimore: Johns Hopkins University Press, 1997).

Greene, Laurie B., John McKiernan-González, and Martin Summers, eds. *Precarious Prescriptions: Contested Histories of Race and Health in North America* (Minneapolis: University of Minnesota Press, 2014).

Greenberg, Daniel S. *The Politics of Pure Science* (Chicago: University of Chicago Press, 1999).

———. *Science for Sale: The Perils, Rewards, and Delusions of Campus Capitalism* (Chicago: University of Chicago Press, 2007).

Hammonds, Evelynn M., and Rebecca Herzig, eds. *The Nature of Difference: Sciences of Race in the United States from Jefferson to Genomics* (Cambridge, MA: MIT Press, 2008).

Harding, Sandra. *The Science Question in Feminism* (Ithaca, NY: Cornell University Press, 1986).

———. *Whose Science? Whose Knowledge? Thinking from Women's Lives* (Ithaca, NY: Cornell University Press, 1991).

———. *Science and Social Inequality: Feminist and Postcolonial Issues* (Urbana: University of Illinois Press, 2006).

———, ed. *The Postcolonial Science and Technology Studies Reader* (Durham, NC: Duke University Press, 2011).

Haraway, Donna. *Primate Visions: Gender, Race and Nature in the World of Modern Science* (New York: Routledge, 1989).

Harwood, Jonathan. "Engineering Education between Science and Practice: Rethinking the Historiography." *History and Technology* (2006) 22(1): 53–79.

———. "Understanding Academic Drift: On the Institutional Dynamics of Higher Technical and Professional Education." *Minerva* (2010) 48: 413–427.

Herman, Ellen. *The Romance of American Psychology: Political Culture in the Age of Experts* (Berkeley: University of California Press, 1995).

Higby, Gregory J. "From Compounding to Caring: An Abridged History of American Pharmacy." In Calvin Knowlton and Richard Penna (eds.), *Pharmaceutical Care: A Primer on the Pharmacist's Changing Role in Patient Care.* 2nd ed. (Bethesda, MD: American Society of Health-System Pharmacists, 2003), pp. 19–42.

Hine, Darlene Clark. *Black Women in White* (Bloomington: Indiana University Press, 1989).

Hoffman, Beatrix. "Scientific Racism, Insurance, and Opposition to the Welfare State: Frederick L. Hoffman's Transatlantic Journey." *Journal of the Gilded Age and Progressive Era* (2003) 2: 150–190.

———. *Health Care for Some: Rights and Rationing in the United States since 1930* (Chicago: University of Chicago Press, 2012).

Hogan, Andrew. "The 'Two Cultures' in Clinical Psychology: Constructing Disciplinary Divides in the Management of Mental Retardation." *ISIS* (2018) 109(4): 695–719.

Howell, Joel D. *Technology in the Hospital: Transforming Patient Care in the Early Twentieth Century* (Baltimore: Johns Hopkins University Press, 1995).

Jones, David S., and Scott H. Podolsky. "The History and Fate of the Gold Standard." *Lancet* (2015) 385: 1502–1503.

Keeling, Arlene W., "Blurring the Boundaries between Medicine and Nursing: Coronary Care Nursing, circa the 1960s." *Nursing History Review* (2005) 13: 139–164.

———. *Nursing and the Privilege of Prescription, 1893–2000* (Columbus: Ohio State University Press, 2007).

Keeling, Arlene W., Barbara Brodie, and John Kirchgessner. *The Voice of Professional Nursing Education: A 40-Year History of the American Association of Colleges of Nursing* (Washington, DC: American Association of Colleges of Nursing, 2010).

Keller, Evelyn Fox. "Women Scientists and Feminist Critics of Science." *Daedalus* (1987) 116(4): 77–91.

Kerr, Clark. *The Uses of the University* (Cambridge, MA: Harvard University Press, 1963).

Klein, Jennifer. *For All These Rights: Business, Labor, and the Shaping of America's Public-Private Welfare State* (Princeton, NJ: Princeton University Press, 2003).

Kleinman, Daniel Lee. *Impure Cultures: University Biology and the World of Commerce* (Madison: University of Wisconsin Press, 2003).

Kline, Wendy. *Bodies of Knowledge: Sexuality, Reproduction, and Women's Health in the Second Wave* (Chicago: University of Chicago Press, 2010).

Leighow, Susan Rimby. "Backrubs vs. Bach: Nursing and the Entry-into-Practice Debate, 1946–1986." *Nursing History Review* (1996) 4: 3–17.

———. *Nurses' Questions / Women's Questions: The Impact of the Demographic Revolution and Feminism on United States Working Women, 1946–1986* (New York: Peter Lang, 1996).

Leslie, Stuart W. *The Cold War and American Science: The Military-Industrial-Academic Complex at MIT and Stanford* (New York: Columbia University Press, 1993).

Loss, Christopher P. *Between Citizens and the State: The Politics of American Higher Education in the 20th Century* (Princeton, NJ: Princeton University Press, 2011).

Lowen, Rebecca S. *Creating the Cold War University: The Transformation of Stanford* (Berkeley: University of California Press, 1997).

Ludmerer, Kenneth M. *Time to Heal: American Medical Education from the Turn of the Century to the Era of Managed Care* (Oxford: Oxford University Press, 1999).

———. *Let Me Heal: The Opportunity to Preserve Excellence in American Medicine* (New York: Oxford University Press, 2014).

Lynaugh, Joan E. Academic Nursing Practice: Looking Back." In Lois K. Evans and Norma M. Lang (eds.) *Academic Nursing Practice: Helping to Share the Future of Health Care* (New York: Springer, 2004), pp. 20–37.

———. "Mildred Tuttle: Private Initiative and Public Response in Nursing Education after World War II." *Nursing History Review* (2006) 14: 203–211.

———. "Nursing the Great Society: The Impact of the Nurse Training Act of 1964." *Nursing History Review* (2008) 16: 13–28.

Lynaugh, Joan, and Barbara Brush. *American Nursing: From Hospitals to Health Systems* (Malden, MA: Blackwell Publishers, 1996).

Malka, Susan Gelfand. *Daring to Care: American Nursing and Second-Wave Feminism* (Chicago: University of Illinois Press, 2007).

Marks, Harry. *The Progress of Experiment: Science and Therapeutic Reform in the United States, 1900–1990* (New York: Cambridge University Press, 1997).

McLeod, Don C. "Clinical Pharmacy: The Past, Present and Future." *American Journal of Hospital Pharmacy* (1976) 33: 29–38.

Melhado, Evan. "Health Planning in the United States and the Decline of Public-Interest Policymaking." *Milbank Quarterly* (2006) 84(2): 359–440.

Melosh, Barbara. *"The Physician's Hand": Work Culture and Conflict in American Nursing* (Philadelphia: Temple University Press, 1982).

Merton, Robert K. "The Search for Professional Status: Sources, Costs, and Consequences." *American Journal of Nursing* (1960) 60(5): 662–664.

Millenson, Michael L. *Demanding Medical Excellence: Doctors and Accountability in the Information Age* (Chicago: University of Chicago Press, 1997).

Millett, John D. *Conflict in Higher Education: State Government Coordination Versus Institutional Independence* (San Francisco: Jossey-Bass Publishers, 1984).

Mukerji, Chandra, *A Fragile Power: Scientists and the State* (Princeton, NJ: Princeton University Press, 1990).

Murray, Margaret A. M. *Women Becoming Mathematicians: Creating a Professional Identity in Post-World War II America* (Cambridge, MA: MIT Press, 2000).

Nelson, Alondra. *Body and Soul: The Black Panther Party and the Fight against Medical Discrimination* (Minneapolis: University of Minnesota Press, 2011).

Noddings, Nel. *Caring: A Feminine Approach to Ethics and Moral Education* (Berkeley: University of California Press, 1984).

Nuriddin, Ayah, Graham Mooney, and Alexandre I. R. White. "Reckoning with Histories of Medical Racism and Violence in the USA." *Lancet* (2020) 396: 949–951.

Olson, Keith W. *The G.I. Bill, the Veterans, and the Colleges* (Lexington: University Press of Kentucky, 1974).

O'Mara, Margaret Pugh. *Cities of Knowledge: Cold War Science and the Search for the Next Silicon Valley* (Princeton, NJ: Princeton University Press, 2005).

Owens, Deirdre Cooper. *Medical Bondage: Race, Gender, and the Origins of American Gynecology* (Athens: University of Georgia Press, 2017).

Owens, Deirdre Cooper, and Sharla M. Fett. "Black Maternal and Infant Health: Historical Legacies of Slavery." *American Journal of Public Health* (2019) 109(1): 1342–1345.

Pickren, Wade, "Tension and Opportunity in Post–World War II American Psychology." *History of Psychology* (2007) 10(3): 279–299.

Pollock, Anne, and Banu Subramaniam. "Resisting Power, Retooling Justice: Promises of Feminist Postcolonial Technosciences." *Science, Technology, and Human Values* (2014) 41(6): 951–966.

Porter, Theodore M., *Trust in Numbers: The Pursuit of Objectivity in Science and Public Life* (Princeton, NJ: Princeton University Press, 1995).

Reverby, Susan. *Ordered to Care: The Dilemma of American Nursing, 1850–1945* (New York: Cambridge University Press, 1987).

———. "A Legitimate Relationship: Nursing, Hospitals, and Science in the Twentieth Century." In Diana Elizabeth Long and Janet Golden (eds.) *The American General Hospital: Communities and Social Contexts* (Ithaca, NY: Cornell University Press, 1989), 135–156.

Roberts, Dorothy. *Fatal Invention: How Science, Politics, and Big Business Re-Create Race in the Twenty-First Century* (New York: New Press, 2011).

Rohde, Joy. *Armed with Expertise: The Militarization of American Social Research during the Cold War* (Ithaca, NY: Cornell University Press, 2013).

Rose, Hilary. "Hand, Brain, and Heart: A Feminist Epistemology for the Natural Sciences." *Signs* (1983) 9(1): 73–90.

Rossiter, Margaret. *Women Scientists in America: Struggles and Strategies to 1940* (Baltimore: Johns Hopkins University Press, 1982).

———. *Women Scientists in America: Before Affirmative Action, 1940–1972* (Baltimore: Johns Hopkins University Press, 1998).

Ruddick, Sara. *Maternal Thinking: Toward a Politics of Peace* (Boston: Beacon Press, 1989).

Ruzek, Sheryl B. *The Women's Health Movement: Feminist Alternatives to Medical Control* (New York: Praeger, 1978).

Sandelowski, Margarete, *Devices and Desires: Gender, Technology, and American Nursing* (Chapel Hill: University of North Carolina Press, 2000).

Schiebinger, Londa, *Has Feminism Changed Science?* (Cambridge, MA: Harvard University Press, 1999).

Shermer, Elizabeth Tandy. *Sunbelt Capitalism: Phoenix and the Transformation of American Politics* (Philadelphia: University of Pennsylvania Press, 2013).

Seely, Bruce E. "Research, Engineering, and Science in American Engineering Colleges: 1900–1960." *Technology and Culture* (1993) 34(2): 344–386.

———. "The Other Re-engineering of Engineering Education, 1900–1965." *Journal of Engineering Education* (July 1999): 285–294.

Smith, Gloria R. "From Invisibility to Blackness: The Story of the National Black Nurses' Association." *Nursing Outlook* (1975) 23: 225–229.

Smith, Kylie. *Talking Therapy: Knowledge and Power in American Psychiatric Nursing* (New Brunswick, NJ: Rutgers University Press, 2020).

Stevens, Rosemary A. *In Sickness and in Wealth: American Hospitals in the Twentieth Century* (Baltimore: Johns Hopkins University Press, 1999).

———. "History and Health Policy in the United States: The Making of a Health Care Industry, 1948–2008." *Social History of Medicine* (2008) 21(3): 461–483.

Stevens, Rosemary A., Charles E. Rosenberg, and Lawton R. Burns, eds. *History and Health Policy in the United States: Putting the Past Back In* (New Brunswick, NJ: Rutgers University Press, 2006).

Strickland, Stephen P. *Politics, Science, and Dread Disease: A Short History of United States Medical Research Policy* (Cambridge, MA: Harvard University Press, 1972).

———. *The History of Regional Medical Programs: The Life and Death of a Small Initiative of the Great Society* (Lanham, MD: University Press of America, 2000).

Thomasson, Melissa A. "Racial Differences in Health Insurance Coverage and Medical Expenditures in the United States: A Historical Perspective." *Social Science History* (2006) 30(4): 529–550.

Threat, Charissa J. *Nursing Civil Rights: Gender and Race in the Army Nurse Corps* (Urbana: University of Illinois Press, 2015).

Timmermans, Stefan, and Marc Berg. *The Gold Standard: The Challenge of Evidence-Based Medicine and Standardization in Health Care* (Philadelphia: Temple University Press, 2003).

Tobbell, Dominique A. *Pills, Power, and Policy: The Struggle for Drug Reform in Cold War America and its Consequences* (Berkeley: University of California Press and Milbank Books on Health and the Public, 2012).

———. "'Eroding the Physician's Control of Therapy': The Postwar Politics of the Prescription." In Jeremy A. Greene and Elizabeth Siegel Watkins (eds.), *Prescribed: Writing, Filling, Using, and Abusing the Prescription in Modern America* (Baltimore: Johns Hopkins University Press, 2012), pp. 66–90.

———. "Plow, Town, and Gown: The Politics of Family Practice in 1960s America." *Bulletin of the History of Medicine* (2013) 87(4): 648–680.

———. "'Coming to Grips with the Nursing Question': The Politics of Nursing Education Reform in 1960s America." *Nursing History Review* (2014) 22: 37–60.

———. "Clinical Pharmacy: An Example of Interprofessional Education in the Late 1960s and 1970s." *Nursing History Review* (2016) 24: 98–102.

Tomes, Nancy. "The Development of Clinical Psychology, Social Work, and Psychiatric Nursing: 1900–1980." In Edwin R. Wallace and John Gach (eds.) *History of Psychiatry and Medical Psychology* (New York: Springer, 2008): 657–682.

———. *Remaking the American Patient: How Madison Avenue and Modern Medicine Turned Patients into Consumers* (Chapel Hill: University of North Carolina Press, 2016).

Wailoo, Keith. *Dying in the City of the Blues: Sickle Cell Anemia and the Politics of Race and Health* (Chapel Hill: University of North Carolina Press, 2001).

Wall, Barbra Mann, and Billye J. Brown. *Through the Eyes of Nursing: Educational Reform at the University of Texas School of Nursing, 1890–1989* (Austin, TX: Austin Books Consortium, 2017).

Watkins, Elizabeth Siegel. *On the Pill: A Social History of Oral Contraceptives, 1950–1970* (Baltimore: Johns Hopkins University Press, 2001).

———. "Deciphering the Prescription: Pharmacists and the Patient Package Insert." In Jeremy A. Greene and Elizabeth Siegel Watkins (eds.) *Prescribed: Writing, Filling, Using, and Abusing the Prescription in Modern America* (Baltimore: Johns Hopkins University Press, 2012), 91–116.

Whelan, Jean C. *Nursing the Nation: Building the Nursing Labor Force* (New Brunswick, NJ: Rutgers University Press, 2021).

Wilson, Elizabeth. *Gut Feminism* (Durham, NC: Duke University Press, 2015),

Zimmerman, Mary K. "The Women's Health Movement: A Critique of Medical Enterprise and the Position of Women." In Beth B. Hess and Myra Marx Ferree (eds.) *Analyzing Gender: A Handbook of Social Science Research* (Newbury Park, CA: Sage, 1987), pp. 442–472.

Zola, Irving Kenneth. "Medicine as an Institution of Social Control." *Sociological Review* (1972) 20(4): 487–504

Index

AACN. *See* American Association of Colleges of Nursing

Abbott, Andrew, 7, 59, 64, 83, 117, 191–92

Abdellah, Faye, 64

abortion, 104

academic health centers (AHCs): administration of, 37, 97–98, 164, 172; characteristics of, 2–3, 36; delivery and governance of health care in, 19, 157, 170, 180; education policy and practice in, 19; emergence of, 2–3, 6, 17, 36–38; essential functions of, 15, 19, 157–58; faculty roles and responsibilities in, 157–58, 201; gendered hierarchies within, 16, 53, 98, 159; interdisciplinary character of, 3, 36; organization linked to, 51; physicians in, 159; politics and tensions in, 2–3, 12, 20, 38–44, 95, 97, 102, 114, 154; revenue-generating capacities of, 159; state funding and oversight of, 15, 193. *See also* research universities

academic leadership in nursing, 11–12, 19, 155–56, 158, 171–73, 176–80

academic medical centers, 36

academic medicine model. *See* medical model of professional education

academic nursing practice, 19, 158, 170–84

academic project of nursing: achievements of, 186–87; and clinical nurse specialists, 160–62; components of, 6–12; debates and tensions in, 10, 18, 19, 22, 53, 119–21, 125; defined, 1; distinctive character of, 14; gendered politics and, 15–16; health planning and, 134–56; interdisciplinary character of, 6, 15, 25, 27–28, 60, 123; mixed results of, 187–90; nursing model of care as basis of, 6, 15, 28–29; other practice professions compared to, 12–14, 55, 111–12, 117–18, 216n71; political context of, 5–6, 14–18, 190–91;

promotion of, 5–12, 32; as racialized project, 11; racist outcomes of, 90, 130; rationales for, 2, 5–6, 11–12, 54–55, 190, 198; research universities and, 92–121; reunification of education and service in, 11–12, 158–62, 164–80, 195; separation of nursing education from practice base in, 11, 15–16, 155, 157–58, 162–64; shortcomings of, 19; workforce needs as factor in, 9–10, 14–15, 47, 124–25, 154. *See also* academic leadership in nursing; bachelor of science in nursing (BSN) programs; nursing education; nursing research; nursing science; PhD programs; practice doctorates

accreditation, 33, 49, 52, 83, 135, 137

Ackell, Edmund, 169–70

activism. *See* health activism

advanced nursing practice, 14, 16, 155, 173, 194, 197, 199

Advances in Nursing Science (journal), 62

AHCs. *See* academic health centers

Aiken, Linda, 78

AMA. *See* American Medical Association

American Academy of Nursing, 180

American Association of Colleges of Nursing (AACN), 51–52, 158, 180, 196–97, 201; *Advancing Healthcare Transformation*, 189; *Essentials*, 52

American Association of Deans of College and University Schools of Nursing, 51, 158

American Journal of Nursing, 55, 117, 136

American Medical Association (AMA), 33, 35, 199; Commission on Graduate Education in Medicine, 50

American Nurses Association (ANA), 10, 32, 35–36, 49, 52, 62, 85, 129, 138, 180, 253n60; Council on State Boards, 152

American Nurses Foundation, 88, 100, 106, 253n60